ANNALS OF THE NEW YORK ACADEMY OF SCIENCES

Volume 693

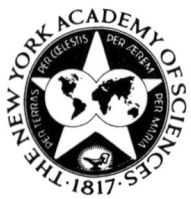

EDITORIAL STAFF

Executive Editor
BILL BOLAND

Managing Editor
JUSTINE CULLINAN

Associate Editor
LINDA HOTCHKISS MEHTA

The New York Academy of Sciences
2 East 63rd Street
New York, New York 10021

THE NEW YORK ACADEMY OF SCIENCES
(Founded in 1817)

BOARD OF GOVERNORS, July 1993–June 1994

CYRIL M. HARRIS, *Chairman of the Board*
JOSHUA LEDERBERG, *President*
HENRY M. GREENBERG, *President-Elect*

Honorary Life Governor
WILLIAM T. GOLDEN

Vice-Presidents
EDWARD COHEN   JERROLD WILLIAM MABEN   MARTIN L. LEIBOWITZ

Secretary-Treasurer
HENRY A. LICHSTEIN

Governors-at-Large

BARRY R. BLOOM   RONALD BRESLOW
SUSANNA CUNNINGHAM-RUNDLES
MARTHA R. MATTEO   DOROTHY NELKIN   RICHARD A. RIFKIND
DAVID E. SHAW   WILLIAM C. STEERE, JR.   SHMUEL WINOGRAD

CHARLES A. SANDERS, *Past Chairman*   HELENE L. KAPLAN, *General Counsel* [ex officio]

RODNEY W. NICHOLS, *Chief Executive Officer* [ex officio]

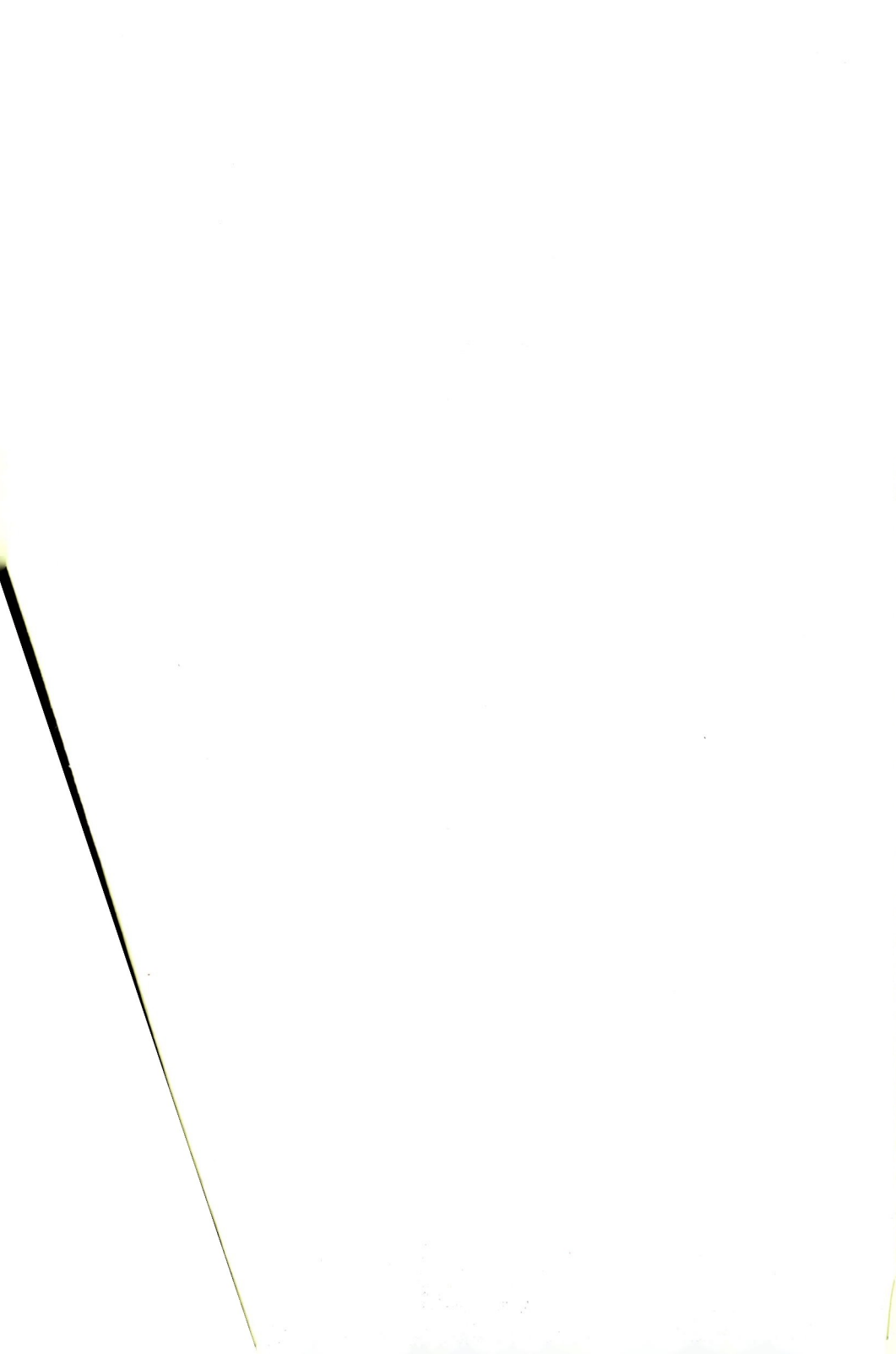

PEDIATRIC AIDS: CLINICAL, PATHOLOGIC, AND BASIC SCIENCE PERSPECTIVES

ANNALS OF THE NEW YORK ACADEMY OF SCIENCES
Volume 693

PEDIATRIC AIDS: CLINICAL, PATHOLOGIC, AND BASIC SCIENCE PERSPECTIVES

Edited by William D. Lyman and Arye Rubinstein

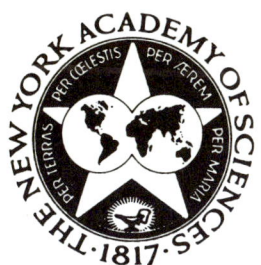

The New York Academy of Sciences
New York, New York
1993

Copyright © 1993 by the New York Academy of Sciences. All rights reserved. Under the provisions of the United States Copyright Act of 1976, individual readers of the Annals are permitted to make fair use of them for teaching or research. Permission is granted to quote from the Annals provided that the customary acknowledgment is made of the source. Material in the Annals may be republished only by permission of the Academy. Address inquiries to the Executive Editor at the New York Academy of Sciences.

Copying fees: For each copy of an article made beyond the free copying permitted under Section 107 or 108 of the 1976 Copyright Act, a fee should be paid through the Copyright Clearance Center Inc., 27 Congress St., Salem, MA 01970. For articles of more than 3 pages, the copying fee is $1.75.

∞ The paper used in this publication meets the minimum requirements of American National Standard for Information Sciences—Permanence of Paper for Printed Library Materials, ANSI Z39.48-1984.

Cover art is a reproduction of Pablo Picasso's *The Tragedy* (1903), Chester Dale Collection, © 1993 National Gallery of Art, Washington, DC.

The Tragedy does not refer to any specific event or specific persons; the figures in the painting are symbols of sorrow and resignation in the face of human imperfectability and misery.

Library of Congress Cataloging-in-Publication Data

Pediatric AIDS : clinical, pathologic, and basic science perspectives
  / edited by William D. Lyman and Arye Rubinstein.
     p.   cm. — (Annals of the New York Academy of Sciences, ISSN 0077-8923 ; v. 693)
  Includes bibliographical references and index.
  ISBN 0-89766-791-3 (cloth). — ISBN 0-89766-792-1 (paper)
  1. AIDS (Disease) in children—Congresses. 2. AIDS (Disease) in children—Pathogenesis—Congresses. I. Lyman, William David. II. Rubinstein, Arye. III. Series
  [DNLM: 1. Acquired Immunodeficiency Syndrome—in infancy & childhood—congresses. W1 AN626YL v. 693 1993 / WD 308 P3705 1993]
Q11.N5 vol. 693
[RJ387.A25]
500 s—dc20
[618.92'9792]
DNLM/DLC
for Library of Congress   93-37011
                                                               CIP

MC/PCP
Printed in the United States of America
ISBN 0-89766-791-3 (cloth)
ISBN 0-89766-792-1 (paper)
ISSN 0077-8923

ANNALS OF THE NEW YORK ACADEMY OF SCIENCES

Volume 693
October 29, 1993

PEDIATRIC AIDS: CLINICAL, PATHOLOGIC, AND BASIC SCIENCE PERSPECTIVES[a]

Editors and Conference Organizers
WILLIAM D. LYMAN AND ARYE RUBINSTEIN

CONTENTS

Preface. *By* WILLIAM D. LYMAN xi

Introductory Remarks. *By* ARYE RUBINSTEIN 1

Part I. Epidemiology and Clinical Diagnosis of Pediatric HIV Infection

Epidemiology of Pediatric Human Immunodeficiency Virus Infection in the United States. *By* MARTHA F. ROGERS, M. BLAKE CALDWELL, MARTA L. GWINN, AND R. J. SIMONDS 4

Antibody in Human Immunodeficiency Virus Infection. *By* PHILIP A. BRUNELL 9

Part II. Cellular Targets of HIV Infection

Maternal Transmission and Diagnosis of Human Immunodeficiency Virus during Infancy. *By* DIANE W. WARA, KATHERINE LUZURIAGA, NATASHA L. MARTIN, JOHN L. SULLIVAN, AND YVONNE J. BRYSON 14

Human Immune Development: Implications for Congenital HIV Infection. *By* SUSANNA CUNNINGHAM-RUNDLES, CINDY (XIN) CHEN, JAMES B. BUSSEL, CLAUDIA BLANKENSHIP, MIRTA B. VEBER, DEBORAH SANDERS-LAUFER, TONY HINDS, JOSEPH S. CERVIA, AND PAUL EDELSON 20

---

[a] This volume is the result of a conference entitled **Pediatric AIDS: Clinical, Pathologic, and Basic Science Perspectives,** which was held by the New York Academy of Sciences on November 18 through 21, 1992 in Washington, D.C.

Immunologic Targets of HIV Infection: T Cells. *By*
WILLIAM T. SHEARER, HOWARD M. ROSENBLATT,
MARK D. SCHLUCHTER, LYNNE M. MOFENSON,
THOMAS N. DENNY, THE NICHD IVIG CLINICAL TRIAL
GROUP, AND THE NHLBI P^{2}C^2 PEDIATRIC PULMONARY AND
CARDIAC COMPLICATIONS OF HIV INFECTION STUDY GROUP . . 35

Reservoirs of HIV Infection or Carriage: Monocytic, Dendritic,
Follicular Dendritic, and B Cells. *By* JEFFREY LAURENCE . . . 52

Part III. Pathogenesis of HIV Diseases: Perspectives for the Pathologist and Basic Scientist

HIV-1 Reverse Transcriptase: A Diversity Generator and
Quasispecies Regulator. *By* JOSÉ L. MUÑOZ, WADE P. PARKS,
STEVEN M. WOLINSKY, BETTE T. M. KORBER,
AND CECELIA HUTTO 65

Pathology of Pediatric AIDS: Overview, Update, and Future
Direction. *By* VIJAY V. JOSHI 71

Central Nervous System Pathology in Pediatric AIDS. *By*
DENNIS W. DICKSON, JOSEFINA F. LLENA,
STEPHEN J. NELSON, AND KAREN M. WEIDENHEIM 93

Neurologic Syndromes. *By* ANITA L. BELMAN 107

Reliability of Neurologic Assessment in a Collaborative Study
of HIV Infection in Children. *By* RAM KAIRAM, JENNIE KLINE,
BRUCE LEVIN, DONALD BRAMBILLA, DAVID COULTER,
KARL KUBAN, LESTER LANSKY, PAUL MARSHALL,
JESUS VELEZ-BORRAS, AND EVELYN RODRIGUEZ 123

Assessing Neurobehavioral Changes in HIV$^+$ Infants and
Children: A Methodological Approach. *By*
EILEEN B. FENNELL 141

Part IV. Clinical Management and Current Treatment

Intravenous Gammaglobulin for Pediatric HIV-1 Infection:
Effects on Infectious Complications, Circulating Immune
Complexes, and CD4 Cell Decline. *By* ARYE RUBINSTEIN,
THERESA CALVELLI, AND R. RUBINSTEIN 151

Opportunistic Infections in Pediatric HIV Disease. *By*
RUSSELL B. VAN DYKE 158

Antiviral Therapy for HIV Infection in Infants and Children.
By ANNE A. GERSHON 166

Part V. Future Perspectives for Treatment

The Clinical Evaluation of Cytokines and Immunomodulators in HIV Infection. *By* ARTHUR J. AMMANN 178

Passive Immunity in the Prevention of Maternal-Fetal Transmission of Human Immunodeficiency Virus Infection. *By* JOHN S. LAMBERT AND E. RICHARD STIEHM 186

Prospects for Prevention of Vertical Transmission of Human Immunodeficiency Virus by Immunization. *By* S. J. CRYZ, JR., H. GOLDSTEIN, E. FÜRER, J. U. QUE, T. HASLER, B. ALTHAUS, AND A. RUBINSTEIN 194

Part VI. Models for Pediatric HIV Infection

Tissue Culture Models of HIV-1 Infection. *By* WILLIAM D. LYMAN, WILLIAM C. HATCH, JORGE N. LAROCCA, AND WILLIAM K. RASHBAUM 202

Animal Models for Perinatal Transmission of Pathogenic Viruses. *By* R. M. RUPRECHT, C. FRATAZZI, P. L. SHARMA, M. F. GREENE, D. PENNINCK, AND M. WYAND 213

AIDS and the Central Nervous System: Examining Pathobiology and Testing Therapeutic Strategies in the SIV-Infected Rhesus Monkey. *By* LEE E. EIDEN, DIANNE M. RAUSCH, ANNA DA CUNHA, ELISABETH A. MURRAY, MELVYN HEYES, LEROY SHARER, DONATUS NOHR, AND EBERHARD WEIHE 229

Part VII. Poster Papers

Maternal Drug Use in Perinatal HIV Studies: The Women and Infants Transmission Study. *By* EVELYN M. RODRIGUEZ, HERMANN MENDEZ, KENNETH RICH, AMY SHEON, HAROLD FOX, KAREN GREEN, CLEMENTE DIAZ, DONALD BRAMBILLA, AND LYNNE MOFENSON 245

A Controlled Study of Cognitive and Language Function in School-Aged HIV-Infected Children. *By* J. HAVENS, A. WHITAKER, J. FELDMAN, L. ALVARADO, AND A. EHRHARDT 249

Elective Pregnancy Terminations and HIV-1. *By* WILLIAM K. RASHBAUM AND WILLIAM D. LYMAN 252

Use of PCR for Detection of HIV-1 Sequences in Babies Born to Seropositive Mothers. *By* Mark M. Manak, James V. Snider, David Petersen, Winston Frederick, Sandra Barnes, and Dao-Pei Huang 255

Diagnosis and Quantitation of HIV-1 Infection in Infants and Children by Whole-Blood Culture. *By* William V. Raszka, Jr., Merlin L. Robb, Arnold K. Fowler, Chester R. Roberts, Norman J. Waecker, David P. Ascher, Richard A. Moriarty, David Goldberg, and Gerald W. Fischer 258

HIV-Specific IgG3 in Cord Blood: Predictive Value for Seroreversion. *By* D. Caselli, M. Marconi, A. Maccabruni, G. Bossi, G. Pasinetti, M. Stronati, and M. Aricò 262

A Rapid, Sensitive, PCR-Based Method for Detection of HIV-1 Specific Nucleic Acid in the Culture Supernatant of Infected Cells. *By* Indira K. Hewlett, Bharat Joshi, Gary Riordan, Laurie Pollock, and Jay S. Epstein 264

HIV-1 Specific IgG Capture Enzyme Immunoassay to Study the Dynamics of HIV-1 Antibody and to Diagnose HIV-1 Infection in Infants. *By* Bharat Parekh, N. Shaffer, G. Schochetman, R. T. Coughlin, C.-H. Hung, J. R. George, and NYC Perinatal HIV Transmission Collaborative Study Group 268

Detection of HIV-1 IgA by an IgA Capture Enzyme Immunoassay for Early Diagnosis in Infants. *By* J. Richard George, B. S. Parekh, N. Shaffer, R. T. Coughlin, C.-H. Hung, M. Rogers, G. Schochetman, and NYC Perinatal HIV Transmission Collaborative Study Group 272

Indeterminate Western Blot in Children Who Serorevert for HIV. *By* D. Caselli, A. Maccabruni, A. Deicas, G. Bossi, M. Degioanni, G. Achilli, and M. Aricò 275

Analysis of the HIV-1 Envelope V3-Loop Sequences from Ten Mother–Child Pairs. *By* Gabriella Scarlatti, Thomas Leitner, Eva Halapi, Johan Wahlberg, Marianne Jansson, Hans Wigzell, Eva Maria Fenyö, Jan Albert, Mathias Uhlén, and Paolo Rossi 277

The Presence of Cryptococcal Capsular Polysaccharide Increases the Sensitivity of HIV-1 Coculture in Children. *By* Massimo Pettoello-Mantovani, Arturo Casadevall, and Harris Goldstein 281

HCV Vertical Transmission in Infants Born to HIV-HCV Seropositive Mothers. *By* A. MACCABRUNI, D. CASELLI, AND M. DEGIOANNI 284

Preliminary Data on *Chlamydia pneumoniae* Seroprevalence in HIV-1 Infected Children. *By* A. PLEBANI, M. CLERICI SCHOELLER, F. BLASI, AND R. COSENTINI 286

Mycobacterium avium Complex in HIV-Infected Children. *By* DEBORAH GLEASON-MORGAN, JOSEPH A. CHURCH, AND LAWRENCE A. ROSS 288

Peripheral B-Cell Activation and Immaturity in HIV-Infected Children. *By* C. RODRIGUEZ, E. RICHARD STIEHM, AND S. PLAEGER-MARSHALL 291

Central Nervous System in Pediatric AIDS: Results from Neuropathologic Pediatric AIDS Registry. *By* P. B. KOZLOWSKY, J. H. SHER, C. RAO, P. A. ANZIL, M. A. WRZOLEK, L. SHARER, E-S. CHO, D. W. DICKSON, K. M. WEIDENHEIM, J. F. LLENA, S. J. NELSON, AND M. D. KANZER 295

Image Analysis of Myelination in Second-Trimester Human Fetal Spinal Cords at Risk for HIV-1 Infection. *By* K. M. WEIDENHEIM, I. EPSHTEYN, W. K. RASHBAUM, J. F. MCGURK, AND W. D. LYMAN 297

Administration of Aerosolized Pentamidine to HIV-Infected Infants. *By* IVAN L. HAND, ANDREW WIZNIA, AND MAURA PORRICOLA 300

Pharmacokinetics of Trimetrexate Glucuronate in Infants with AIDS and *Pneumocystis carinii* Pneumonia. *By* BISHARA J. FREIJ, RAOUL L. WIENTZEN, JR., GAYLE HAYEK, AND LLOYD R. WHITFIELD 302

Evaluation of Anti-HIV Agents *in Vitro* by Quantitative PCR. *By* BHARAT JOSHI, JAY EPSTEIN, SHERWIN F. LEE, RON MAYNER, AND INDIRA K. HEWLETT 306

Immunoregulation of Tumor Necrosis Factor Production by HIV-1 gp-120 in Neonates and Adults. *By* MADHAVAN P. N. NAIR, ANN M. SWEET, AND STANLEY A. SCHWARTZ 309

Different Strains of HIV-1 Infect Distinct Human Fetal Neural Cells. *By* WILLIAM C. HATCH, E. POUSADA, L. LOSEV, AND W. D. LYMAN 312

Productive Infection of Human Fetal Microglia *in Vitro* by HIV-1. *By* SUNHEE C. LEE, WILLIAM C. HATCH, WEI LIU, CELIA F. BROSNAN, AND DENNIS W. DICKSON 314

HIV Infection of Human Cortical Neuronal Cells: Enhancement by Differentiating Growth Factor. *By* R. RODRIGUEZ, S. RENNE, D. J. VOLSKY, AND Y. MIZRACHI 317

Neural Cell Receptor for HIV-1: Initial Biochemical Characterization. *By* Y. MIZRACHI 320

HIV-1 mRNA Transcripts from Persistently Infected Human Fetal Astrocytes. *By* WALTER J. ATWOOD, CARLO S. TORNATORE, KAREN MEYERS, AND EUGENE O. MAJOR 324

Index of Contributors 327

Financial assistance was received from:

Supporter
- WYETH PEDIATRICS

Contributors
- ABBOTT LABORATORIES
- AMERICAN CYANAMID COMPANY, MEDICAL RESEARCH DIVISION
- AMGEN
- ARMOUR PHARMACEUTICAL COMPANY
- BURROUGHS WELLCOME COMPANY
- DU PONT MERCK PHARMACEUTICAL COMPANY
- GENENTECH, INC.
- GLAZO INC. RESEARCH INSTITUTE
- HOECHST-ROUSSEL PHARMACEUTICALS INC.
- HOFFMANN-LA ROCHE INC.
- MERCK RESEARCH LABORATORIES
- NATIONAL INSTITUTE OF MENTAL HEALTH
- PFIZER INC.
- R. W. JOHNSON PHARMACEUTICAL RESEARCH INSTITUTE
- UPJOHN COMPANY
- UPJOHN LABORATORIES

The New York Academy of Sciences believes it has a responsibility to provide an open forum for discussion of scientific questions. The positions taken by the participants in the reported conferences are their own and not necessarily those of the Academy. The Academy has no intent to influence legislation by providing such forums.

Preface

WILLIAM D. LYMAN

*Departments of Pathology, Neuroscience, and
Obstetrics and Gynecology
Albert Einstein College of Medicine
Bronx, New York 10461*

Since the first description of pediatric AIDS in 1982, the understanding of this syndrome in children has advanced rapidly. Only some of this progress has been the product of knowledge gained about its adult counterpart. Because AIDS in children has unique aspects, some of the most important advances in its understanding came from the efforts of a group of scientists and clinicians dedicated to pediatric and maternal–fetal medicine.

The proceedings of the meeting reported in this volume of the *Annals of the New York Academy of Sciences* represent the efforts of many of these individuals. We are especially proud to recognize their achievements and provide a forum for information exchange, facilitate additional collaborations, and educate medical practitioners and interested scientists. As demonstrated by the diversity of papers in this volume, this meeting followed a logical sequence of topics beginning with epidemiology and extending to the cellular targets and pathology associated with HIV-1 infection in children. This is complemented by a consideration of the benefits and pitfalls of current treatments. New therapeutic strategies for children and the latest models of pediatric AIDS are also discussed. Because of the recognized importance of poster sessions, organized discussions of these presentations and a state-of-the-art roundtable completed the program for this three-day meeting.

Unlike many other scientific conferences wherein prompt translation of recent laboratory advances to patient care is not possible, it was our combined hope that, in fact, this transition for pediatric AIDS patients would be facilitated by this meeting. Nevertheless, even if the efficiency of converting laboratory data to treatment protocols is not achieved, it is our belief that the exchange of basic knowledge about pediatric AIDS will, in fact, provide a substrate for additional advances in the treatment and prevention of this disease.

We wish to thank the New York Academy of Sciences for its help and support in organizing this meeting. Special thanks go to Geraldine Busacco, Sherryl Greenberg, and the rest of the Conference Department staff for extraordinary professionalism in logistical, secretarial, and financial matters. We also want to thank Agnes Geoghan and Barbara Shea for help with the initial work and correspondence in putting this conference together. We also wish to acknowledge the sustained help of the members of the Editorial Department in seeing this volume through the press. Special thanks in this regard are owed to Mrs. Linda Mehta, who gave generously of her time and talent in the expeditious production and editing of this volume. Lastly, we want to thank the speakers and session chairs who sparked lively discussions and maintained a smooth and stimulating exchange of ideas.

Introductory Remarks

ARYE RUBINSTEIN

Departments of Pediatrics and Microbiology and Immunology
Albert Einstein College of Medicine
Bronx, New York 10461

This volume contains the proceedings of a conference organized under the auspices of the New York Academy of Sciences and the National Institutes of Health. The topics to be discussed cover a broad spectrum of the problematic issue of human immunodeficiency virus type I (HIV-1) infection in infants and children. Current statistics indicate that, worldwide, hundreds of thousands of children are HIV-1 infected, and the projections of the World Health Organization indicate that millions of children will be afflicted with this disease by the end of this century.

This conference took place, almost exactly to the day, fourteen years after the first HIV-1 infected infant was referred to our immunodeficiency clinic at the Albert Einstein College of Medicine.[1,2] Although the correct diagnosis could not be made in the first patient in 1978, it was already then obvious that this child represented a new entity of immunodeficiency. The first abstract that my collaborators and I submitted in 1981 for the annual spring conference of the American Academy of Pediatrics included many elements of the disease spectrum and its immunopathology.

RECURRENT INFECTIONS, INTERSTITIAL PNEUMONIA, HYPERGAMMAGLOBULINEMIA, AND REVERSED T_4/T_8 RATIO IN CHILDREN WITH HIGH ANTIBODY LEVELS TO EPSTEIN-BARR VIRUS

Five black infants were treated for recurrent bacterial and viral (Herpes simplex, severe varicella) infections, chronic interstitial pneumonia and generalized lymphadenopathy. The histology of lymph-node biopsies resembled angioimmunoblastic lymphadenopathy. The immunological workup revealed high antibody titers (VCA) to Epstein-Barr virus, a hypergammaglobulinemia (mainly IgG, up to 5,400 mg% with a monoclonal spike in one patient) and a reversed T_4/T_8 ratio. The T_8 cells were Ia negative and exhibited no suppressor activity on B cells. The clinical and immunological picture was similar to that observed in adult drug abusers and homosexual men. Mothers of three of the infants were promiscuous and drug abusers.

A few months after submission of this abstract, the mothers of these children were also found to be immunodeficient and to have low CD4 cell counts.[2] Although the hallmarks of the disease in our first patients focused on recurrent bacterial infections, other investigators began to observe children with opportunistic infections similar to those reported in adult AIDS. Dr. Ammann and co-workers[3] described a child who developed the disease after a blood transfusion. Dr. Oleske's[4] first cases were children who have died from opportunistic infections.

The common denominator between all these pediatric cases and AIDS in adults was described by us in *Acquired Immune Deficiency Syndrome, Annals of the New York Academy of Sciences* in 1984, even before the etiologic agent, HIV-1, was identified.[5] Sera of infected children contained an "autoantibody" that reacted exclusively with lymphocytes obtained from patients with AIDS at all ages. Two years later, after the causative agent of the disease (HIV-1) was discovered, it was shown that this "autoantibody" reacted with the envelope of HIV-1.

Full-blown AIDS in adults was considered to be the "tip of the iceberg" with many more HIV-1 infected persons remaining asymptomatic for years. To date, it is still unclear how many HIV-1 infected children remain asymptomatic and for how long. In this conference "long-term survivors" are described, some of whom were born in 1978 to 1979.

There is no doubt that HIV-1 infection in children is closely linked to the infection of their mothers. In order to develop meaningful preventative strategies, it is necessary to determine the timing of infection—whether early fetal, late fetal, perinatal, or postnatal. Earlier studies have identified genomic imprints of HIV-1 in fetuses at gestational ages of 11 to 24 weeks.[6,7] Recent investigations have shown that HIV-1 cannot be identified by a variety of methods (viral culture, PCR, p24) in the peripheral blood of about one-half of all infected newborns.[8-10] Whether the undetectability of HIV-1 in the peripheral blood of newborns actually denotes recent (perinatal) infection with low virus load or is due to selective sequestration of the virus in fetal central lymphoid organs or other organs[7] is unknown. Studies of organotypic cultures of fetal central nervous system elements, presented at this conference, demonstrate that fetal tissues are extremely vulnerable to HIV-1 through direct infection or as an "innocent bystander" of an immunologic assault on the virus.

This conference also brings together scientists from a broad range of areas in drug and vaccine research. New drug trials, passive and active immunotherapies, targeted at prevention of HIV-1 transmission from mother to fetus/newborn are in progress. It appears that vigorous maternal neutralizing antibody responses to viral envelope glycoproteins are associated with reduced transmission rates, albeit the virus may evade this immune response and selected "escape mutants" may then infect the fetus. New vaccines designed to boost and broaden maternal humoral and cellular immune responses in order to prevent the emergence of escape mutants are discussed.

In spite of seemingly insurmountable obstacles, we have come a long way. A new disease was characterized; its etiology, epidemiology, and spectrum are now well understood. Exciting new therapies and preventive measures are on the horizon. Our hope is that this conference will bring together and encourage scientists to accelerate the momentum of progress in conquering this dreadful disease.

REFERENCES

1. RUBINSTEIN, A. 1983. Acquired immunodeficiency syndrome in infants. Editorial: Am. J. Dis. Child. **137:** 825.

2. RUBINSTEIN, A., M. SICKLICK, A. GUPTA, L. BERNSTEIN, et al. 1983. Acquired immunodeficiency with reversed T4/T8 ratios in infants born to promiscuous and drug-addicted mothers. JAMA **249:** 2350.
3. AMMANN, A. J., M. J. COWAN, D. W. WARA, et al. 1983. Acquired immunodeficiency in an infant: Possible transmission by means of blood product administration. Lancet **1:** 956–958.
4. OLESKE, J., A. MINNEROR, R. COOPER, JR., et al. 1983. Immune deficiency syndrome in children. JAMA **249:** 2345–2349.
5. RUBINSTEIN, A., C. BUTKUS-SMALL & L. J. BERNSTEIN. 1984. Autoantibodies to T cells in adult and pediatic AIDS. Ann. N.Y. Acad. Sci. **437:** 508–512.
6. CORNGNAUD, V., F. LAURE, A. BROUSARD, et al. 1991. Frequent and early in utero HIV-1 infection. AIDS Res. Hum. Retrovir. **7:** 337–341.
7. SOEIRO, R., A. RUBINSTEIN, W. K. RASHBAUM & W. D. LYMAN. 1992. Maternofetal transmission of AIDS: Frequency of human immunodeficiency virus type-1 nucleic acid sequences in human fetal DNA. J. Infect. Dis. **166:** 699–703.
8. EHRNST, A., S. LONDGREN, M. DICTOR, B. JOHANNSON, A. SONNERBORG, J. CZAJKOWSKI, G. SUNDIN & A. B. BOKLIN. 1991. HIV in pregnant women and their offspring: Evidence for late transmission. Lancet **337:** 253–260.
9. CONCENSUS WORKSHOP, SIENA, ITALY. 1992. Maternal factors involved in mother-to-child transmission of HIV-1. J. AIDS **5:** 1019–1029.
10. BRYSON, Y. J., K. LUZURIAGA, J. L. SULLIVAN & D. W. WARA. 1992. Establishment of a definition of the timing of vertical HIV-1 infection. N. Engl. J. Med. **327(17):** 1246–1247.

Epidemiology of Pediatric Human Immunodeficiency Virus Infection in the United States

MARTHA F. ROGERS,[a] M. BLAKE CALDWELL,
MARTA L. GWINN, AND R. J. SIMONDS

Division of HIV/AIDS
National Center for Infectious Diseases
Centers for Disease Control and Prevention
U.S. Public Health Service
U.S. Department of Health and Human Services
Atlanta, Georgia 30333

THE SCOPE OF THE PROBLEM

Human immunodeficiency virus (HIV) infection is a growing problem facing providers of health care to children. As of December 31, 1992, 4,249 children under 13 years of age had been reported with AIDS to the Centers for Disease Control and Prevention (CDC); 771 were reported in 1992 alone. Acquired immunodeficiency syndrome (AIDS) is the eighth leading cause of death in children ages 1 to 4 years nationwide and ranks among the top five causes of death in some locations.

Each year since 1988, approximately 6,000 to 7,000 HIV-infected women have given birth to a live-born infant in the United States, for a prevalence of 1.5 HIV-infected women per 1,000 women with live births. This estimate is based on data from the National Survey of Childbearing Women, a blinded seroprevalence survey using blood routinely collected from infants for metabolic testing (i.e., phenylketonuria).[1] Although infants' blood is tested, the prevalence reflects HIV infection in their mothers, since all infants born to these mothers will have maternal antibody to HIV for up to 15 to 18 months after birth. Most states that have conducted the survey for multiple years have stable prevalence rates, although seroprevalence is rising in a few areas.[2]

---

[a] Address for correspondence: Martha F. Rogers, M.D., Mailstop E45, Centers for Disease Control and Prevention, Atlanta, GA 30333.

MODES OF TRANSMISSION

HIV is transmitted to children predominantly from their mothers (perinatal or vertical transmission). Other modes of transmission to children include blood or blood product transfusion, sexual abuse,[3] and other parenteral exposure to HIV-infected blood.[4] Among children with AIDS reported to CDC in 1992, 90% acquired HIV through perinatal exposure. Most of their mothers acquired HIV through injection drug use (35%) or heterosexual transmission (34%). A small percentage (3%) of mothers acquired the virus from blood or blood product transfusion, and for some mothers (27%), the mode of transmission is undetermined.

Among the 4,249 reported pediatric AIDS cases, 494 (12%) were attributed to transfusion of contaminated blood or blood products. Nearly all of these transfusions occurred before donor-screening practices were implemented in March 1985. Only two of these children received blood or blood products that had been screened for HIV antibody, indicating the tremendous success of this prevention policy. Most transfusion-associated AIDS cases currently being diagnosed represent long incubation periods for HIV from the time of transfusion and infection (before 1985) to onset of AIDS.

THE NEED FOR FOSTER CARE

Children with HIV infection often come from disrupted families. Many of these children cannot be cared for by their biologic mothers because of the mother's drug use, sickness, or death. In a large CDC surveillance study of 1,683 children born to HIV-infected mothers, 55% of the children were living with a biologic parent, 10% lived with another relative, 28% were in foster care, 3% had been adopted, and 4% lived in group settings or with other caregivers.[5] Children of mothers who were or had been injecting drug users were more likely to be living with an alternative caregiver than were children whose mothers were not injecting drug users (61% vs. 22%).[5]

HIV AND SYPHILIS

During the early and middle 1980s, pediatric HIV infection most often affected inner-city residents of large metropolitan areas. Over the past few years, however, infection has spread to smaller cities and rural areas, particularly in the southeastern United States, the region with the largest percent increase in AIDS cases in 1991.[6]

The states with the highest syphilis rates in 1991 were also in the Southeast. FIGURE 1 shows U.S. counties with primary and secondary syphilis rates of greater than 10 per 100,000 population,[7] and FIGURE 2 shows counties or state regions with rates of HIV infection in childbearing women.[8] The similarity in distribution is striking. HIV and syphilis are both sexually transmitted diseases. Syphilis and other genital ulcer diseases have been associated with an increased risk of acquiring HIV infection[9]; they are thought to facilitate transmission of HIV by disrupting

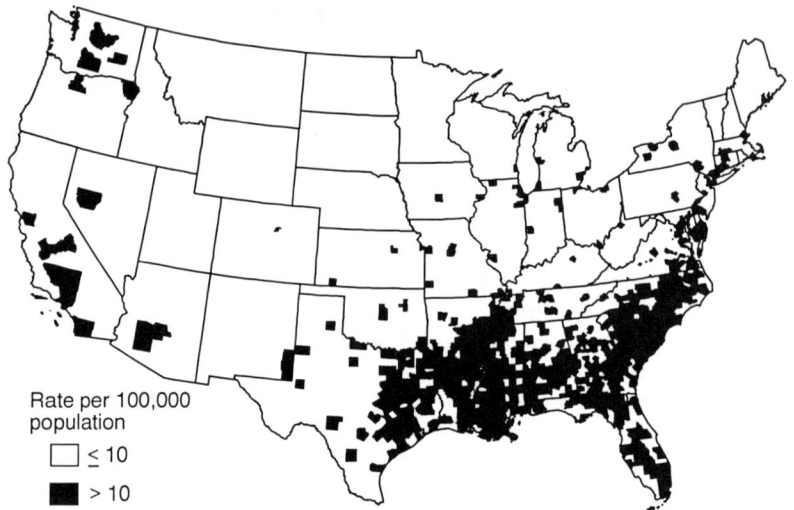

FIGURE 1. Cases of syphilis (primary and secondary) reported in 1991 from U.S. counties. Shading highlights those counties with rates above 10.0 per 100,000 population.[7]

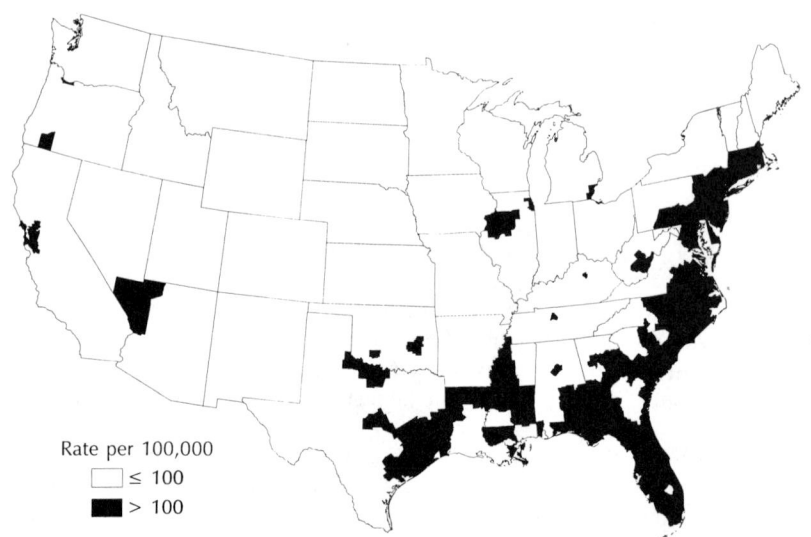

FIGURE 2. Prevalence of HIV in childbearing women in health districts in the United States. Surveys were conducted in 1991.

the mucosal surfaces and providing increased numbers of potential target cells (CD4+ lymphocytes or macrophages) close to the site of HIV entry. HIV prevention programs in areas with high rates of syphilis will need to address both epidemics.

PREVENTION OF OPPORTUNISTIC INFECTIONS

Despite recent advances in antiretroviral and prophylactic therapy for opportunistic infections, *Pneumocystis carinii* pneumonia (PCP) remains the most common AIDS-defining illness in children. Among 697 children with perinatally acquired AIDS reported to CDC in 1992, 239 (34%) had PCP. The peak incidence of PCP among children with AIDS occurs at three to six months of age. Over half the cases of PCP associated with perinatally acquired AIDS were in children in this age group. If these cases are to be prevented with prophylactic antibiotic therapy, children born to HIV-infected mothers will need to be identified early, preferably around the time of birth. These children must then be monitored for CD4+ cell count levels to determine their need for prophylaxis.[10]

The CDC Pediatric Spectrum of Disease Project, conducted in six geographic areas (Los Angeles County, San Francisco Bay area, Washington, D.C., three cities in Texas, Massachusetts, and New York City), examined the timing of diagnosis of HIV infection or exposure with respect to PCP diagnosis. Only 35% of children five months of age or younger at the time of PCP diagnosis had been evaluated for HIV infection before onset of PCP. This finding points out the need for early evaluation for HIV infection, appropriate monitoring of CD4+ counts, and use of prophylactic therapy when indicated.[10]

Tuberculosis is an increasingly common infection in HIV-infected persons, particularly injecting drug users. Cases of tuberculosis are now being reported in children as well.[11] Diagnosis is difficult because HIV-infected immunosuppressed adults and children are anergic. Uninfected children living in households with HIV-infected adults with tuberculosis are at risk of acquiring tuberculosis and developing active disease.[11] Multidrug-resistant *Mycobacterium tuberculosis* has also been reported.[12] Clearly, heightened awareness of the problem, better diagnostic tests, prompt identification and treatment of contacts of active tuberculosis cases, and appropriate therapy aimed at drug-resistant organisms are important for stemming the spread of tuberculosis in the HIV-infected population and their contacts.

SUMMARY

HIV infection is an important cause of morbidity and mortality in the pediatric population. Providers of heath care to children need to be aware of the problem and the characteristics of the most affected populations. Early diagnosis of HIV infection is critical for initiating appropriate antiviral therapy and prophylactic treatment for opportunistic infections. Attending to the myriad of social problems these families face is equally important for providing an optimal chance for prolonged survival and a reasonably high quality of life.

REFERENCES

1. GWINN, M., M. PAPPAIOANOU, R. GEORGE, et al. 1991. Prevalence of HIV infection in childbearing women in the United States: Surveillance using newborn blood samples. JAMA **265:** 1704–1708.
2. CLARK, J-P., A. S. ROGERS, M. HAIMES & S. PANNY. 1992. HIV seroprevalence among childbearing women in Maryland: An analysis of trends. Pediatr. AIDS HIV Infect. Fetus Adolesc. **3:** 68–72.
3. GELLERT, G. A., M. J. DURFEE, C. D. BERKOWITZ, K. V. HIGGENS & V. C. TUBIOLO. 1993. Situational and sociodemographic characteristics of children infected with human immunodeficiency virus from pediatric sexual abuse. Pediatrics **91:** 39–44.
4. CENTERS FOR DISEASE CONTROL. 1992. HIV infection in two brothers receiving intravenous therapy for hemophilia. Morbid. Mortal. Wkly. Rpt. **41:** 228–231.
5. CALDWELL, M. B., L. MASCOLA, W. SMITH, et al. 1992. Biologic, foster, and adoptive parents: Care givers of children exposed perinatally to human immunodeficiency virus in the United States. Pediatrics **90:** 603–607.
6. CENTERS FOR DISEASE CONTROL. 1992. Update: Acquired immunodeficiency syndrome—United States, 1991. Morbid. Mortal. Wkly. Rpt. **41:** 463–468.
7. CENTERS FOR DISEASE CONTROL. 1992. Summary of notifiable diseases, United States, 1991. Morbid. Mortal. Wkly. Rpt. **40:** 45.
8. WASSER, S., M. GWINN & P. FLEMING. 1993. Urban–nonurban distribution of HIV infection in childbearing women in the United States. J. Acquir. Immune. Defic. Syndr. In press.
9. PLUMMER, F. A., J. N. SIMONSEN, D. W. CAMERON, et al. 1991. Cofactors in male-female sexual transmission of human immunodeficiency virus type 1. J. Infect. Dis **163:** 233–239.
10. CENTERS FOR DISEASE CONTROL. 1991. Guidelines for prophylaxis against *Pneumocystis carinii* pneumonia for children infected with human immunodeficiency virus. Morbid. Mortal. Wkly. Rpt. **40(RR-2):** 1–13.
11. JONES, D. S., J. M. MALECKI, W. J. BIGLER, J. J. WITTE & M. J. OXTOBY. 1992. Pediatric tuberculosis and human immunodeficiency virus infection in Palm Beach County, Florida. Am. J Dis. Child. **146:** 1166–1170.
12. EDLIN, B. R., J. I. TOKARS, M. GRIECO, et al. 1992. An outbreak of multidrug-resistant tuberculosis among hospitalized patients with the acquired immunodeficiency syndrome. N. Engl. J. Med. **326:** 1514–1521.

Antibody in Human Immunodeficiency Virus Infection[a]

PHILIP A. BRUNELL[b]

*The Division of Infectious Diseases
Ahmanson Pediatric Centers
Cedars–Sinai Medical Center
UCLA School of Medicine
Los Angeles, California 90048*

As the name of the disease, acquired immunodeficiency syndrome, suggests, there are significant immunologic abnormalities in patients infected with human immunodeficiency virus (HIV). The occurrence of opportunistic infections and the occurrence of more frequent and more severe common infections are clinical manifestations of these abnormalities in children infected with HIV. Indeed, the occurrence of these clinical events is used in clinical staging of HIV infection. The precise immunologic abnormalities in HIV-infected individuals are still being elucidated, but clearly both cellular and humoral factors are affected.

Measles provides a paradigm for the study of abnormalities of humoral function. In normal children, administration of immune globulin at the time of exposure has been shown to modify or prevent measles. In addition, the presence of measles antibody before exposure has been found to predict protection against measles.[1] The infants of HIV-infected women have been found to have a higher risk of developing measles during the early months of life than the infants of uninfected women. This is true regardless of whether the infants themselves are HIV infected.[2,3] This observation suggests that these women may have lower levels of measles antibody with which to endow their fetuses. Thus, their infants lose their passively acquired protective antibody earlier and become infected sooner than the infants of uninfected women. Measles has been reported to be more severe in HIV-infected children—even those who have been immunized against the disease.[4–7] Immunization of these children provides an opportunity to study the antibody response to vaccine virus in a carefully controlled fashion.

Measles antibody levels and seronegativity were reported to be lower in normal controls than in a group of children infected by blood transfusion during infancy.[8]

[a] Supported in part by the Centers for Disease Control's Cooperative Agreement Number U64/CCU90451.
[b] Address for correspondence: Dr. Philip A. Brunell, Division of Pediatric Infectious Diseases, Ahmanson Pediatric Center, Cedars–Sinai Medical Center, 8700 Beverly Blvd., Room 4310, Los Angeles, CA 90048.

Although no apparent abnormalities were found in immunoglobin levels or B-cell numbers, other studies have revealed profound intrinsic defects in B-cell function that were reported to be independent of T cells.[9] In addition to the lower antibody levels in these HIV-infected children, reimmunization with measles vaccine failed to prevent a relentless decline in antibody levels in these children during the ensuing period of observation. Antibody elevations following reimmunization were observed in a smaller proportion of HIV-infected children than had been reported previously in normal vaccinees.[10] In contrast to the normal children who had persistence of measles antibody following reimmunization, HIV-infected children who did respond tended to have a blunted or transitory rise in measles antibody. Thus, their immunologic recall appeared to be defective. In addition to declining antibody levels in HIV-infected children, there appeared to be an inability to synthesize high-avidity antibody. Chaotropic agents, for example, have been used to distinguish primary infection from reexposure for a variety of infectious agents.[11-13] Thus, although one might have expected an increase in urea-resistant, high-avidity antibody after reimmunization with measles vaccine, this was found in only a few HIV-infected children who received an additional dose of vaccine. In addition, a progressive decline in high-avidity antibody was found in these HIV-infected children.[8]

The inability to sustain adequate levels of measles antibody, respond to reimmunization, or synthesize high-avidity antibody appropriately are all evidence of defective immunologic memory. No obvious relationship was found in these children between competency of these functions and the total number or percent of CD4 cells or CD8 cells or clinical stage of illness. Adoptive transfer experiments, however, have demonstrated the role of two different clones of CD4 cells, one secreting IL-4 and IL-5 and the other IL-2 and IFN-γ on terminal differentiation of B cells into antibody-producing cells as well as inducing both memory and affinity maturation.[14] It also is of interest that the $CD29^+/CD45RO^+$ subset of CD4 cells, which provides helper functions and participates in response to recall antigens, has been reported to be preferentially infected by HIV.[15] Thus, abnormalities in critical subsets of CD4 cells may not be reflected by the parameters measured.

The identification of deficiencies of specific subsets of cells that are associated with abnormalities of antibody production in HIV-infected persons would be of great potential usefulness. CD4 cells have been a helpful but imperfect measure of disease progression and for predicting increased risk of pneumocystis infection.[16] It would be preferable, however, to identify a deficiency of a specific subset of cells that might presage the occurrence of opportunistic or more frequent common infections. This would not only allow for more accurate clinical staging but also it would facilitate the timely use of prophylactic measures, for example, the use of IVIG or antipneumocystis prophylaxis. The observation that, in mice, antibody production and avidity maturation can be blocked by antibody against mediators secreted by specific clones of CD4 cells[14] suggests that it might be possible to restore some of these functions in HIV-infected patients by providing mediators secreted by subsets found to be deficient.

Changes in antibody avidity in HIV-infected patients may be of significance in a variety of ways. It may influence both the choice and interpretation of serologic assays that are used in these patients. In assays, for example, neutralization tests or the hemagglutination inhibition test (HAI), antibody and live organisms or antigen, respectively, are incubated under conditions optimal for their combination. Then, the uncombined antigen or unneutralized organism is detected by an indicator system. In other types of assays, for example, ELISA or fluorescence antibody assays, which are based on detection of reactions between antibody and antigen, there are frequent washings to remove unreacted antibody. The washing fluid, which is devoid of reactants, may permit a reequilibration that could result in the loss of lower avidity antibody. The use of the latter type of assay in HIV-infected patients who may have lost their ability to produce high-avidity antibody may lead to false negatives in diagnostic serologic tests. This may be more critical in antibody-capture ELISA such as those used to detect IgM. In these assays, multiple reagents are used, each followed by many washings. This may account for the relatively low sensitivity of these assays. The particular assay used to assess protection conferred by vaccines also may be important in the interpretation of the data. It is of interest that the HAI was reported to be much more sensitive when compared to an ELISA in normal measles vaccine recipients,[17,18] while the reverse was true in HIV-infected children.[7] This is consistent with the observation that HIV-infected children tend to lose their ability to synthesize high-avidity measles antibody. Thus, they would have been found to have lower titers by ELISA *using low concentrations of both antigen and antibody* which would have been less capable of detecting low-avidity antibody than the HAI.

As the relationship of avidity to protection has not been established for measles, it cannot be stated which assay is optimal for measuring protection. It has been reported that high-avidity antibody against *Hemophilus influenzae* type b has greater bactericidal activity than low-avidity antibody.[19] Detection of protection of baby rats against infection with streptococcus is dependent upon the *avidity* of the antibody.[20] There have been many efforts to define protective levels of antibody against measles, but little attention paid to the relationship of antibody avidity to protection. In normal children, seronegativity as defined by ELISA predicted the outcome of exposure; cases occurred only in the seronegatives, and none occurred in those found to be seropositive.[1] Similar efforts have been made for the neutralizing antibody assay.[21] In comparing the two assays, the neutralizing antibody assay was more sensitive for detecting antibody three weeks after immunization, at which time more low-avidity antibody would be expected to be present than later. Mean ELISA titers were lower at this time than they were eight months post immunization.[18]

The implication of these findings on immunization of patients who are HIV infected may be significant. They will not be fully apparent, however, until the relationship between antibody avidity and protection is better defined. If avidity is found to be a determinant of protection, the timing of immunization, the characteristics of vaccines used to immunize, and how the response to immunization is assayed will be important. Children who are infected around the time of birth may retain their ability to produce high-avidity antibody long enough to respond normally to routine immunizations. Thus they can be immunized with measles vaccine[22] without suffering the severe side effects observed in children with leukemia.[23] If high-avidity antibody is found to be essential for protection, it would be useful to determine how long this capability is retained in order to establish the optimal timing of immunization in HIV-infected children. The significance of the progressive loss of ability to synthesize high-avidity antibody is uncertain at the present time. Restoration of high-avidity measles antibody by reimmunization does not appear to be effective as the disease progresses. Adults who were infected with HIV following their infection with measles virus or measles vaccine virus presumably would already have been programmed to produce high-avidity antibody. Thus, the effect of HIV infection on measles antibody synthesis would be expected to be less profound than in children. There has been considerable variation in the reports of persistence of measles antibody in HIV-infected adults.[2,24,25] These may reflect the assays used, the stage of infection, and the frequency of reexposure to measles. In normal children reexposure to measles results in a higher antibody titer in measles vaccinees.[26] Our data indicate, however, that recall may be defective in HIV-infected persons so that reexposure may not have the same booster effects as in normal persons. Finally, the success of attempts to affect the progression of HIV infection by boosting immunity by immunization may be dependent on the timing and type of immunization.

REFERENCES

1. GUSTAFSON, T. L., A. W. LIEVENS, P. A. BRUNELL, R. G. MOELLENBERG, et al. 1987. Measles outbreak in a fully immunized secondary-school population. N. Engl. J. Med. **316**: 771–774.
2. EMBREE, J. E., P. DATTA, W. STACKIW, et al. 1992. Increased risk of early measles in infants of human immunodeficiency virus type 1–seropositive mothers. J. Infect. Dis. **165**: 262–267.
3. LEPAGE, P., F. DABIS, P. MSELLATI, et al. 1992. Safety and immunogenicity of high dose Edmonston-Zagreb measles vaccine in children with HIV-1 infection. Am. J. Dis. Child **146**: 550–555.
4. SENSION, M. G., T. C. QUINN, L. E. MARKOWITZ, M. J. LINNAN, et al. 1988. Measles in hospitalized African children with human immunodeficiency virus. Am. J. Dis. Child. **142**: 1271–1272.
5. MORBIDITY AND MORTALITY WEEKLY REPORT. 1988. Measles in HIV-infected children, United States. JAMA (April 22/29) **259(16)**: 2352–2357.
6. KAPLAN, L. J., R. S. DAUM, M. SMARON & C. A. MCCARTHY. 1992. Severe measles in immunocompromised patients. JAMA (March 4) **267(9)**: 1237–1241.
7. KRASINSKI, K. & W. BORKOWSKY. 1989. Measles and measles immunity in children infected with human immunodeficiency virus. JAMA **261(17)**: 2512–2516.
8. BRUNELL, P. A., V. VIMAL, T. COURVILLE, I. SRUGO & V. ISRAELE. 1992. The accelerated decline of antibody in HIV infected measles vaccinees. VIII International Conference on AIDS/III STD World Congress. Amsterdam, the Netherlands. Poster Abstracts **2**: A20.
9. LANE H. C., H. MASUR, L. C. EDGAR, G. WHALEN, et al. 1983. Abnormalities of B-cell activation and immunoregulation in patients with the acquired immunodeficiency syndrome. N. Engl. J. Med. **309(8)**: 453–458.
10. MARKOWITZ, L. E., P. ALBRECHT, W. A. ORENSTEIN, S. M. LETT, et al. 1992. Persistence of measles antibody after revaccination. J. Infect. Dis. **166**: 205–208.
11. BLACKBURN, N. K., T. G. BESSELAAR, B. D. SCHOUB & K. F. O'CONNELL. 1991. Differentiation of primary cytomegalovirus infection from reactivation using the urea denaturation test for measuring antibody avidity. J. Med. Virol. **33**: 6–9.
12. HEDMAN, K. & S. A. ROUSSEAU 1989. Measurement of avidity of specific IgG for verification of recent primary rubella. J. Med. Virol. **27**: 288–292.

13. THOMAS, H. I. J. & P. MORGAN-CAPNER. 1988. Rubella-specific IgG subclass avidity ELISA and its role in the differentiation between primary rubella and rubella reinfection. Epidem. Inf. **101:** 591–598.
14. RIZZO, L. V., R. H. DEKRUYFF & D. T. UMETSU. 1992. Generation of B cell memory and affinity maturation. Induction with Th1 and Th2 T cell clones. J. Immunol. **148(12):** 3733–3739.
15. FAUCI, A. S., S. M. SCHNITTMAN, G. POLI, et al. 1991. Immunopathogenic mechanisms in human immunodeficiency virus (HIV) infection. Ann. Intern. Med. **114(8):** 679–693.
16. LEADS FROM THE MORBIDITY AND MORTALITY WEEKLY REPORT. 1991. Guidelines for prophylaxis against *Pneumocystis carinii* pneumonia for children infected with human immunodeficiency virus. JAMA **265(13):** 1637–1644.
17. WEIGLE, K. A., M. D. MURPHY & P. A. BRUNELL. 1984. Enzyme-linked immunosorbent assay for evaluation of immunity to measles virus. J. Clin. Microbiol. **19(3):** 376–379.
18. STETLER, H. C., W. A. ORENSTEIN, R. H. BERNIER, et al. 1986. Impact of revaccinating children who initially received measles vaccine before ten months of age. Pediatrics **77(4):** 471–476.
19. SCHLESINGER, Y., D. M. GRANOFF & VACCINE STUDY GROUP. 1992. Avidity and bactericidal activity of antibody elicited by different *Haemophilus influenzae* type b conjugate vaccines. JAMA **267(11):** 1489–1494.
20. PINCUS, S. H., A. O. SHIGEOKA, A. A. MOE, L. P. EWING & H. R. HILL. 1988. Protective efficacy of IgM monoclonal antibodies in experimental group B streptococcal infection is a function of antibody avidity. J. Immunol. **140(8):** 2779–2785.
21. CHEN, R., L. E. MARKOWITZ, P. ALBRECHT, J. A. STEWART, et al. 1990. Measles antibody: Reevaluation of protective titers. J. Infect. Dis. **162:** 1036–1042.
22. MCLAUGHLIN, M., P. THOMAS, I. ONORATO, et al. 1988. Live virus vaccines in human immunodeficiency virus-infected children: A retrospective survey. Pediatrics **82(2):** 229–233.
23. MITUS, A., A. HOLLOWAY, A. E. EVANS & J. F. ENDERS. 1962. Attenuated measles vaccine in children with acute leukemia. Am. J. Dis. Child. **103:** 243–248.
24. SHA, B. E., A. A. HARRIS, C. A. BENSON, et al. 1991. Prevalence of measles antibodies in asymptomatic human immunodeficiency virus-infected adults. J. Infect. Dis. **164:** 973–975.
25. GLASER, J. B. & R. GREIFINGER. 1992. Measles antibodies in human immunodeficiency virus infected adults. J. Infect. Dis. **165:** 589.
26. KRUGMAN, S. 1977. Present status of measles and rubella immunization in the United States: A medical progress report. J. Pediatr. **90:** 1–12.

Maternal Transmission and Diagnosis of Human Immunodeficiency Virus during Infancy

DIANE W. WARA,[a,b] KATHERINE LUZURIAGA,[c]
NATASHA L. MARTIN,[a] JOHN L. SULLIVAN,[c] AND
YVONNE J. BRYSON[d]

[a] Department of Pediatrics
UCSF, School of Medicine
San Francisco, California 95143

[c] Department of Pediatrics
University of Massachusetts Medical School
Worcester, Massachusetts 01605

[d] Department of Pediatrics
UCLA School of Medicine
Los Angeles, California 90024-1752

Over 90% of children infected with human immunodeficiency virus type 1 (HIV-1) in the United States acquire their infection from their mothers. Transmission may occur *in utero*[1-3] or postpartum (through breast milk).[4,5] Increasing evidence, however, supports the transmission of HIV-1 during the peripartum period.[6-10] In the United States, the majority of infants acquire HIV-1 by *in utero* or peripartum transmission. Of infants born to HIV-infected women, only a subgroup eventually prove infected. The risk of transmission varies throughout the world from 14.4% in the European Collaborative Study,[11] 28% in New York City,[12] 31% in San Francisco, to 45% in areas of Kenya. The risk factors for perinatal transmission, its timing, and the early diagnosis of HIV-1-infected infants are under active investigation.

Several factors contribute to the variable rates of HIV-1 perinatal transmission. It is likely that many or all will eventually prove important. The duration of the epidemic may contribute to the severity of illness among HIV-infected pregnant women. In the European Collaborative Study, which was based on 721 children

---

[b] Address for correspondence: Diane W. Wara, M.D., Department of Pediatrics, UCSF, School of Medicine, Box 0105, 505 Parnassus, San Francisco, CA 94143.

born to 701 mothers, the rate of vertical transmission was 14.4%.[11] The most significant predictor of transmission was the stage of maternal infection. Four infants born to 13 women with clinical AIDS were infected (31%); 14 infants born to 602 women without signs or symptoms of HIV infection were infected (14%). The immunologic and virologic correlates of progressive HIV infection also predicted perinatal transmission. The transmission rate was threefold higher in those with CD4 cell counts below 400/μl (19%) than in those with CD4 cell counts above 700/μl (6%). The presence of p24 antigen during the third trimester or at the time of delivery increased the risk of transmission from 10% to 29%. The ability to detect virus in the peripheral blood of a pregnant woman, as well as the presence of rapidly proliferating virus with high copy numbers (> 500), increased the risk of transmission. It is likely that a minor subset of maternal virus is transmitted to the infant and possible that a specific capsular epitope within the V3 region protects against transmission of the virus.[13]

The maternal immune response to her own (autologous) virus influences transmission. The presence of neutralizing antibodies in the mother directed against her own virus appears to decrease transmission.[14–16] For unknown reasons, not all women form these antibodies. The presence of neutralizing antibody directed against heterologous virus does not decrease viral transmission. It is likely that the role of other immune responses, such as antibody-dependent cellular cytotoxicity or the presence of cytotoxic T lymphocytes, will be shown to modify perinatal transmission.

The infant's gestational age, mode of delivery, and breast feeding also affect the risk of perinatal transmission. In the European Collaborative Trial, the relationship between transmission rate and gestational age was nonlinear, with a higher risk of transmission to infants born before 34 weeks' gestational age (33%) than to those born after 34 weeks' gestation (14%). There was little additional reduction in the risk of transmission to infants born between 34 and 40 weeks' gestation.[11] Maternal intravenous drug use was a risk factor for prematurity; however, the increased risk of transmission persisted after allowing for this fact. It is possible that infants born before 34 weeks' gestational age acquire inadequate IgG maternal antibody directed against HIV. Active transplacental transfer of IgG from mother to fetus occurs between 32 weeks' gestational age and term.

The mode of delivery may influence perinatal transmission. Although several studies have shown equivalent transmission to infants born vaginally or by cesarian section, the European Collaborative Study results suggest that emergency cesarean section may protect against perinatal transmission. The majority of infants (76%) were delivered vaginally, and the transmission rate for delivery vaginally (16%) and by elective cesarean section (13%) were similar. Nevertheless, delivery by emergency cesarean section correlated with a reduced risk of transmission (7%).[11] The relationship between perinatal transmission and cesarean section merits further attention.

HIV-1 has been detected in breast milk and colostrum both by culture and polymerase chain reaction (PCR). Its presence does not necessarily mean that breast feeding is a significant mode of transmission. Several case reports[4] as well as a review of experience in Kigali, Rwanda[5] strongly suggest that HIV-1 can be transmitted by breast milk from mother to infant. Dunn *et al.* reviewed five previ-

TABLE 1. Estimates of Additional Risk of HIV-1 Transmission through Breast-Feeding

Location	Rate of Transmission	
	Ever Breast-Fed n (%)	Never Breast-Fed n (%)
Europe	13/41 (32)	110/767 (14)
Miami	7/25 (28)	18/54 (33)
France	7/16 (44)	101/590 (17)
Switzerland	2/13 (15)	21/128 (16)
Kinshasa, Zaire	19/96 (20)	0/10 (0)
Australia	7/14 (50)	3/18 (17)

NOTE: Modified from Dunn et al.[17]

ously published studies and estimated an incremental risk of HIV-1 transmission through breast-feeding, above perinatal transmission, of 14%[17] (TABLE 1). The European Collaborative Study results reflected an increment of 15% transmission to infants if ever breast-fed.[11] The combined results of these studies support the recommendation that HIV-1-infected women in the United States not breast-feed their infants.

The subgroup of infants (14%–45%) who prove to be HIV-1 infected may acquire their infection *in utero*, intrapartum, or postpartum through breast-feeding. The *in utero* model, similar to transmission of rubella virus, is supported by the identification of HIV in fetal tissue as early as 12 to 15 weeks' gestation[1,2] and abnormalities of fetal thymus by 15 to 30 weeks' gestation.[3] Placental abnormalities, including funisitis and chorioamnionitis, suggest HIV-1 infection before the perinatal period. Finally, the ability to isolate virus and/or to demonstrate its presence by PCR or immune-complex-dissociated HIV p24 antigen (ICD p24) at or within the first week of birth in approximately 50% of infants who eventually prove infected supports *in utero* acquisition of virus in some infants.[10,17–20]

The intrapartum transmission of HIV-1, similar to the transmission of hepatitis B, is supported by the *inability* to isolate virus or to demonstrate its presence by PCR or ICD p24 antigen in at least 50% of infants who eventually prove infected. Both in adults and children, virus cannot be cultured from the peripheral blood for approximately six weeks following the time of transmission. Three infants with prospective studies were reported with negative cord blood PCR, p24 antigen and cultures, and with positive PCR and cultures by 2 months of age. The sequence of virus identification in these patients suggests that they were infected perinatally; the increase and decline of the HIV-1 titer and serum p24 level may represent primary viremia.[7,8]

It is probable that perinatal transmission of HIV-1 occurs by exposure to virus in blood and/or amniotic fluid during delivery. HIV may enter the systemic circulation by the mucosal route (mouth, stomach, intestine), the skin, or the conjunctivae. Stomach pH is neutral during the first 24 hours of life and so could sustain HIV-1. Abrasions of skin, through fetal scalp monitoring or delivery, have been associated with transmission. The finding that in twin births the first-born twin was more frequently infected than the second born provides further evidence of intrapartum infection.[21] It is likely that the first-born twin encounters higher concentrations of virus in the birth canal than the second, more quickly born.

The bimodal onset of HIV-related disease in infants and children further supports both *in utero* and intrapartum transmission. A retrospective chart review of 238 children with AIDS whose only known route of infection was maternal revealed two populations of children.[22] Approximately 20% developed AIDS during their first year of life with a median incubation period of 4.1 months. A second, and larger, cohort developed signs or symptoms of AIDS at a rate of 8% per year, with a median onset of disease at 4.8 years. It is possible that those infants with early-onset disease were infected *in utero*, while those with a longer incubation period were infected perinatally. Burgard *et al.* reported that the presence of p24 antigen at birth in seven infants was associated with the development of early and rapidly progressive HIV-related disease.[18] It is likely that newborns with p24 antigen at birth were infected *in utero* and represent those at risk for early-onset disease. The correlation between the culture of virus and/or detection of p24 antigen at birth and the early onset of rapidly progressive disease will require a larger, prospective study.

The timing of HIV acquisition, the active transport of IgG across the placenta, and the relative immaturity of the newborn's immune system influence our ability to distinguish an infected from an uninfected infant. All infants born to HIV-infected women have circulating IgG antibody to HIV. IgG actively crosses the placenta between 30 and 32 weeks' gestation, and its presence in the newborn mirrors the mother's immune response rather than documenting infection in the infant. Therefore, until age 18 months, an infant's HIV status is determined by documenting virus in the peripheral blood by culture, PCR, or ICD p24. Recently, a sensitive and specific assay for IgA anti-HIV has been developed. IgA does not cross the placenta, and the presence of IgA anti-HIV may provide a serological tool for early diagnosis.[23,24] However, the sensitivity of the IgA assay is only 77% by age 12 weeks; it is possible that HIV-infected infants have an incomplete early immune response to the virus. IgA anti-HIV is produced by age six months by over 90% of infected children.

We hypothesize that infants infected *in utero* have either HIV genome detected by PCR or HIV isolated from blood within 48 hours of birth. In contrast, those infected intrapartum undergo a primary viremia and only subsequently (days 7 to 90) can virus be detected.[25] The identification of virus by culture of peripheral blood mononuclear cells (PBMC) remains the "gold standard" for diagnosis of infection in infants younger than age 18 months. Frequently, PBMC cultures and PCR are negative, even in infants eventually proven to be infected during the first month of life; both approaches to diagnosis offer greater than 90% sensitivity by age six months (TABLE 2). The diagnostic value of viral culture in 181 infants at birth revealed 48% sensitivity but 100% specificity.[18] Others have shown that PCR also is approximately 50% sensitive at birth. p24 antigen is less sensitive than culture or PCR for diagnosis of HIV infection at birth. ICD p24, however, which disrupts potential immune complexes between circulating viral antigen and maternal antibody, was 63% sensitive and 91% specific for infection in cord blood.[10] This study was limited to the prospective evaluation of eight infected neonates; five of the eight had ICD p24 present in cord blood. The ICD p24 assay appears

TABLE 2. Comparison of Methods Used for Early Diagnosis in Infected Infants: Sensitivity (%)

Method	Age[a]				
	1 week	4 weeks	2 months	3–6 months	>6 months
Culture	30–50	50	70–90	>90	>90
PCR	30–50	50	70–90	>90	>90
p24 ag	10–25	20–50	30–60	30–50	20–40
ICD p24 ag	63	100	ND	ND	ND
IgA anti-HIV	<10	10–30	20–50	50–80	>90

[a] Results expressed as percent sensitivity.

rapid, simple, relative accurate, and inexpensive for the diagnosis of HIV infection in neonates.

The current challenge is to translate these research findings into a practical, cost-effective algorithm for the diagnosis of HIV during infancy in a range of clinical settings. Current recommendations include obtaining HIV culture and PCR from infants born to HIV-1-infected mothers as close to birth as is possible. If there is no evidence of virus, both should be repeated at the ages of 3 and 6 months. The initial presence of virus should be interpreted as probable infection, and HIV-1 infection should be confirmed by a second culture or PCR. The recent report of the sensitivity and specificity of ICD p24 is encouraging, and additional neonates should be evaluated; it is possible that ICD p24 will soon replace the more costly PBMC culture and PCR for diagnosis of HIV during the first few months of life. The combination of culture and PCR are sufficiently sensitive for the diagnosis of HIV by age 6 months. If there is no evidence of virus after two or more cultures are obtained around age 6 months, further evaluation should use IgG anti-HIV; ELISA and, if positive, Western blot, should be obtained at the ages of 12 and 18 months. It is unlikely that an infant with no virologic, serologic, immunologic, or clinical evidence of HIV infection by age 18 months is infected.

Establishing the diagnosis of HIV infection with confidence early in life is difficult. Nevertheless, relieving the family's anxiety if the infant is not infected and establishing a beneficial medical regimen if the infant is infected support an aggressive approach to early diagnosis. It is probable that a simplified approach to early diagnosis will be established within the next few years.

REFERENCES

1. SPRECHER, S., G. SOUMENKOFF, F. PUISSANT & M. DE GUELDRA. 1985. Vertical transmission of HIV in 15-week fetus. Lancet 2: 288–289.
2. JOVAISAS, E., M. A. KOCH & A. SCHAFER. 1985. LAV/HTLV III in 20-week fetus. Lancet 2: 1129.
3. PAPIERNIK, M., Y. BROSSARD, N. MULLIEZ, et al. 1992. Thymic abnormalities in fetuses aborted from human immunodeficiency virus type 1 seropositive women. Pediatrics 89: 297–301.
4. ZIEGLER, J., R. JOHNSON, D. COOPER, et al. 1985. Postnatal transmission of AIDS-associated retrovirus from mother to infant. Lancet 1: 896.
5. VAN DE PERRE, P., A. SIMONON, P. MSELLATI, et al. 1991. Postnatal transmission of

human immunodeficiency virus type 1 from mother to infant. N. Engl. J. Med. **325:** 594–598.
6. EHRNST, A., S. LINDGRAN, M. DICTOR, et al. 1991. HIV in pregnant women and their offspring: Evidence for late transmission. Lancet **338:** 203–207.
7. ALIMENTI, A., K. LUZURIAGA, B. STECHENBERG & J. L. SULLIVAN. 1991. Quantitation of human immunodeficiency virus in vertically infected infants and children. J. Pediatr. **119:** 225–229.
8. LUZURIAGA, K., P. MCQUILKIN & A. ALIMENTI. 1993. Early viremia and immune responses in vertical human immunodeficiency virus type 1 infection. J. Inf. Dis. In press.
9. KRIVINE, A., G. FIRTION, L. CAO, et al. 1992. HIV replication during the first weeks of life. Lancet **339:** 1187–1189.
10. MILES, S., E. BALDEN, L. MAGPANTAY, et al. 1993. Rapid serologic testing with immune-complex-dissociated HIV p24 antigen for early detection of HIV infection in neonates. N. Engl. J. Med. **328:** 297–302.
11. EUROPEAN COLLABORATIVE STUDY. 1992. Risk factors for mother-to-child transmission of HIV-1. Lancet **339:** 1007–1012.
12. THOMAS, P., J. WEEDON & NEW YORK CITY PERINATAL HIV TRANSMISSION COLLABORATIVE STUDY GROUP. 1992. Maternal predictors of perinatal HIV transmission. VIII International Conference on AIDS, Amsterdam. Abst # WeC 1059: We56.
13. WOLINSKY, S., C. WIKE, B. KORBER, et al. 1992. Selective transmission of human immunodeficiency virus type-1 variants from mothers to infants. Science **255:** 1134–1137.
14. SCARLATTI, G., J. ALBERT & P. ROSSI. 1992. Homologus and heterologous neutralization activity in sera of HIV-1 infected mothers: Correlation to transmission. VIII International Conference on AIDS, Amsterdam. Abst # WeC 1061.
15. KLIKS, S., M. FADEM, D. WARA & J. LEVY. 1992. Evidence for the maternal transfer of neutralization-escape or enhancement variants into newborn infants. VIII International Conference on AIDS.
16. LEHMAN, D., E. GARRATTY, S. PLAEGER-MARSHALL & Y. BRYSON. 1992. Neutralizing antibody to autologous HIV virus isolates in asymptomatic mothers. Presented at the Society for Pediatric Research, Baltimore, Maryland. April, 1992.
17. DUNN, D., M. NEWELL, A. ADES & C. PECKHAM. 1992. Risk of human immunodeficiency virus type 1 transmission through breastfeeding. Lancet **340:** 585–588.
18. BURGARD, M., M. MAYAYX & S. BLANCHE. 1992. The use of viral culture and p24 antigen testing to diagnose human immunodeficiency virus infection in neonates. N. Engl. J. Med. **327:** 1192–1197.
19. ROGERS, M., C-Y. OU, M. RAYFIELD, et al. 1989. Use of the polymerase chain reaction for the early detection of the proviral sequences of human immunodeficiency virus in infants born to seropositive mothers. N. Engl. J. Med. **320:** 1649–1654.
20. BRYSON, Y., I. CHEN, S. MILES, et al. 1992. A prospective evaluation of HIV co-culture for early diagnosis of perinatal HIV infection. Presented at the 7th International Conference on AIDS, Florence, Italy, June 1992.
21. GOEDERT, J., A. DULIEGE, C. AMOS, et al. 1991. High risk of HIV-1 infection for first-born twins. Lancet **338:** 1471–1475.
22. AUGER, I., P. THOMAS, V. DE GRUTTOLA, et al. 1988. Incubation periods for paediatric AIDS patients. Nature **336:** 575–577.
23. MARTIN N., J. LEVY, H. LEGG, et al. Detection of infection with human immunodeficiency virus (HIV) type 1 in infants by an anti-HIV immunoglobulin A assay using recombinant proteins. J. Pediatr. **118:** 354–358.
24. QUINN, T., R. KLINE, N. HALSEY, et al. 1991. Early diagnosis of perinatal HIV infection by detection of viral-specific IgA antibodies. JAMA **266:** 3439–3442.
25. BRYSON, Y., K. LUZURIAGA, J. SULLIVAN & D. WARA. 1992. Establishment of a definition of the timing of vertical HIV-1 infection. N. Engl. J. Med. **327(17):** 1246–1247.

Human Immune Development: Implications for Congenital HIV Infection[a]

SUSANNA CUNNINGHAM-RUNDLES,[b,c,d]
CINDY (XIN) CHEN,[c,d] JAMES B. BUSSEL,[a]
CLAUDIA BLANKENSHIP,[e] MIRTA B. VEBER,[c]
DEBORAH SANDERS-LAUFER,[e] TONY HINDS,[e]
JOSEPH S. CERVIA,[e] AND PAUL EDELSON[e]

[c] *The Immunology Research Laboratory*
[d] *Division of Hematology/Oncology*
[e] *Division of Infectious Disease*
Department of Pediatrics
The New York Hospital
Cornell University Medical Center
New York, New York 10021

INTRODUCTION

Knowledge of the normal human immune system and its potential vulnerability at different stages of development is important for study of the human immunodeficiency virus (HIV)-infected infant. Because clinical latency is often prolonged in adults with HIV infection, immune defense mechanisms are thought to provide effective, if transient, protection. Studies suggest that host defense mechanisms are gradually overwhelmed by the generation of viral diversity[1] in the context of gradual CD4 depletion.[2] In contrast, however, in children, the rate of progression is much faster, and latency much briefer.[3] The reasons for this are not known, but are assumed to be related to general immaturity of the host defense system during fetal life and at birth. The possible mechanisms of normal fetal and neonatal hyporesponsiveness include direct downregulation (associated with maternal-fetal tolerance), incomplete differentiation of immune cells, and lack of exposure to antigens of the external world.[4,5] Change in immune processing appears to occur in association with development and aging throughout life. As a consequence

---

[a] This work was supported by National Institutes of Health Grants R01 525851 and CA 29502.

[b] Address for correspondence: Dr. S. Cunningham-Rundles, The New York Hospital-Cornell University Medical Center, 1300 York Avenue, New York, NY 10021.

of aging, specific lymphocyte subpopulations needed to mediate host defense may become depleted.[6] Changes in the thymus occur from the time of birth and accompany the transition to adulthood.[7] Current evidence suggests that the period around 21 years of age is an important transition period that may affect response to HIV viral infection. In a large epidemiological study of 300 hemophiliacs exposed to HIV through blood product transfusion before 1985, Goedert et al.[8] found that hemophiliacs younger than 21 years of age at the time of seroconversion showed better retention of $CD4^+$ T-cell number during the succeeding five-year period compared to those who were older. The potential relevance of this is suggested from the fact that it was possible to confirm these findings in a study of a single, smaller, homogeneous clinic population of 40 hemophiliacs in which the median age difference between the two groups was only about six years.[9] It seems likely that thymic change, which enters a new phase of more rapid involution, characterized by reduced serum level of thymic hormone at approximately 16 years[10] may be involved in this difference. If the thymus of the HIV-infected host contains a substantial population of infected cells, as has been shown for the lymph node,[11] infected cells would potentially be flushed into the circulation with involution. When thymic involution undergoes normal speeding up, loss of the thymus as a barrier to passage of infected cells into the peripheral blood compartment would add to viral load.

In contrast to the positive effect of younger age on host response in late adolescence, congenital HIV infection confers the greatest risk of progression: almost 50% at two years compared to any other risk group.[3] Several studies have suggested that the $CD4^+$ T lymphocyte subpopulation that has memory function may be more susceptible to HIV infection.[12] Function of this population of cells is important for normal response to newly encountered environmental pathogens. Since the memory T-cell population is smaller at birth than in later life, it may be depleted more rapidly than in adults.[13,14] Thus, transition points between stages of immune development may be associated with selective vulnerability to HIV. Study of these stages could provide clues to the interaction of HIV with the developing host.

Normal immune development at birth has been fairly well characterized for the humoral arm of immune response in terms of the delayed switch from IgM to IgG antibodies and the increased frequency of low or absent antibody response, while the cellular immune response has been much less well characterized.[4,15,16] Recent studies using monoclonal antibodies and flow cytometry have shown that lymphocyte subpopulations from the full-term infant of normal gestational age are similar to adults and have similar proliferative response to T- and B-cell mitogens.[17–19] Although cytokines such as interleukin-1 and interleukin-2 are made normally by the neonate,[20,21] interferon γ production has been found to be deficient,[22] and neonates have been shown to have reduced response to interferon γ.[23] In general, it has seemed that the nonresponsiveness of the neonate is caused by immaturity. Nevertheless, several lines of inquiry, including data presented here, indicate that in some fundamental instances this nonresponsiveness is an effect of specific downregulation, perhaps related to the late or waning effect of mechanisms needed during *in utero* life to maintain maternal–fetal tolerance. In studies presented here, we discuss the normal development of the human immune system, investigated during gestation by means of periumbilical blood sampling (PUBS), in comparison with the premature infant of comparable gestational age. We also discuss patterns of development relevant to infants exposed during gestation or at birth to HIV.

CD4+ LYMPHOCYTE SUBSET DEVELOPMENT

Infection of the CD4+ T lymphocyte is central to the development of HIV disease. It seems logical that the relative availability of these cells in an appropriate activation state is important for the establishment of infection. From the studies of Haynes *et al.*, it is known that T cells expressing the α, β heterodimeric form of the T-cell receptor appear in significant number after about 12 weeks of gestation.[24] By means of PUBS sampling, Rainaut *et al.*[25] have shown that mature T cells are easily identified in peripheral blood circulation by 20 to 26 weeks. Longitudinal study of the relative percentage of these cells during gestation by PUBS sampling suggests that there are significant and previously unrecognized changes during fetal development. As shown in FIGURE 1 for three fetuses studied sequentially and in data presented in TABLE 1 for a large number of fetuses studied at specific times during gestation, we have found that the percentage of CD4+ T cells declined transiently but significantly in late gestation (weeks 35 to 37) compared to levels in the previous period of fetal life (weeks 28 to 30) and compared

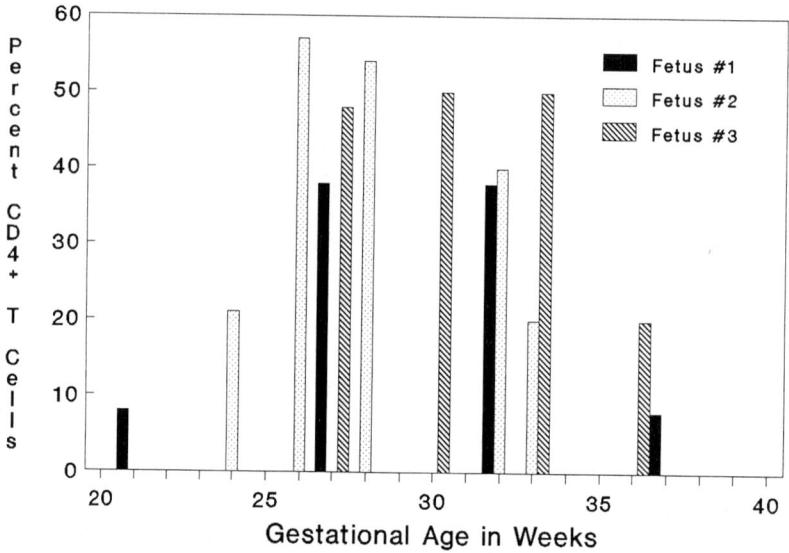

FIGURE 1. Data show change in percent CD4+ T cells as measured by flow cytometry using anti-CD8 monoclonal antibody conjugated to FITC compared with change in gestational age for three infants sampled periumbilically during fetal life.

to normal adult controls. At birth, cord blood studies of these infants showed that CD4+ T cell percentages had normalized to adult levels. Cord blood studies of full-term infants by others have shown that lymphocytosis at birth[26] is generally, although not universally, observed, so that there is a relatively increased number of CD4+ T lymphocytes at this point.[18] Changes such as these might be reflected in greater or lesser risk of infection for the HIV-exposed infant depending on the activation state of these cells.

After birth, marked changes in lymphocyte subsets occur in the peripheral blood T-cell compartment, particularly during the first five years of life. These changes have been recognized only recently by new studies that have established normal ranges.[27] The need for accurate, age-adjusted normal ranges in evaluation of pediatric HIV disease is particularly important, since at least one-half of infants born to HIV-infected mothers with antibody to HIV are not infected and eventually lose this maternal antibody (seroreverts), but this may take more than a year.[28] Since HIV-infected mothers also have increased risk for other infections, susceptibility to opportunistic infections, or may undergo reactivation of latent infections, it has not been clear whether the immune system of HIV-exposed, noninfected, seroreverting infants is actually developmentally equivalent to that of non-HIV-exposed infants. To examine this, we compared non-HIV-exposed infants to both infected and noninfected HIV-exposed infants as determined retrospectively. As shown in FIGURE 2, there was no difference in CD4+ T cell percentage or absolute number between HIV-negative, age-matched infant groups exposed or unexposed

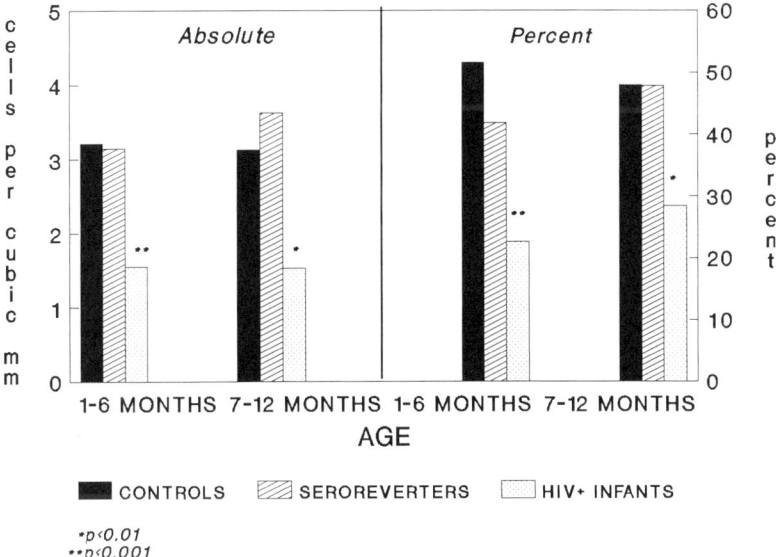

FIGURE 2. Data show relationship between percent and absolute CD4+ T cell number and age in seroreverting, HIV− infants of HIV+ mothers in comparison with HIV+ infants and HIV−-nonexposed infants.

TABLE 1. Fetal CD4$^+$ T-Lymphocyte Development: Effect of Gestational Age on Relative Percentage

	Fetal 28–30 Weeks (9)[a]	Fetal 35–37 Weeks (9)	Adults (112)
Min	22.4	7.4	23.9
Max	55.5	50.6	68.1
Mean	43.4	30.5	46.5
SD	11.7	14.3	8.0
p	ns[b]	$p < 0.01$	

[a] N given in parentheses.
[b] Not significant.

to HIV at one to five months or at six to nine months of age. These data suggest that at least with respect to CD4, seroreverting infants show normal development of the peripheral T-cell compartment despite being born to HIV-infected mothers.

DEVELOPMENT OF FUNCTIONAL T-CELL RESPONSE

The normal neonatal CD4$^+$ T-cell population is similar in relative proportion (percent) of lymphocytes, but increased in number compared to that of adults. Recent studies have suggested that there are important intrinsic differences in subpopulations of CD4$^+$ T cells identifiable by surface antigen differences. The neonatal T-cell population has been found to contain relatively few "memory" T cells expressing CD29 compared to adults and relatively more cells of "naive" phenotype expressing CD4 5RA.[13] The significance of this is related to differences in the capacity of these populations to respond to antigens and produce cytokines. Previous studies have shown that fetal T cells can respond to some activation signals even at 7 to 10 weeks of gestation.[29] Although the B-cell proliferative response also appears early in development, there is only limited differentiation into immunoglobulin-producing plasma cells, and production of antibodies is essentially restricted to the IgM subclass.[30] Cytotoxic activity of the fetal lymphocyte has been found to be markedly limited.[29] In the case of natural killer (NK) cell activity discussed below, this is attributable to very much lower levels of NK cells during fetal life and at birth. Several lines of investigation have shown that cytokine production in fetal life is more limited than in adults. Thymic epithelial cells produce IL-1, IL-6, G-CSF, M-CSF, and GM-CSF, which are essential for maturation,[31] but production of interferon γ by lymphocytes and tumor necrosis factor (TNF) by monocytes is reduced or absent. Previous studies have suggested that while T cells from the neonate have adult responsiveness to T-cell mitogens, there is poor responsiveness to antigens encountered normally postnatally.[5] Indeed, the poor responsiveness of cord blood lymphocytes to substances that readily stimulate lymphocytes from adults has been used to define a substance as an antigen.

Although most previous studies on fetal and neonatal immune response have used traditional plant lectins such as phytohemagglutinin (PHA) as lymphocyte mitogens, we became interested in using potentially physiological signals, specifically microbial antigens, toward which exposure might occur *in utero*. Sequential study of comparative immune responsiveness during fetal life to PHA, a typical T cell mitogen, and *Staphylococcus epidermadis*, which causes clinically significant illness in premature infants, is shown in FIGURE 3. In contrast to responsiveness to PHA, which remained relatively constant throughout gestation, activation toward *S. epidermadis* was greatest at 28 to 30 weeks of gestation and stronger than that of adult controls. In parallel studies, we examined responsiveness of infants of appropriate size for gestational age born prematurely at 27 to 30 weeks for responsiveness to microbial activators including *S. epidermadis*.[32] On the first day of life, these infants showed significantly stronger ($p < 0.01$) responsiveness to several microbial activators compared to cord blood of full-term infants or adult controls. Data is shown in FIGURE 4. Longitudinal studies of these infants over 10 to 14 days showed that this hyperresponsiveness was rapidly downregulated after birth, although response to PHA did not change over this period. Infants' lymphocyte responses declined significantly compared to their own response to the same microbial activator at birth. These effects were unrelated to sepsis, since septic infants were found to have generalized anergy to all activators.[32] These

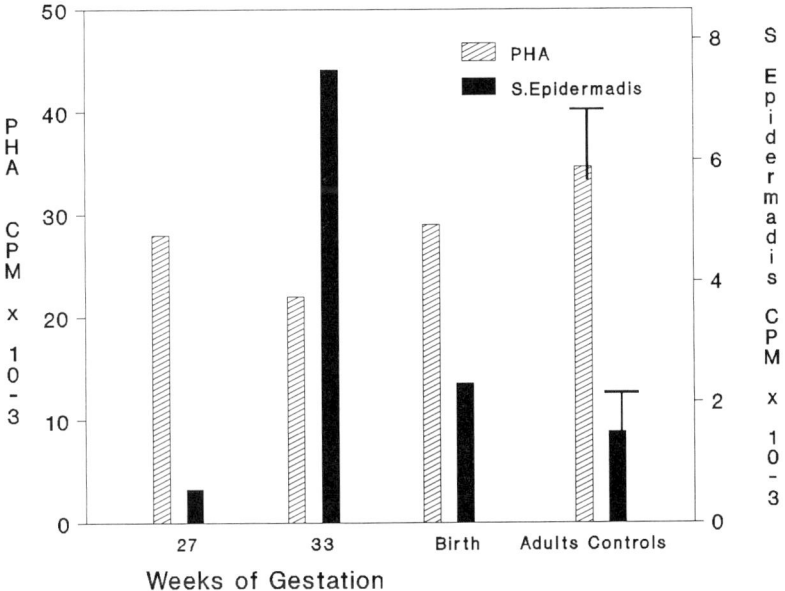

FIGURE 3. Fetal lymphocyte proliferative response to PHA and *S. epidermis* are shown for one fetus sampled longitudinally. Mononuclear cells were cultured at a lymphocyte density of 5×10^4 in microtiter plates for three or five days as appropriate for each activator, and proliferation was assessed by [^{14}C]thymidine incorporation. Data obtained for adult controls are shown in parallel.

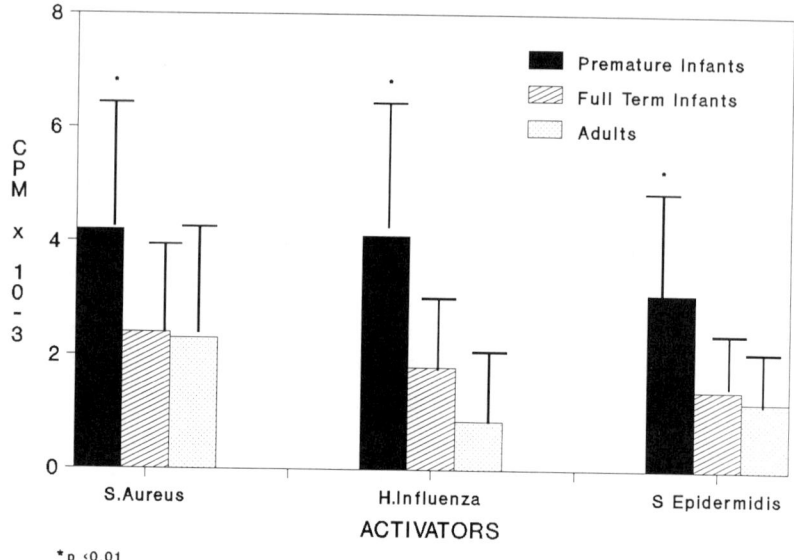

FIGURE 4. Proliferative response to three microbial activators is shown for premature infants (27 to 30 weeks gestation), full-term infants, and adult controls. Data were obtained by culture of mononuclear cells as described in legend to FIGURE 3.

data suggest that during late gestation there is a period of hyperresponsiveness to microbial signals *in vitro*. It is likely, therefore, that equivalent lymphocyte activation could occur *in utero* with relative ease at this stage. Because cellular activation is important in HIV infection for integration of the provirus, this developmental state could be associated with a period of vulnerability to HIV at around 27 to 30 weeks of gestation.

HOMOLOGY BETWEEN FETAL AND HIV$^+$ INFANT CD8$^+$ T CELLS

As noted above, the neonate has a relative lymphocytosis compared to adults. Within the T-cell compartment, this is characterized by a relatively increased ratio of CD4$^+$ T cells to CD8$^+$ T cells (CD4/CD8 ratio) because of the relatively low percentage of CD8$^+$ T cells. We have observed previously that the premature infant shows a rapid increase in CD8$^+$ T cells in association with sepsis,[33] suggesting that CD8$^+$ T cells respond to environmental stimulus. Data shown in FIGURE 5 show relative mean percentages of CD8$^+$ T cells in fetal life, at birth, and in adults. Related studies showed that fetal CD8$^+$ T cells more frequently co-expressed CD38 than did adults ($p < 0.001$). This coexpressing population of CD8$^+$ T cells normally declines in late gestation as shown for one single representative fetus studied longitudinally (FIG. 6). The fetal CD8$^+$ T cell therefore appears to be similar to the CD8$^+$ T cell seen in HIV-infected persons in that both coexpress

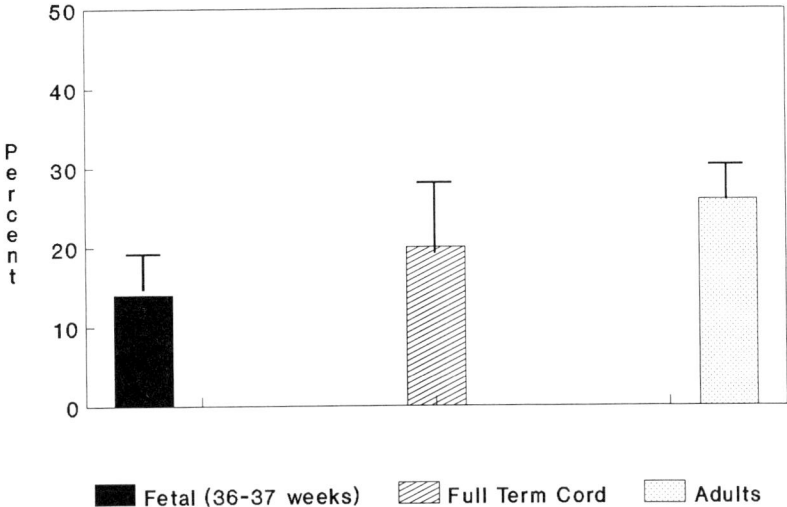

FIGURE 5. Relative percentage of $CD8^+$ T cells in peripheral blood as assessed by flow cytometry is shown for fetal life ($n = 12$) in comparison with full-term infants ($n = 10$) in comparison with adults ($n = 40$).

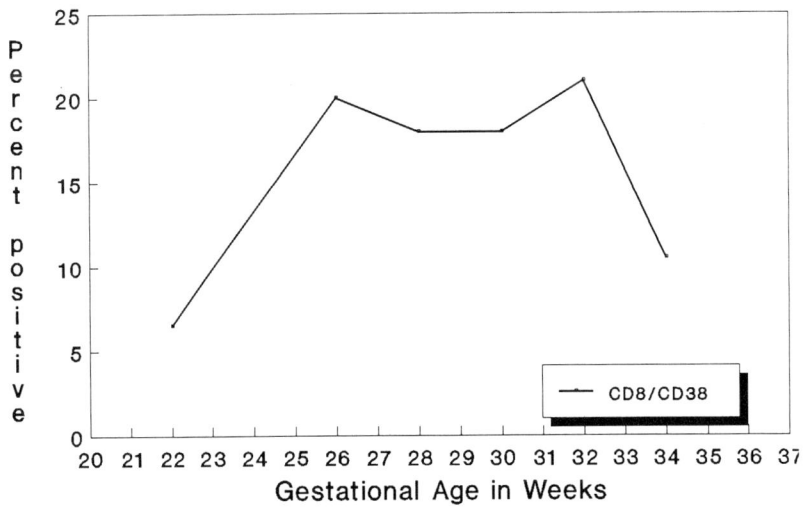

FIGURE 6. Expression of $CD8^+$ T cells coexpressing CD_{38} during fetal life is shown for one fetus sampled six times by periumbilical blood sampling during gestation. Data were obtained by dual fluorescence flow cytometry using monoclonal antibodies against CD8 (FITC) and CD38 (PE). Data are given as percentages.

CD38.[34] Expansion of this subpopulation of cells has been observed to be directly associated with decline in CD4$^+$ T cells in HIV$^+$ hemophiliacs.[9] We have recently observed significant expansion of these cells in HIV$^+$ infants compared with age-matched controls.

DIFFERENTIATION OF THE NATURAL KILLER CELL SYSTEM AND HIV INFECTION

The role of the natural killer (NK) cell system as a relatively primitive, first-line defense against viruses, bacteria, and tumors has been suggested by numerous human and animal studies.[35] A specific relationship between NK cells and opportunistic pathogens has been suggested by studies in the C57BL/6 beige mutant mouse, which are congenitally NK cell deficient and have increased susceptibility to *M. avium* complex infections.[36] Furthermore, *in vivo* depletion of NK cell activity in normal C57BL/6 mice also led to rapid development of severe and disseminated *Mycobacterium avium* disease.[37] A link may exist between loss of NK cells and susceptibility to opportunistic infections in adults with HIV disease, since the NK cell system normally provides surveillance against pathogens that can activate the HIV-1 tat infectivity gene.[38] Direct infection of NK cells by HIV has been recently been demonstrated.[39] Interestingly, infection did not prevent cytotoxic activity against NK-sensitive targets. Therefore, direct intracellular effects of HIV on NK function appear to be ruled out. In contrast, HIV gp120 may be able to modulate NK cell activity, since homologous synthetic peptides have been shown to have inhibitory activity *in vitro*.[40]

When NK cell activity diminishes in HIV$^+$ adults, the first observed loss is response to interferon α *in vitro*.[41] Later, there is loss of endogenous activity. Large granular lymphocytes (LGL), NK cells expressing CD16, are not diminished in patients with AIDS. In fact, Leu 7$^+$(CD57)-expressing NK cells are highly increased in adult HIV disease[41] and may increase before loss of functional activity. Although in normal persons these cells do not coexpress CD8, among persons with HIV disease, CD57$^+$-coexpressing CD8$^+$ T cells are strikingly increased.[34] NK cells are not usually active at birth (see FIG. 7); however, rapid maturation of cells and function does occur. In the developing fetus, we noted few NK cells bearing the CD57 phenotype (range: 0–4%; mean: 2%, $n = 7$). Yabuhara *et al.*[42] have found that the immaturity of the normal neonatal NK system is reflected at the level of binding, lysis, and recycling, which are reduced. NK cell number increased most significantly during early childhood, suggesting that this system may provide an important aspect of host defense before specific immune response is fully developed.

Immaturity of the lymphoid system at birth may alter the level at which indirect effects of the HIV virus might affect immune response through impact on developing cells such as B cells or NK cells. Impact on the NK cell system may be dependent on time of infection. We have observed that HIV$^+$ infants who have had no significant loss of CD4$^+$ T cells and yet developed AIDS-related pneumonia had highly reduced or no NK activity.[43] To study this further, NK activity in HIV-exposed infants was examined in comparison with healthy infants under the age of one year. Among HIV⁺ infants (less than 1 year) NK cell activity was significantly reduced ($p < 0.01$) compared to age-matched, unexposed infants (FIG. 8). A significant lack of response to interferon α *in vitro* ($p < 0.01$) was also observed, as shown in FIGURE 9. Lack of response to interferon α *in vitro* also occurs in adult HIV disease, typically occurring before loss of endogenous activity. When the percentage of NK cells expressing CD57 was compared among full-term healthy infants at birth (cord blood), HIV⁺ infants, and HIV⁻ infants, all of whom were five months to one year, both groups of older infants had significantly more NK cells than the newly born, showing that NK cell number alone did not explain reduced function. Nevertheless, although the HIV⁺ infants did not have statistically fewer NK cells than HIV⁻ infants as a group, some infants were clearly deficient. Interestingly, expansion of CD8⁺ CD57⁺ cells did not occur in infants with defective NK cell function and PCP.

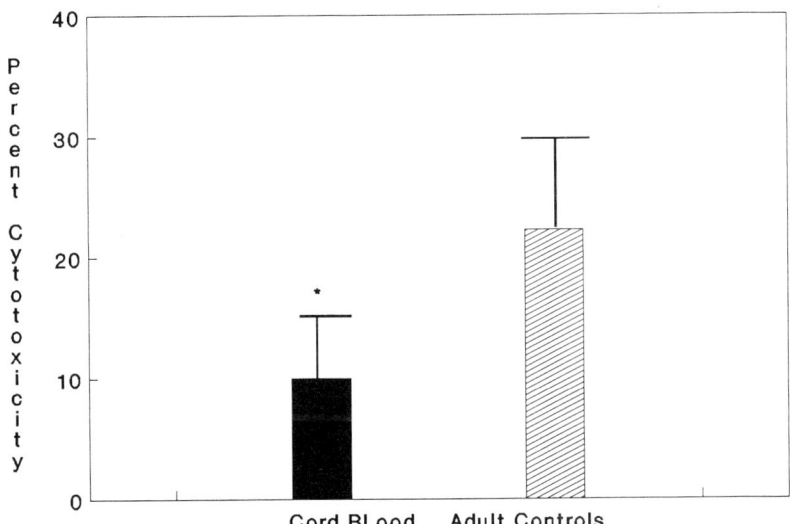

FIGURE 7. Data show natural killer (NK) cell activity of mononuclear cells from full-term infants obtained from cord blood and adult controls. Effector cells were assayed for cytotoxicity directed against chromium-51-labeled K562 tumor cell targets in a short-term chromium release assay. Data are for an effector to target ratio of 50:1; $p < 0.03$.

Regulation of the NK cell system at birth in the normal neonate has been also found to be different than that of adults in being more highly responsive to, and therefore more dependent on, IL-2[42] and less responsive to interferon α. It appears from other evidence that IL-2 can affect both lytic and binding activity,[44] and interferon α potentiates binding alone.[45] Since IL-2 induces interferon γ production, interferon γ may be the key mediator of this effect. This specific dependence of the neonatal NK system on IL-2 may have particular importance for the HIV-infected neonate, because HIV appears to block upregulation of IL-2 (and transferrin) receptors[46] and would interfere with signaling. Because preferential infection of CD4⁺ memory cells by HIV may cause selective loss[12] and these cells are

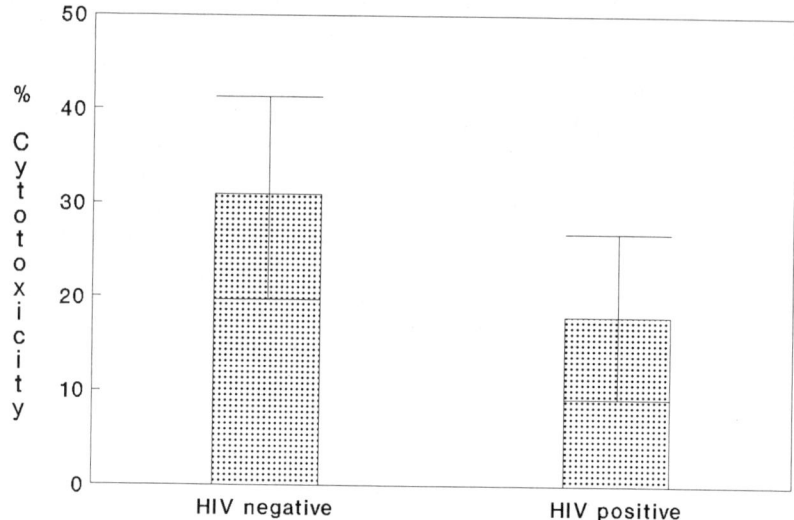

FIGURE 8. Data show relative NK cell activity of mononuclear cells isolated from peripheral blood of HIV⁺ infants (< 1 year) compared to age-matched controls. Method is briefly described in legend to FIGURE 7.

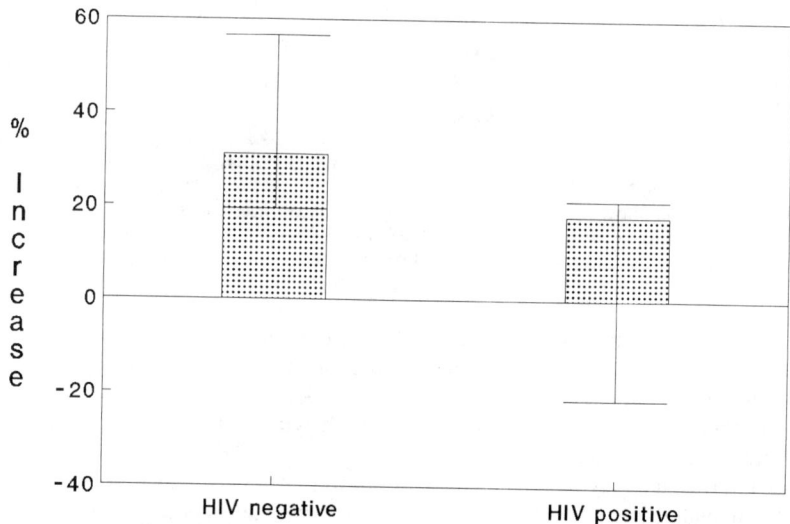

FIGURE 9. Relative effect of interferon α (800 U per well) on NK cell activity *in vitro* for HIV⁺ infants (< 1 year) compared to HIV⁻ age-matched controls is shown. Data are given as percent increment over endogenous cytotoxicity in the absence of INFα addition.

the major producers of interferon γ,[47] the NK cell system may be deprived of maturation factors. Also, impairment of this subset of $CD4^+$ T cells not associated with gross, observable loss of cells might be sufficient to impede development of the NK system. In addition, to direct effect of NK cell deficiency on susceptibility to opportunistic pathogens, it is likely that loss of cytokines produced by NK cells, such as interferon,[48] may affect host defense in the HIV-infected infant.

The lack of NK cell function in the normal neonate can be attributed to a lack of interferon γ production controlled at the level of gene activation. However, an alternative hypothesis based on suppressor activity may be suggested from the work of Seki et al.,[49] who demonstrated existence of a naturally occurring, radiosensitive suppressor T cell activated by plant lectins in vitro in the neonate. This suppressor cell could be bypassed if microbial antigens were used to elicit a response that led to normal interferon γ production. Recent data from our laboratory[50] confirm that the same activators used to upregulate interferon γ production in the Seki study could also be used to induce NK cell activity in the neonate with parallel induction of interferon γ. In related studies, we found that asymptomatic HIV^+ hemophiliacs with highly reduced NK cell activity and no response to interferon α were able to respond to this type of signal by means of direct triggering of interferon γ through the FcRIII on NK cells. These observations also point to the possibility of regulatory differences at the cytokine level in fetal and neonatal life compared to childhood or adult life. A common thread appears to be that there is a selectively different effect of microbial activators compared to that of plant lectins. This heightened responsiveness to microbial activators may reflect incomplete elimination of relevant clones responding to super antigens, incomplete development of tolerance to such specificities, or pathway activation differences governed by other undefined regulatory elements.

CONCLUSIONS

An apparent mimicry between the mechanisms associated with normal fetal immune development that, of necessity, involve downregulation and the effects of HIV infection itself appear to coincide in the congenitally exposed infant. The studies presented here and those of others indicate major differences in immune response related to development and maturation of the immune system during fetal life and after birth. The rapid progression of HIV disease in the infant has sometimes appeared to be a telescoping of events also seen in adults. Nevertheless substantial evidence exists that the immune systems of the fetus and infant respond differently and have different affinities for activating signals than does the adult immune system. Clarification of these differences is critical for the development of appropriate treatment strategies for infants with HIV infection.

ACKNOWLEDGMENTS

The authors are grateful for the technical assistance of C. Poggenberg, T. Manalo, and D. Ehleiter.

REFERENCES

1. HAHN, B. H., G. M. SHAW, M. E. TAYLOR, R. R. REDFIELD, P. D. MARKHAM, S. Z. SALAHUDDIN, F. WONG-STAAL, R. C. GALLO, E. S. PARKS & W. P. PARKS. 1986. Genetic variation in HTLV-III/LAV over time in patients with AIDS or at risk for AIDS. Science **232:** 1548.
2. FAUCI, A. S. 1988. The human immunodeficiency virus: Infectivity and mechanisms of pathogenesis. Science **239:** 617.
3. SCOTT, G. B., C. HUTTO, R. W. MAKUCH, M. T. MASTRUCCI, T. O'CONNOR, C. D. MITCHELL, E. J. TRAPIDO & W. P. PARKS. 1989. Survival in children with perinatally acquired human immunodeficiency virus type-1 infection. N. Engl. J. Med. **321:** 1791.
4. ANDERSON, U., A. G. BAIRD, S. BRITTON & R. PALACIOS. 1981. Humoral and cellular immunity in humans studied at the cell level from birth to two years of age. Immunol. Rev. **57:** 5.
5. JACOBY, D. R., L. B. OLDING & M. B. A. OLDSTONE. 1984. Immunologic regulation of fetal–maternal balance. Adv. Immunol. **35:** 157.
6. HICKS, M. J., J. F. JONES, L. L. MINNICH, K. A. WEIGLE, A. C. THIES & J. M. LAYTON. 1983. Age-related changes in T- and B-lymphocyte subpopulations in the peripheral blood. Arch. Pathol. Lab. Med. **107:** 518.
7. CLARKE, A. G. & K. A. MACLENNAN. 1986. The many facets of thymic involution. Immunol. Today **7:** 204.
8. GOEDERT, J. J., C. M. KESSELER, L. M. ALEDORT, R. J. BIGGAR, W. A. ANDES, G. C. WHITE, J. E. DRUMMOND, K. VAIDYA, D. L. MANN, M. E. EYSTER, M. V. RAGNI, M. M. LEDERMAN, A. R. COHEN, G. L. BRAY, P. S. ROSENBERT, R. M. FRIEDMAN, M. W. HILGARTNER, W. A. BLATTER, B. KRONER & M. H. GAIL. 1989. A prospective study of human immunodeficiency virus type 1 infection and the development of AIDS in subjects with hemophilia. N. Engl. J. Med. **321:** 1141.
9. CUNNINGHAM-RUNDLES, S., M. W. HILGARTNER, T. H. TARTAR & S. H. KOIDE. 1991. Cofactors in the latency and progression of human immunodeficiency virus disease. J. Immunol. Res. **3:** 31.
10. IWATA, T., G. S. INCEFY, S. CUNNINGHAM-RUNDLES, C. CUNNINGHAM-RUNDLES, E. SMITHWICK, N. GELLER, R. O'REILLY & R. A. GOOD. 1981. Circulating thymic hormone activity in patients with primary and secondary immune-deficiency diseases. Am. J. Med. **71:** 385.
11. PANTALEO, G., C. GRAZIOSI, L. BUTINI, P. PIZZO, S. M. SCHNITTMAN, D. M. KOTLER & A. S. FAUCI. 1988. Lymphoid organs function as major reservoirs for human immunodeficiency virus. Proc. Natl. Acad. Sci. USA **88:** 9838.
12. SCHNITTMAN, S. M., H. C. LANE, J. GREENHOUSE, J. S. JUSTEMENT, M. BASELER & A. S. FAUCI. 1990. Preferential infection of CD4$^+$ memory T cells by human immunodeficiency virus type 1: Evidence for a role in the selective T-cell functional defects observed in infected individuals. Proc. Natl. Acad. Sci. **87:** 6058.
13. DE PAOLI, P., S. BATTISTIN & G. T. SANTINI. 1988. Age-related changes in human lymphocyte subsets: Progressive reduction of the CD4, CD45 R (suppressor inducer) population. Clin. Immunol. Immunopathol. **48:** 290.
14. FLETCHER, M. A., J. W. MOSELEY, J. HASSETT, G. F. GJERSET, J. KAPLAN, J. W. PARKER, E. DONEGAN, J. W. LUSHER, H. LEE & THE TRANSFUSION SAFETY STUDY GROUP. 1992. Effect of age on human immunodeficiency virus type-1 induced changes in lymphocyte populations among patients with congenital clotting disorders. Blood **80:** 831.
15. HAYWARD, A. R. 1981. Development of lymphocyte responses and interactions in the human fetus and newborn. Immunol. Rev. **57:** 39.
16. MIYAWAKI, T., N. MORIYA, T. NAGAOKI & N. TANIGUCHI. 1981. Maturation of B-cell differentiation ability and T-cell regulatory function in infancy and childhood. Immunol. Rev. **57:** 61.
17. ZOLA, H., H. A. MOORE, J. BRADLEY, J. A. NEED & P. C. L. BEVERLEY. 1983. Lympho-

cyte subpopulations in human cord blood: Analysis with monoclonal antibodies. J. Reprod. Immunol. **5:** 311.
18. THOMAS, R. M. & D. C. LINCH. 1983. Identification of lymphocyte subsets in the newborn using a variety of monoclonal antibodies. Arch. Dis. Child. **58:** 34.
19. PITTARD, W. B., III, K. MILLER & R. U. SORENSEN. 1984. Normal lymphocyte responses to mitogens in term and premature infants following normal and abnormal intrauterine growth. Clin. Immunol. Immunopathol. **30:** 178.
20. WEATHERSTONE, K. B. & E. A. RICH. 1989. Tumor necrosis factor/cachechtin and interleukin-1 secretion by cord blood monocytes from premature and term infants. Ped. Res. **25:** 342–346.
21. SAITO, S., M. SAITO, V. KATO, I. MORIYAMA & M. ICHIJO. 1988. Interleukin 2 production by human fetal lymphocytes. J. Reprod. Immunol. **14:** 247.
22. LEWIS, D. A., A. LARSEN & C. B. WILSON. 1986. Reduced interferon γ mRNA levels in human neonates. J. Exp. Med. **163:** 1018.
23. OH, S. H., B. GONIK, S. B. GREENBERG & S. KOHL. 1986. Enhancement of human neonatal natural killer cytotoxicity to herpes simplex virus with use of recombinant human interferons: Lack of neonatal response to γ interferons. J. Infect. Dis. **153:** 791.
24. HAYNES, B. F., K. H. SINGER, S M. DENNING & M. E. MARTIN. 1988. Analysis of expression of CD2, CD3 and T-cell antigen receptor molecules during early human fetal thymic development. J. Immunol. **141:** 3776.
25. RAINAUT, M., M. PAGNEZ, T. HERCEND, F. DAFFOS & F. FORESTIER. 1987. Characterization of mononuclear cell subpopulations of normal fetal peripheral blood. Hum. Immunol. **18:** 331.
26. WARA, D. & D. J. BARNETT. 1979. Cell-mediated immunity in the newborn: Clinical aspects. Pediatrics **64:** 822.
27. DENNY, T., R. YOGEU, R. GELMAN, C. SKUZA, J. OLESKE, E. CHADWICK, S. C. CHENGI & E. CONNOR. 1992. Lymphocyte subsets in healthy children during the first 5 years of life. JAMA **267:** 1484.
28. THE EUROPEAN COLLABORATIVE STUDY. 1988. Mother to child transmission of HIV infection. Lancet **2:** 1039.
29. TOIVANEN, P., J. UKSILA, A. LEINO, O. LASSILA, T. HIRVONEN & O. RUUSKANEN. 1981. Development of mitogen responding T cells and natural killer cells in the human fetus. Immun. Rev. **57:** 89.
30. HAYWARD, A. & J. KURNICK. 1980. Development of lymphocyte responses and regulatory mechanisms. Inserm. Symp. **16:** 23.
31. HAYNES, B. F., S. M. DENNING, P. T. LE & K. H. SINGER. 1990. Human intrathymic T cell differentiation Sem. Immunol. **2:** 67.
32. VEBER, M. B., S. CUNNINGHAM-RUNDLES, M. SCHULMAN, F. MANDELL & P. A. M. AULT. 1991. Clin. Exp. Immunol. **83:** 391. Acute shift in response to microbial activators in very-low-birthweight infants. Clin. Exp. Immunol. **83:** 391.
33. BUSSEL, J. B., S. CUNNINGHAM-RUNDLES, E. F. LA GAMMA & M. SHELLABARGER. 1989. Analysis of lymphocyte proliferative response and subpopulations in very low-birthweight infants during first 8 weeks of life. Ped. Res. **23:** 457.
34. GIORGI, J. V. & B. DETELS. 1989. T-cell subset alteration in HIV-infected homosexual men. NIAID multicenter AIDS cohort study. Clin. Immunol. Immunopathol. **52:** 10.
35. HERBERMAN, R. B. & J. R. ORTALDO. 1981. Natural killer cells: Their role in defenses against disease. Science **214:** 24.
36. GANGADHARAM, P. R. J., C. K. EDWARDS, P. S. MURPHY & P. F. PRATT. 1983. An acute infection model for *Mycobacterium intracellulare* disease using beige mice: Preliminary results. Am. Rev. Respir. Dis. **127:** 648.
37. KALATARDI, V. H. & P. R. J. GANGADHARAM. 1991. In vivo depletion of natural killer cell activity leads to enhanced multiplication of *Mycobacterium avium* complex in mice. Infect. Immun. **59:** 2818.
38. POLI, G., M. INTRONA, F. ZANABONI, G. PERI, M. CARBONARI, F. AIUTI, A. LAZZARIN, M. MORONI & A. MANTOVANI. 1985. Natural killer cells in intravenous drug abuses with lymphadenopathy syndrome. Clin. Exp. Immunol. **62:** 128.

39. CHEHEMI, J., S. BANDYOPADHYAY, K. PRAKASH, B. PERUSSIA, N. F. HASSAN, H. KAWASHINA, D. CAMPBELL, J. KORNBLUTH & S. E. STARR. 1991. In vitro infection of natural killer cells with different human immunodeficiency virus type 1 isolates. J. Virol. **65:** 1812.
40. CAUDA, R., M. TUMBORELLA, L. ORTONO, P. KANDA & R. C. KENNEDY. 1988. Inhibition of normal human natural killer cell activity by human immunodeficiency virus synthetic transmembrane peptides. Cell Immunol. **115:** 57.
41. CUNNINGHAM-RUNDLES, S., R. BEDFORD & C. E. METROKA. 1988. Cellular cytotoxicity in AIDS. In AIDS and Other Manifestations of HIV Infection. G. Wormer, R. Staal & E. Bottone, Eds.: #331. Noyes Press. Park Ridge, NJ.
42. YABUHARA, A., H. KAWAI & A. KAMIYAMA. 1990. Development of natural killer cytotoxicity during childhood: Marked increases in number of natural killer cells with adequate cytotoxic abilities during infancy to early childhood. Ped. Res. **28:** 316.
43. BONAGURA, V. P., S. CUNNINGHAM-RUNDLES & S. SCHUVAL. 1992. Natural killer cell dysfunction in HIV$^+$ infants with *Pneumocystis carinii* pneumonia. J. Ped. **121:** 195.
44. ROTHLEIN, R. & T. A. SPRINGER. 1986. The requirement for lymphocyte function associated antigen 1 in homotypic leukocyte adhesion stimulated by phorbol ester. J. Exp. Med. **163:** 1132.
45. KATZ, P., A. M. ZAYTOUN & A. S. FAUCI. 1982. Deficiency of active natural killer cells in the Chediak-Higashi syndrome: Localization of the defect using a single cell cytotoxicity assay. J. Clin. Invest. **69:** 1231.
46. HOFMANN, B., P. NISHANIAN, R. L. BALDWIN, P. INSIXIENGMAY, A. NELL & J. L. FAHEY. 1990. HIV inhibits the early steps of lymphocyte activation including initiation of inositol phospholipid metabolism. J. Immunol. **145:** 3699.
47. SANDERS, M. E., M. W. MAKGOBA, C. H. JONE, H. A. YOUNG & S. SHAW. 1989. Enhanced responsiveness of human memory T cell to CD2 and CD3 receptor-mediated activation. Eur. J. Immunol. **19:** 803.
48. BIRON, C. A., G. SONNENFELD & R. M. WELSH. 1984. Interferon induces natural killer cell blastogenesis in vivo. J. Leuk. Biol. **35:** 31–37.
49. SEKI, H., K. TAGA, A. MATSUDA, N. UWADANA, M. HASAI, T. MIHYAWAKI & N. TANIGUCHI. 1986. Phenotypic and functional characteristics of active suppressor cells against IFN-γ production in PHA-stimulated cord blood lymphocytes. J. Immunol. **137:** 3158.
50. CUNNINGHAM-RUNDLES, S. & F. P. J. PEARSON. 1990. ImuVert activation of natural killer cytotoxicity and interferon-γ production via CD16 triggering. Internatl. J. Immunopharmacol. **12:** 589.

Immunologic Targets of HIV Infection: T Cells[a]

WILLIAM T. SHEARER,[b,c,d] HOWARD M. ROSENBLATT,[b]
MARK D. SCHLUCHTER,[e] LYNNE M. MOFENSON,[f]
THOMAS N. DENNY,[g] THE NICHD IVIG CLINICAL
TRIAL GROUP,[f] AND THE NHLBI P²C² PEDIATRIC
PULMONARY AND CARDIAC COMPLICATIONS OF HIV
INFECTION STUDY GROUP[h]

One of the principal targets of human immunodeficiency virus-1 (HIV-1) is the human T lymphocyte (T cell) owing to tropism of the glycoprotein (gp) 160 for the $CD4^+$ molecule on the helper T cell ($CD4^+$ cell).[1,2] The best documented surrogate marker of clinical disease progression, decline in $CD4^+$ cell count, has been shown to predict the stage of illness in adults with HIV-1. It is now well known that following an early viremic phase,[3,4] a prolonged stage of viral latency exists (at least within the peripheral blood compartment), lasting up to 10 years in adults infected by HIV.[5] Invariably, however, when the $CD4^+$ cell count begins to decline, there is a substantial decline in health experienced in patients, usually in the form of opportunistic infections and cancers. In children, the period of latency is shorter and symptomatic infants usually expire by 3 years of age.[6]

Multiple pathologic mechanisms are thought to contribute to $CD4^+$ cell death: programmed cell death (apoptosis),[8] antibody and complement-mediated cyto-

---

[a] This work was supported by National Institutes of Health Grants HR-96040, AI-27551, HD-26603, AI-32466, and a contract from the National Institute of Child Health and Human Development, the Women and Infants HIV Transmision Study, and the Immunology Research Fund of Texas Children's Hospital.

[b] Address for correspondence: William T. Shearer, M.D., Ph.D., Department of Allergy & Immunology, Texas Children's Hospital, 6621 Fannin, MS 1-3291, Houston, TX 77030.

[c] Departments of Pediatrics, Microbiology, and Immunology, Baylor College of Medicine, Houston, Texas 77030.

[d] Department of Pediatrics, Baylor College of Medicine, Houston, Texas 77030.

[e] Department of Biostatistics/Epidemiology, Cleveland Clinic Foundation, Cleveland, Ohio 44195.

[f] National Institute of Child Health and Human Development, Rockville, Maryland 20892.

[g] Department of Pediatrics, New Jersey Medical School and Children's Hospital of New Jersey, Newark, New Jersey 07103.

[h] National Heart, Lung and Blood Institute, Bethesda, Maryland 20892.

lysis,[9] Vβ gene deletion of the T-cell receptor due to superantigen activation,[10] $CD4^+$ cell syncytium formation,[11] and autoimmune reactions.[12] With HIV-infected adults, analysis of $CD4^+$ cell decline is straightforward, because there is an essentially stable level of $CD4^+$ cells in normal young adults (15–45 years).[13] In infants and young children, however, $CD4^+$ cell analysis in HIV-1 infection is hampered by an incomplete understanding of $CD4^+$ cell production and appearance in the peripheral blood in infants, as well as changes in $CD4^+$ lymphocyte number with age.[14]

Several investigators have begun to describe important age-related changes in $CD4^+$ cell counts during infancy and early childhood in HIV-infected and uninfected children.[15–22] No single investigation is complete in the sense of possessing adequate numbers of uninfected control and HIV-infected pediatric patient $CD4^+$ cell counts assessed in a prospective longitudinal fashion. Therefore, this review will attempt to summarize both published research data[14–22] and that being accrued both in individual laboratories and in large clinical trials on $CD4^+$ lymphocyte counts in HIV-infected and uninfected children in different age groups. We will correlate $CD4^+$ cell counts in HIV-infected infants and children with clinical disease status and with mortality. When better understood, assessment of $CD4^+$ cell number in HIV-infected children is expected to be as informative as $CD4^+$ values are currently in the assessment of clinical stage of HIV disease, determination of initiation of HIV-related therapies, and prognosis in adults with HIV-1 infection.

MATERIALS AND METHODS

Subjects and Blood Samples

Subjects were recruited from the National Institutes of Health–sponsored pediatric HIV-1 clinical trials: National Heart, Lung and Blood Institute: Pediatric Pulmonary and Cardiovascular Complications of Vertically Transmitted Human Immunodeficiency Virus Infection (NHLBI P^2C^2 HIV) Study;[i] National Institute of Child Health and Human Development: Clinical Trial of the Efficacy of Intravenous Gamma Globulin in Treatment of Symptomatic Children Infected with HIV (NICHD IVIG Clinical Trial[i]); National Institute of Allergy and Infections Diseases: Pediatric AIDS Clinical Trials Group and the Women and Infants HIV Transmission Study; and the Centers for Disease Control (CDC)-sponsored Natural History Study of HIV-Infected Children; Baylor College of Medicine and Texas Children's Hospital, Houston, TX; and New Jersey Medical School and Children's Hospital of New Jersey, Newark, NJ.

Blood samples were obtained with informed consent using forms approved by institutional review boards in a 5-year time period (1988 to 1992). All lymphocyte subset analyses were performed in laboratories approved by the Pediatric AIDS Clinical Trial Group Quality Control Program (Fast Systems, Inc., Rockville,

---

[i] Members and institutions are listed in the Appendix.

MD) and the NIAID Division of AIDS Flow Cytometry Advisory Committee or by the NICHD IVIG Clinical Trial Study Group. Samples were excluded if they were clotted or if they were more than 24 hours old.

Patient Population

P^2C^2 HIV Study

As of November 30, 1992, this ongoing prospective NHLBI study of children born to HIV-infected women is following two groups of children: Group I, 185 children already HIV infected (vertical transmission) and Group II, children enrolled before or at birth who are born to HIV-infected women. A total of 389 infants have been enrolled in Group II. Target enrollments are 200 Group I and 500 Group II children by January 31, 1993. In Group II children, lymphocyte subset ($CD4^+$, $CD8^+$ cell counts) determinations are made at birth, 3, 9, 15, 21, 30, 36, 42, and 48 months. Group I children, who may be any age with documented HIV infection, are being studied as well. The study is being conducted in five clinical centers.

IVIG Clinical Trial

The NICHD IVIG Clinical Trial was a randomized, double-blind, placebo-controlled outpatient study conducted in 28 clinical centers in the mainland United States and Puerto Rico to determine whether IVIG would reduce the risk of infections in HIV-infected children. Eligible patients were asymptomatic but immunologically abnormal or clinically symptomatic HIV-infected nonhemophiliac children younger than 13 years. Between March 1988 and study termination in January 1991, 376 patients were enrolled; 92% had vertically acquired HIV infection, and 78% were under age 5 years. At entry, the majority had clinical evidence of HIV disease, Centers for Disease Control (CDC) Pediatric Class P-2; however, 32% of children had nonspecific symptoms of class P-2-A only, and 7% had only lymphoid interstitial pneumonitis (LIP) (class P-2-C). Thirteen percent were asymptomatic with abnormal immune function, class P-1-B.

Of the 376 patients enrolled, 313 had a $CD4^+$ count of at least $200/mm^3$ and 50 had a $CD4^+$ count of less than $200/mm^3$; 13 patients lacked an entry $CD4^+$ count. $CD4^+$ cell counts were monitored in patients every 12 weeks during the trial.

Pediatric HIV/AIDS Program at Baylor College of Medicine, Texas Children's Hospital, Department of Pediatrics, Houston, Texas

HIV-infected infants and children were recruited for lymphocyte subset determination. One hundred thirty-one subjects with vertically acquired HIV infection (20 P1, 111 P2) were studied. Lymphocyte phenotyping using standard two-color-fluorescence flow cytometry was performed on these 131 HIV-infected children. Absolute CD4+ lymphocyte counts were expressed as cells/mm^3.

New Jersey Medical School, Children's Hospital of New Jersey, Newark, NJ

Normal children's lymphocytes,[14] HIV seroreverter's lymphocytes, and HIV-infected children's lymphocytes were determined using recruitment mechanisms of the HIV/AIDS program. For purposes of this manuscript, 16 known HIV-infected children and 70 HIV-seroreverting children were studied.

Lymphocyte Subset Analysis

The P^{2}C^2 HIV Study, the Pediatric HIV/AIDS Program at Baylor College of Medicine/Texas Children's Hospital, and the New Jersey Medical School/Children's Hospital of New Jersey used the lymphocyte subset analysis approved by the Pediatric AIDS Clinical Trial Group Quality Control Program. The NICHD IVIG Clinical Trial Study Group utilized recognized clinical immunology laboratories to perform lymphocyte subset analysis.

Periodic anticoagulated blood specimens were obtained and lymphocyte subset analysis was performed within 24 hours, using whole blood lysis (ACTG and the majority of NICHD laboratories) and/or density gradient centrifugation (three NICHD laboratories) and commercially available antihuman CD-specific antibodies conjugated to fluorescein isothiocyanate or phycoerythrin. Details of instrumentation, gating, and population analysis have been previously described.[14,24]

RESULTS

CD4+ Cell Counts in HIV-Infected Infants and Children

The CD4+ (T-helper) lymphocyte counts for Group I and Group II on the P^{2}C^2 HIV Study are presented in FIGURE 1. Group I patients (known to be HIV-infected) display a general overall decline in CD4+ lymphocyte numbers with increasing age, with the median absolute CD4+ lymphocyte number dropping to less than 1000 cells/mm in the patients 36 months of age or older (FIG. 1A). In Group II patients studied sequentially from birth, in whom the HIV status is unknown ($n = 258$), there is a wide variation in CD4+ lymphocyte counts with no set pattern, as might be expected in a mixed population of HIV-infected and HIV-noninfected children (FIG. 1B). In the Group II children ($n = 31$) whose HIV infection status became identified as positive (Group IIa), longitudinal CD4+ evaluations demonstrated a clear pattern of lower sequential CD4+ lymphocyte counts (FIG. 1C) compared to Group II children who were proven to be HIV-negative ($n = 28$) (Group IIb) (FIG. 1D). In addition to this total lymphocyte count data presented in FIGURE 1, similar differences in the percentage of CD4+ lymphocyte populations in Group I, Group II undetermined HIV status, Group IIa, and Group IIb patients were obtained (data not shown).

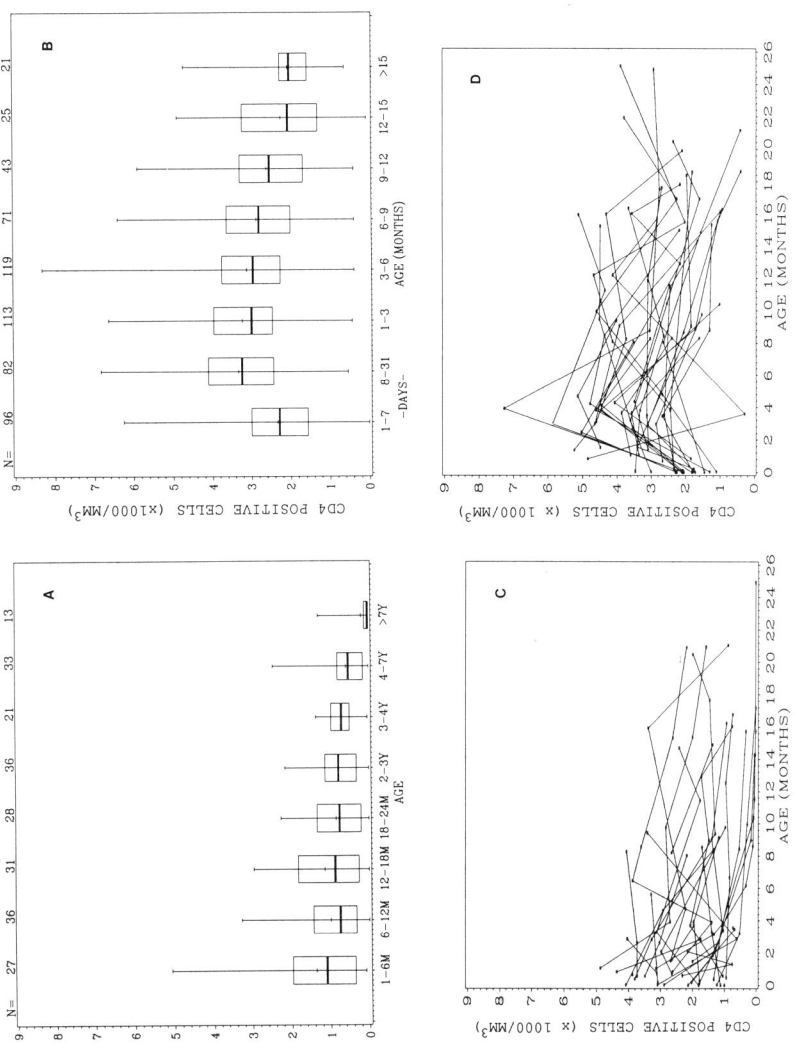

FIGURE 1. Box plots (median, interquartile range, and range) for CD4+ lymphocytes (T-helper cells × 10³/mm³) in the P²C² HIV Study. (A) Symptomatic Group I patients; (B) Group II (HIV-undeclared) patients; (C) Group IIa (HIV-infected) patients; (D) Group IIb (HIV-noninfected) patients. In A and B, the number of patients (n) is given at the top over the columns, and patients may be included in more than one box plot; in C and D, sequential CD4+ lymphocyte counts per patient are connected by lines.

FIGURE 2 illustrates the sequential mean CD4+ lymphocyte counts for Group IIa and Group IIb children in the P²C² HIV Study. It is clear that in HIV-infected children there is a progressive loss of CD4+ lymphocytes from the peripheral blood compartment, whereas noninfected children born to HIV-infected mothers show an entirely different pattern. From the 1.5- to 3-month time points, the noninfected children actually show an increase in CD4+ cell counts and subsequently a decline. In a separate perinatal transmission study at the New Jersey Medical School including many children followed prospectively from birth, this same early rise in the CD4+ cell counts of HIV seroreverters has been seen (FIG. 3). Several studies have shown that normal infants and children have high levels of CD4+ lymphocytes at birth that appear to decline rapidly between birth and the age of approximately 72 months. Mofenson et al.[23] recently used age-related normative CD4+ cell count means and standard deviations obtained from 10 published papers and abstracts to generate a least-squares line with age-related standard deviations to fit the data through application of a cube root transformation to the available data on mean CD4+ measurements and age [mean CD4+ count $= (16.60 - 1.18 \text{ Age}^{1/3})^3$]. The formula for the slope of this line can then be used to calculate the expected decline in CD4+ cell count over time by age in children not infected with HIV. This was done and compared with the estimated mean CD4+ counts obtained for Group IIa and Group IIb children (FIG. 2). At 1.5, 3,

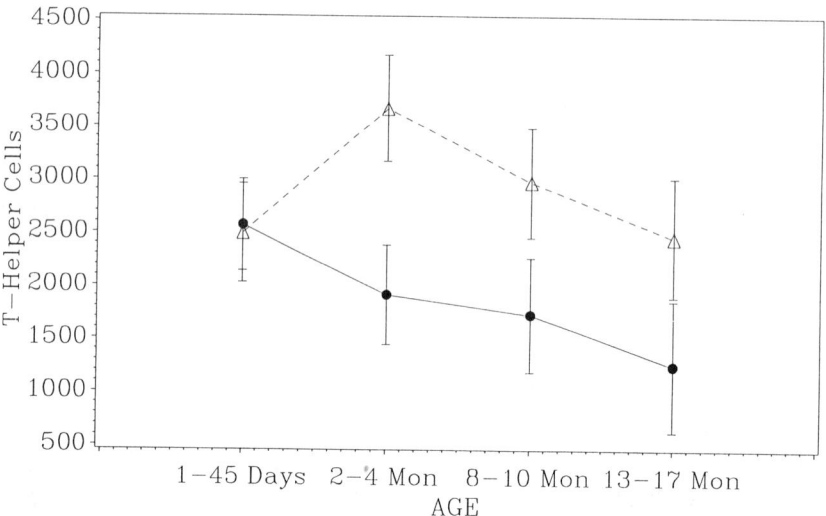

FIGURE 2. Mean and 95% confidence interval for CD4+ lymphocytes (T-helper cells × $10^3/\text{mm}^3$) by HIV status for Group II in the P²C² HIV Study. The *solid circles* represent 31 HIV-infected children; the *open triangles* represent 28 HIV-negative (seroreverting) children. The data is represented as the means ± standard errors. For all data comparisons beyond 45 days, a p value of at least 0.05 exists.

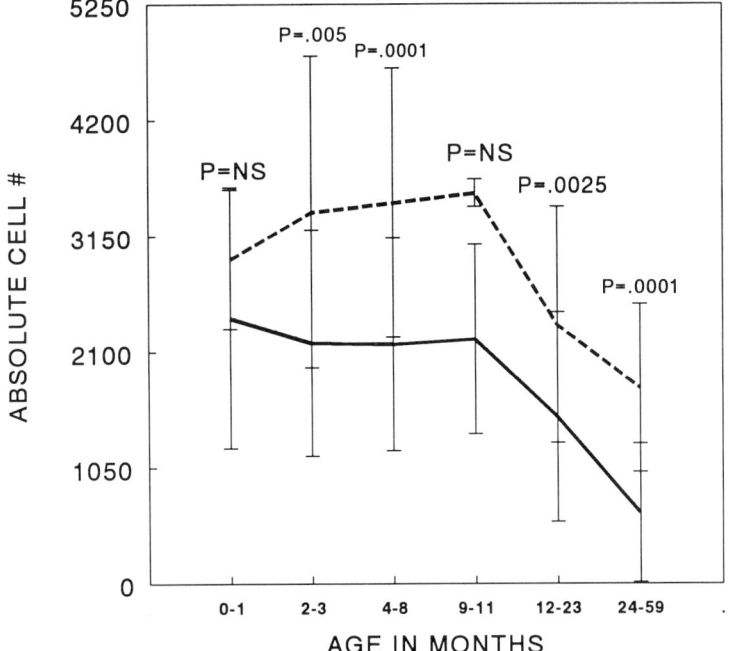

FIGURE 3. Absolute CD4+ lymphocyte values for patients enrolled in the Perinatal Transmission Study at New Jersey Medical School. The *dashed line* represents 70 HIV-seroreverting children and the *solid line* represents 16 HIV-infected children. Data points represent the means ± standard errors; p values were calculated by the Wilcoxon rank sum nonparametric independent t-test.

9, and 17 months, the mean CD4+ cell counts for normal children were calculated to be 3645, 3422, 2985, and 2506, respectively. Aside from the value obtained by these calculations at 1.5 months, these predicted means for normal children agree closely with the actual estimated means for Group IIb patients (FIG. 2).

Differences in CD8+ (suppressor) T lymphocyte populations between these same groups of patients in the P^2C^2 HIV Study are best appreciated from the percentage plots (FIG. 4). Group I patients display a striking imbalance of T lymphocyte subsets, due in large measure to an elevation of CD8+ lymphocyte percentage (Fig. 4A). Group II HIV status-unknown patients have CD8+ lymphocyte percentages with no specific pattern, although the wide range of CD8+ percentages seen in this group most likely is skewed by HIV-infected patients that have not yet been definitively diagnosed (FIG. 4B). Sequential data points for HIV-infected Group II patients (FIG. 4C) show significantly elevated patterns as compared to HIV-noninfected Group II patients (FIG. 4D). CD4+:CD8+ ratio of lymphocytes for the corresponding groups of patients are given in FIGURE 5. There is an impressive decline in the CD4+:CD8+ ratio in Group I patients (FIG. 5A) as compared

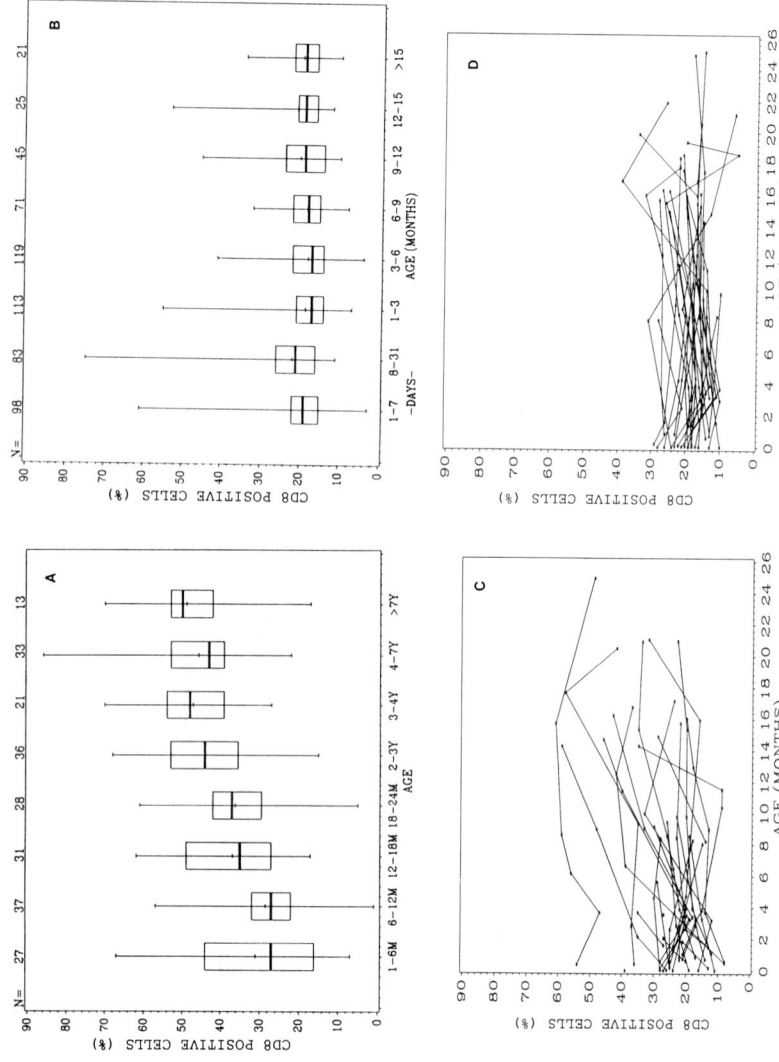

FIGURE 4. CD8+ lymphocyte (T-suppressor cells %) data in the P²C² HIV Study. The groups of patients are the same as in FIGURE 1.

TABLE 1. Absolute CD4+ Counts (cells/mm^3) by Age and Clinical Status in HIV-Infected Infants and Children (Baylor College of Medicine)

Age	P1		P2	
	n	Mean SD	n	Mean SD
<1 Year	8	2189 ± 953	26	1037 ± 795[a]
1–5 Years	6	985 ± 349	48	731 ± 618
>5 Years	6	463 ± 207	37	313 ± 251

[a] $p \leq 0.01$; P1 vs. P2.

to HIV status-unknown Group II patients (FIG. 5B). Group IIa patients (FIG. 5C) exhibit a clear trend toward lower CD4+:CD8+ ratios than Group IIb patients (FIG. 5D).

Association of CD4+ Cell Count and Clinical State of HIV-Infected Infants and Children

To study the association of CD4+ cell level with clinical status of HIV-infected infants and children, CD4+ cell counts were compared in 131 patients from the Baylor College of Medicine with either P1 (Centers for Disease Control Classification System for HIV-infected Children) (asymptomatic) or P2 (symptomatic) classification status (TABLE 1). In children under 1 year of age, there was a statistically significant reduction in the CD4+ cell counts (1037 ± 795) of P2 status compared to those of P1 status (2189 ± 953, $p < 0.01$, two-tailed Student's t test). In the 1 to 5 year age category and in those children greater than 5 years of age, a trend toward an association of P2 status with reduced CD4+ cell numbers was seen, but because of the scatter of the data, no statistical significance was achieved in either case.

Association of CD4+ Cell Count with Mortality of HIV-Infected Infants and Children

Using data gathered during the NICHD IVIG Clinical Trial,[24,25] an evaluation of the association of CD4+ cell count and mortality was undertaken[26] (TABLE 2). Overall study mortality during this 33-month-long trial was 16.8%. Overall survival was not affected by IVIG treatment; however, it was significantly affected by entry CD4+ cell count. Of 50 patients with CD4+ cell counts below 200/mm^3 at entry, 35 patients (70%) died, as compared to 9% of patients (27 of 313 patients) with entry CD4+ count 200/mm^3 or greater. The median entry CD4+ cell count of patients who expired was 157/mm^3 ($n = 63$) as contrasted with the median entry CD4+ cell count of patients overall, 933/mm^3 ($n = 376$).

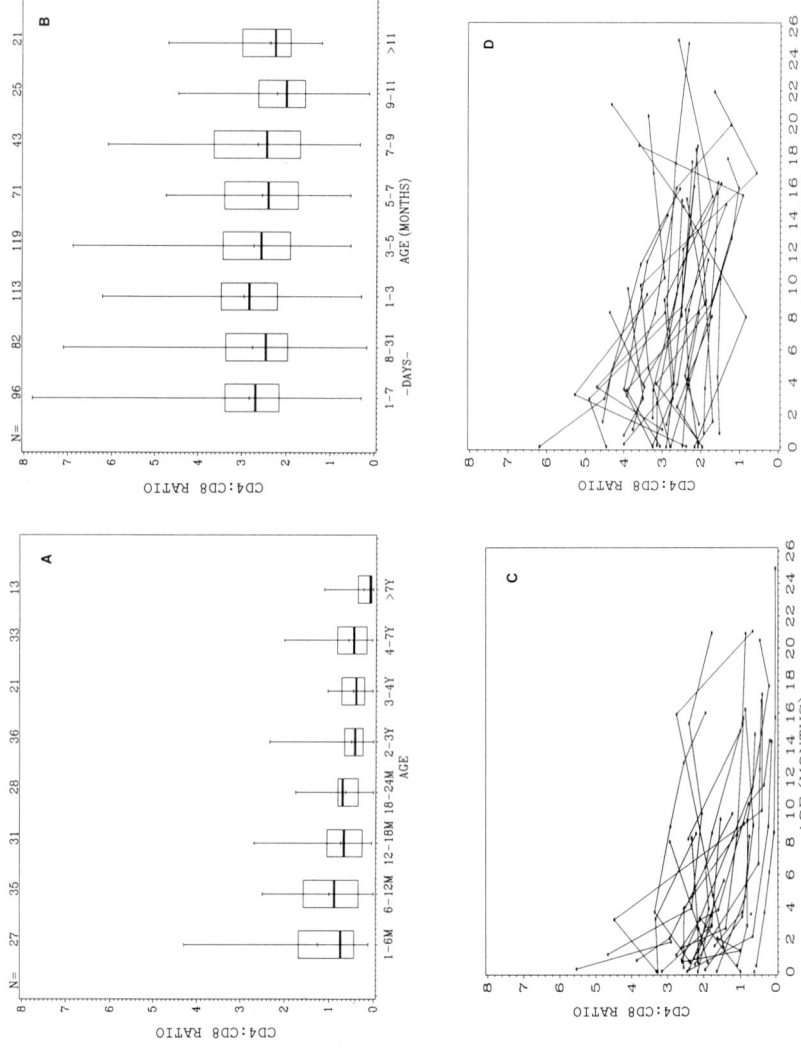

FIGURE 5. Median, interquartile range, and range for the CD4$^+$: CD8$^+$ lymphocyte (T4 : T8) ratio in the P^{2}C^2 HIV Study. The groups of patients are the same as in FIGURES 1 and 4.

TABLE 2. CD4+ Count and Mortality in HIV-Infected Infants and Children (NICHD IVIG Clinical Trial)

Deaths
- Entry CD4+ <200: 35/50 died, 70%
- Entry CD4+ ≥200: 27/313 died, 9%
- Lacked entry CD4+ count: 1/13 died, 8%

CD4+ Counts at Entry
- Median entry CD4+ count of patients who died: 157/mm^3
- Median entry CD4+ count of patients overall: 933/mm^3

CD4+ Counts Falling below 200
- CD4+ within 3 months of death was <200 in 48 (77%)
- In patients with entry CD4+ ≥200, CD4+ fell to <200 before death in 14/22 (64%) who had measurement within 3 months before death

CD4+ cell count fell below 200/mm^3 within 3 months before death in 77% of patients who died; the median CD4+ cell count measured before death was 62/mm^3. In those patients with entry CD4+ cell count 200/mm^3 or above who died and had also had a CD4+ measurement within 3 months before death, CD4+ cell count fell to under 200/mm^3 in 64%.

Evaluation of the NICHD data revealed the conditional probability of dying within 3 months, given a CD4+ cell count within a given range at the beginning of the time interval, as shown in FIGURE 6. Although the risk of death within 3

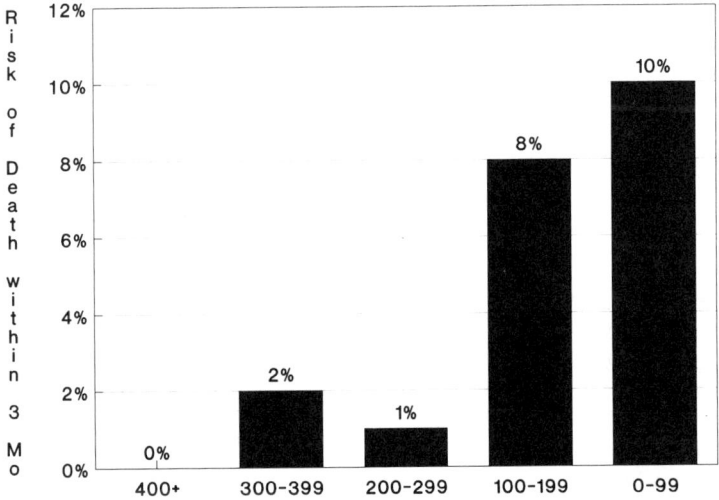

FIGURE 6. Three-month risk of death for patients with CD4+ lymphocyte count within a given range at the beginning of the time interval; based on 376 HIV-infected children in the NICHD IVIG Clinical Trial with 17% study mortality (63 deaths).[23-26]

months given a CD4$^+$ count above 200/mm^3 was low, between 0 and 2%, once the CD4$^+$ count dropped below 200/mm^3 the risk of death increased four- to eightfold, to 8% for CD4$^+$ count that dropped between 100 to 199/mm^3 and was estimated to be 10% once the CD4$^+$ count dropped below 100/mm^3.

In a preliminary analysis, the increased risk of death once the CD4$^+$ count falls below 200/mm^3 appears to be independent of age. Using the PCP-prophylaxis age-related CD4$^+$ cell count guidelines as the age-CD4$^+$ count referent group, we found that regardless of age category the relative risk of death increased most dramatically when CD4$^+$ count dropped between 100 and 199/mm^3. Only minimal additional risk was observed with further decline. For example, under one year of age, the relative risk of death within 3 months of a CD4$^+$ cell count falling between 200 and 1500/mm^3 was 1.4, with approximately a sevenfold increase to 9.2 once CD4$^+$ falls between 100 and 199/mm^3, and a subsequent twofold increase to 19.8 once CD4$^+$ falls below 100 (see Mofenson et al.[27]).

DISCUSSION

It is important for pediatricians clinically managing or maintaining pediatric HIV-infected patients on research protocols to have some easy and quick measure of the patient's immune function. On the basis of the use of the CD4$^+$ cell count and, more importantly, the rate of CD4$^+$ cell decline in assessing clinical status in adult patients with HIV infection, it is reasonable to expect that if the normal pediatric CD4$^+$ cell range could be established for the first 5 years of life, clinical care of infants and children with HIV infection would be greatly facilitated. The primary use of CD4$^+$ cell count would be as an adjunct to clinical symptoms in guiding HIV-related therapeutics. This use has already been implemented in the published guidelines for initiation of prophylaxis with trimethaprin-sulfamethoxazole and other agents for *Pneumocystia carinii* pneumonia in pediatric patients.[28–31] Similar considerations for use of age-related CD4$^+$ cell values are being formulated as guidance for initiation of antiretroviral therapy in infants and children.[32] Secondarily, CD4$^+$ cell decline in HIV-infected children could be used as a measure of prognosis, longevity, and as a surrogate marker for disease progression in clinical therapeutic trials, much like it is in adults. Third, correlations may be able to be made between CD4$^+$ cell count levels and diverse complications of pediatric HIV infection such as lymphoid interstitial pneumonitis, cardiomyopathies, and the wasting syndrome.

The data presented in this manuscript represent a beginning to the understanding of the consequences of HIV infection of T cells in children. Although preliminary in nature, the prospective CD4$^+$ cell measurements made on Group II infants born to HIV-infected women in the P^{2}C^2 HIV Study will enable delineation of the CD4$^+$ peripheral blood profiles of infants with definitive HIV infection and those who eventually serorevert. Further clarification and validation of the apparent increase in absolute CD4$^+$ cell number in P^{2}C^2 HIV Study seroreverters during the first few months of life (1.5 months vs. 3 months) is needed. These early life increases in CD4$^+$ cell counts in non-HIV-infected children have also been documented in at least two other studies of normal children.[16,22]

Correlation of $CD4^+$ cell counts with clinical condition and mortality of HIV-infected children is important to clinicians for eventual use of $CD4^+$ cell count as at least a partial predictor of disease progression in patients. Data presented in this manuscript (TABLE 1) demonstrates that children under 1 year of age at Baylor College of Medicine with advanced HIV infection (P2 CDC classification) had half as many $CD4^+$ cells as asymptomatic HIV-infected children (P1 CDC classification). The manuscript data on $CD4^+$ cell counts and mortality taken from the NICHD IVIG Clinical Trial data show a clear association between $CD4^+$ cell counts (<200 cells/mm^3) and risk of dying (TABLE 2 and FIG. 6). It will be important to establish what proportion of these children were on antiretroviral therapy before a stronger statement can be made about the relationship of a reduced $CD4^+$ cell count and mortality risk. A significant correlation of $CD4^+$ count under 50 cells/mm^3 and mortality has been demonstrated in recent studies of HIV-infected adults taking zidovudine.[33,34] With additional analysis of the association of $CD4^+$ cell count and patient clinical status and/or mortality, it may be possible to provide the physician as well as family members with a general sense of the potential future course of their HIV-infected child and to assist in decisions regarding initiations of therapeutic interventions in children at high risk of disease complications or death. Also, the $CD4^+$ cell counts and the rate of $CD4^+$ cell decline of children to be entered or already enrolled in clinical research protocols may prove invaluable in interpreting clinical events and outcomes when the children are on scientific protocols.

In summary, the data presented in this manuscript illustrates the potential power of using $CD4^+$ lymphocyte number in HIV-infected children to predict clinical outcomes and HIV infection status and begins to correlate low $CD4^+$ cell counts with progression of disease and risk of mortality. Because of the small number of HIV-infected children evaluated in this manner at present, continuation of collaborative studies will be necessary to validate and amplify on these results.

SUMMARY

One of the principal targets of HIV infection is the human peripheral blood $CD4^+$ T cell, resulting in progressive $CD4^+$ lymphocyte loss. Hypothesized mechanisms for this loss include apoptosis, cytolytic reactions, V-β gene deletion of the T-cell receptor (TCR) by superantigens, $CD4^+$ lymphocyte syncytium formation, and autoimmune reactions. In adults with HIV infection, the critical decline in $CD4^+$ lymphocyte number that heralds the onset of AIDS-defining conditions is well characterized, whereas in infants and children the critical level of $CD4^+$ cells predisposing to the development of AIDS-defining conditions or mortality is not fully characterized, due to an incomplete knowledge of $CD4^+$ lymphocyte number and changes with age in normal and HIV-infected children. In a prospective study of 317 infants born to HIV-infected women, early results show that the monthly change in absolute $CD4^+$ lymphocyte number over a 3- to 9-month period in HIV-infected infants was -109 cells/mm^3 per month, at least double the rate of decline measured in HIV-noninfected infants in the study or that calculated from normal infants' values reported in the literature. In other clinical studies in

HIV-infected infants and children, it was possible to study the effect of low $CD4^+$ cell counts on clinical status and mortality. In HIV-infected pediatric patients younger than 1 year, it was possible to correlate low $CD4^+$ cell number with advanced disease status (CDC pediatric class P-2). It was also possible to correlate extremely low $CD4^+$ cell counts (<200 cells/mm^3) in HIV-infected children with a significant risk of mortality within the next 3 months of life. Sequential $CD4^+$ cell analysis of HIV-high-risk infants will delineate the rate of HIV-related decline in $CD4^+$ cells, thus facilitating the diagnosis of HIV infection and aiding in identification of HIV-infected children at high risk of disease progression or death.

REFERENCES

1. KLATZMANN, D., E. CHAMPAGNE, S. CHAMARET, J. GRUEST, D. GUETARD, T. HERCEND, J.-C. GLUCKMAN & L. MONTAGNIER. 1984. T-lymphocyte T4 molecule behaves as the receptor for human retrovirus LAU. Nature **312**: 767–771.
2. DAGLEISH, A. G., B. C. L. BEVERLY, P. R. CLAPHAM, D. H. CRAWFORD, M. F. GREAVES & R. A. WEISS. 1984. The CD4 (T4) antigen is an essential component of the receptor for the AIDS retrovirus. Nature **312**: 763–767.
3. HO, D. D., T. MOUDGIL & M. ALAN. 1989. Quantitation of human immunodeficiency virus type 1 in the blood of infected persons. N. Engl. J. Med. **321**: 1626–1631.
4. COOMBS, R. W., A. C. COLLIER, J. P. ALLAIN, et al. 1989. Plasma viremia in human immunodeficiency virus infection. N. Engl. J. Med. **321**: 1626–1631.
5. PANTALEO, G., C. GRAZIOSI & A. S. FAUCI. 1993. The immunopathogenesis of human immunodeficiency virus infection. N. Engl. J. Med. **328**: 327–335.
6. SCOTT, G. B., C. HUTTO, R. W. MCKUCH, et al. 1989. Survival in children with perinatally acquired human immunodeficiency virus type 1 infection. N. Engl. J. Med. **321**: 1791–1796.
7. HANSON, C. G. & W. T. SHEARER. 1992. Pediatric HIV infection and AIDS. In Textbook of Pediatric Infectious Disease, 3rd edit. R. D. Feigin & J. D. Cherry, Eds.: 990–1011. Saunders. Philadelphia, PA.
8. AMEISEN, J. C. & A. CAPRON. 1991. Cell dysfunction and depletion in AIDS: The programmed cell death hypothesis. Immunol. Today **104**: 101–104.
9. GOLDING, H., F. A. ROBEY, F. T. GATES III, et al. 1988. Identification of homologous regions in human immunodeficiency virus 1 gp 41 and human MHC class II beta 1 domain-1. Monoclonal antibodies against the gp41-derived peptide and patients' sera react with native HLA class II antigens, suggesting a role for autoimmunity in the pathogenesis of acquired immune deficiency syndrome. J. Exp. Med. **167**: 914–923.
10. PRIMI, D. 1992. Mechanisms of CD4 depletion selective Vβ gene depletion, Session 31. In VIII International Conference on AIDS. Amsterdam, the Netherlands. Final Program, Vol. 1: 96. CONGREX Holland BV.
11. KOOT, M. 1992. Mechanisms of CD4 depletion. Phenotype of HIV and syncytia formation, Session 31. VIII International Conferences on AIDS. Amsterdam, the Netherlands. Final Program, Vol. 1: 96. CONGREX Holland BV.
12. WEINHOLD, K. J., H. K. LYERLY, S. D. STANLEY, et al. 1989. HIV-1 GP120-mediated immune suppression and lymphocyte destruction in the absence of viral infection. J. Immunol. **142**: 3091–3097.
13. FAHEY, J. L., J. M. G. TAYLOR & R. DETELS. 1990. The prognostic value of cellular and serologic markers in infection with human immunodeficiency virus type 1. N. Engl. J. Med. **322**: 166–172.
14. DENNY, T., R. YOGEN, R. GELMAN, C. SKUZA, J. OLESKE, E. CHADWICK, S-C. CHENG & E. CONNOR. 1992. Lymphocyte subsets in healthy children during the first 5 years of life. JAMA **267**: 1484–1488.
15. YANASE, Y., T. TANGO, K. OKUMURA, et al. 1986. Lymphocyte subsets identified by monoclonal antibodies in healthy children. Ped. Res. **20**: 1147–1151.

16. FALCAO, R. P., S. J. ISMAEL & E. A. DONADI. 1987. Age-associated changes of T lymphocyte subsets. Diagn. Clin. Immunol. **5:** 205–208.
17. D'ARMINIO MONFORTE, A., R. NOVATI, M. GALLI, et al. 1990. T-cell subsets and serum immunoglobulin levels in infants born to HIV-seropositive mothers: A longitudinal evaluation. AIDS **4:** 1141–1144.
18. BABCOCK, G. F., A. F. TAYLOR, B. A. HYND, R. M. SRAMKOSKI & J. W. ALEXANDER. 1987. Flow cytometric analysis of lymphocyte subset phenotypes comparing normal children and adults. Diagn. Clin. Immunol. **5:** 175–179.
19. DE MARTINO, M., P.-A. TOVO, L. GALLI, et al. 1991. Prognostic significance of immunologic changes in 675 infants perinatally exposed to human immunodeficiency virus. J. Pediatr. **119:** 702–709.
20. HULSTAERT, F., V. DENEYS, A. M. MAZZON, et al. 1991. CD4 T lymphocyte values in pediatric and adult populations. Int. Conf. AIDS **7:** 288.
21. VAN DYKE, R. B., D. CALLIGARO, L. GOMEZ, et al. 1991. (Abstract) CD4 and CD8 lymphocyte profiles in HIV seronegative and uninfected infants born to HIV-1 infected mothers. 11th ACTG NIH. Meeting. March. (AIDS Clinical Trial Group) Washington, D.C.
22. ERKELLER-YUKSEL, F. M., V. DENEYS, B. YUKSEL, et al. 1992. Age-related changes in human blood lymphocyte subpopulations. J. Pediatr. **120:** 216–222.
23. MOFENSON, L. M., J. MOYE & J. BETHEL (for the NICHD IVIG Clinical Trial Study Group). 1992. Effect of intravenous immunoglobulin (IVIG) on CD4$^+$ cell decline in HIV-infected children in a clinical trial of IVIG prophylaxis. In VIII International Conference on AIDS. Poster Abstracts, Vol. 2: B161. CONGREX Holland B.V. Amsterdam, the Netherlands.
24. THE NICHD IVIG CLINICAL TRIAL STUDY GROUP. 1991. Efficacy of intravenous immunoglobulin for the prophylaxis of serious bacterial infections in symptomatic human immunodeficiency virus-infected children. N. Engl. J. Med. **325:** 73–80.
25. MOFENSON, L. M., J. MOYE, J. BETHEL, R. HIRSCHHORN, C. JORDAN & R. NUGENT (for the National Institute of Child Health and Human Development IVIG Clinical Trial Study Group). 1992. Prophylactic intravenous immunoglobulin in HIV-infected children with CD4$^+$ counts of 0.20 × 10^9/L or over: Effect on viral, opportunistic and bacterial infections. JAMA **268:** 483–488.
26. MOFENSON, L. M., J. MOYE, R. NUGENT & P. FLYER. (for the NICHD IVIG Clinical Trial Study Group). 1992. Serious infection and mortality in HIV-infected children in a clinical trial of intravenous immunoglobulin (Abstract No. 908). In Proceedings of the 32nd Interscience Conference on Antimicrobial Agents & Chemotherapy. American Society for Microbiology, Washington, D.C.
27. MOFENSO, L. M., J. BETHEL, J. MOYE, P. FLYER & R. NUGENT (for the NICHD IVIG Clinical Trial Study Group). 1993. Effect of intravenous immunoglobulin on CD4$^+$ lymphocyte decline in HIV-infected children in a clinical trial of IVIG infection prophylaxis. J. AIDS, in press.
28. CONNOR, E., M. BAGARAZZI, G. MCSHERRY, et al. 1991. Clinical and laboratory correlates of *Pneumocystis carinii* pneumonia in children infected with HIV. JAMA **265:** 1693–1697.
29. KOVACS, A., T. FREDERICK, J. CHURCH, A. ELLER, M. OXTOBY & L. MASCOLA. CD4 T-lymphocyte counts and *Pneumocystis carinii* pneumonia in pediatric HIV infection. JAMA **265:** 1698–1703.
30. LIEBOVITZ, E., M. RIGAUD, H. POLLACK, et al. 1990. *Pneumocystis carinii* pneumonia in infants infected with the human immunodeficiency virus with more than 450 CD4 T lymphocytes per cubic millimeter. N. Engl. J. Med. **323:** 531–533.
31. CENTERS FOR DISEASE CONTROL. 1991. Guidelines for prophylaxis against *Pneumocystis carinii* pneumonia for children infected with human immunodeficiency virus. Morbid. Mortal. Wkly. Rep. **40(RR-2):** 1–12.
32. PIZZO, P. A. 1993. Pediatric AIDS: Part I, medical management of HIV-infected children. AIDS Clin. Care **5:** 9–10.
33. YARCHOAN, R., D. G. VENZON, J. M. PLUDA, et al. 1991. CD4 count and the risk for

death in patients infected with HIV receiving antiretroviral therapy. Ann. Intern. Med. **115:** 184–189.
34. PHILLIPS, A. N., J. ELFORD, C. SABIN, M. BOFILL, G. JANOSSY & C. A. LEE. 1992. Immunodeficiency and the risk of death in HIV infection. JAMA **268:** 2662–2666.

APPENDIX 1

The following persons and institutions constituted the National Heart Lung and Blood Institute Pediatric Pulmonary and Cardiac Complications of Vertically Transmitted Human Immunodeficiency Virus Infection Study.

National Heart, Lung and Blood Institute, Bethesda, MD— H. H. Peavy, M. D., A. Kalica, Ph.D., C. Kasten-Sportes, M. D., C. Vreim, Ph.D., C. Weinstein, Ph.D., and M. C. Wu, Ph.D.; *Cleveland Clinic Foundation,* Cleveland, OH—J. Boyett, Ph.D.[*] (through 7/91), M. Schluchter, Ph.D.[*], D. Moodie, M.D., G. Beck, Ph.D., B. Baetz-Greenwalt, M.D., K. Easley, M.S., J. Goldfarb, M.D., L. Gragg, M.S., M. McHugh, M.D., A. Mehta, M.D., M. Meziane, M.D., R. Sterba, M.D.; *Case Western Reserve University,* Cleveland OH—H. Houser, M.D., R. Martin, M.D.; *Baylor College of Medicine, University of Texas Medical School at Houston,* Houston TX—W. Shearer, M.D., Ph.D.[*], N. Ayers, M.D., C. Baker, M.D., T. Bricker, M.D., G. Demmler, M.D., M. Doyle, M.D., M. Dyson, M.D., A. Garson, Jr., M.D., B. Gonik, M.D., H. Hammill, M.D., T. N. Hansen, M.D., I. C. Hanson, M.D., P. Hiatt, M.D., K. Hoots, M.D., R. Jacobson, M.D., D. Kearney, M.D., M. W. Kline, M.D., C. Kozinetz, Ph.D., M.P.H., C. Langston, M.D., C. Lapin, M.D., A. Ludomirsky, M.D., W. Moore, M.D., L. Pickering, M.D., E. Singleton, M.D., L. Taber, M.D.; *The Children's Hospital, Boston/Harvard Medical School,* Boston, MA—S. Lipshultz, M.D.[*], R. Cleveland, M.D., S. Colan, M.D., A. Colin, M.D., E. Cooper, M.D., W. Cranley, M.D., K. McIntosh, M.D., E. J. Orav, Ph.D., A. Perez-Atayde, M.D., S. Pelton, M.D., S. Sanders, M.D., S. Steinbach, M.D., S. T. Treves, M.D., R. Tuomala, M.D., and M. E. B. Wohl, M.D.; *Mount Sinai School of Medicine,* New York, NY—M. Kattan, M.D.[*], R. Dische, M.D., B. Fyfe, M.D., S. Heaton, M.D., D. Hodes, M.D., W. Lai, M.D., K. I. Norton, M.D., V. Peters, M.D., S. Ritter, M.D., J. Rosen, M.D., R. Sperling, M.D.; *Presbyterian Hospital in the City of New York/Columbia University,* New York, NY—F. Bierman, M.D.[*] (through 5/91), R. Mellins, M.D.[*], P. Alderson, M.D., W. E. Berdon, M.D., W. Fleishman, M.D., W. Gersony, M.D., A. C. Koumbourlis, M.D., P. LaRussa, M.D., C. Marboe, M.D., S. Miller, M.D., J. Pitt, M.D., L. M. Quittell, M.D., T. Starc, M.D.; *UCLA School of Medicine,* Los Angeles, CA—S. Kaplan, M.D.[*], Y. Al-Khatib, M.D., I. Boechat, M.D., P. Boyer, M.D., Ph.D., Y. Bryson, M.D., D. Chen, M.D., R. Doroshow, M.D., R. Elashoff, Ph.D., M. Garg, M.D., R. Hawkins, M.D., A. Hohn, M.D., A. Kovacs, M.D., A. Platzker, M.D., R. Settlage, M.D., R. Williams, M.D., M. Woo, M.D., B. P. Wood, M.D.; *The University of Texas Health Science Center at San Antonio,* San Antonio, TX—C. V. Sumaya, M.D.[*] (through 12/92), H. Jenson, M.D.[*]

[*] Principal investigator.

APPENDIX 2

The following persons and institutions constituted the National Institute of Child Health and Human Development Intravenous Immunoglobulin Clinical Trial Study Group.
National Institute of Child Health and Human Development, Bethesda, MD—A. Willoughby, M.D., M.P.H., L. M. Mofenson, M.D., R. Nugent, Ph.D., J. Moye, M.D. (from the Pediatric, Adolescent and Maternal AIDS Branch), and H. W. Berendes, M.D., M.H.S., J. G. Rigau-Perez, M.D., M.P.H. (from the Division of Prevention Research); *Westat, Inc.*, Rockville, MD—S. Durako, C. Jordan, R.N., K. Rust, Ph.D., R. Hirschhorn, M.A., J. Bethel, Ph.D.; *Lincoln Hospital Center*, Bronx, NY—K. Shah, M.D., J. Chow, M.D.; *Cornell Medical Center-New York Hospital*, New York, NY—P. Edelson, M.D., D. Sanders, M.D.; *Schneider Children's Hospital-Queens Hospital Center of Long Island Jewish Medical Center*, New Hyde Park, NY—V. Bonagura, M.D., D. Valacer, M.D.; *Beth Israel Medical Center*, New York, NY—W. Henley, M.D.; *Metropolitan Hospital Center*, New York, NY—M. Bamji, M.D.; *New York Medical College*, Valhalla, NY—A. Gupta, M.D., K. I. Li, M.D.; *Harlem Hospital Center*, New York, NY—E. J. Abrams, M.D.; *State University of New York Health Science Center*, Brooklyn, NY—S. Fikrig, M.D.; *St. Luke's/Roosevelt Hospital Center*, New York, NY—S. S. Bakshi, M.D.; *North Shore University Hospital*, Manhassett, NY—S. Pahwa, M.D.; *New York University Medical Center-Bellevue Hospital Center*, New York, NY—K. Krasinski, M.D.; *Babies Hospital*, New York, NY—J. Pitt, M.D.; *Albert Einstein College of Medicine*, Bronx, NY—L. Bernstein, M.D., A. Rubinstein, M.D.; *University of Connecticut Health Center*, Hartford, CT—G. Johnson, M.D.; *Boston City Hospital*, Boston, MA—E. R. Cooper, M.D.; *University of Medicine and Dentistry of New Jersey-Robert Wood Johnson Medical School*, New Brunswick, NJ—L. Frenkel, M.D.; *St. Christopher's Hospital*, Philadelphia, PA—H. W. Lischner, M.D., S. A. Raphael, M.D.; *University of Maryland*, Baltimore, MD—J. P. Johnson, M.D.; *Children's Hospital National Medical Center*, Washington, DC—T. Rakusan, M.D.; *Emory University School of Medicine*, Atlanta, GA—S. Nesheim, M.D., A. Nahmias, M.D., H. Keyserling, M.D.; *Children's Memorial Hospital*, Chicago, IL—R. Yogev, M.D., E. Chadwick, M.D.; *University of Illinois College of Medicine*, Chicago, IL—K. Rich, M.D.; *Texas Children's Hospital*, Houston, TX—W. T. Shearer, M.D., Ph.D., I. C. Guerra-Hanson, M.D.; *Children's Hospital Medical Center*, Oakland, CA—A. Petru, M.D.; *University of Puerto Rico*, San Juan, PR—C. Diaz, M.D., J. L. Colon Santini, M.D.; *San Juan City Hospital*, San Juan, PR—E. Jimenez, M.D.; *Ramon Ruiz Arnau University Hospital*, Bayamon, PR—D. Garcia-Trias, M.D., C. Acantilado, M.D.; *Cutter Biological, Miles, Inc.*, Berkeley, CA—R. Schwartz, M.D.

Reservoirs of HIV Infection or Carriage: Monocytic, Dendritic, Follicular Dendritic, and B Cells

JEFFREY LAURENCE[a]

Laboratory for AIDS Virus Research
Division of Hematology/Oncology
Department of Medicine
Cornell University Medical College
New York, New York 10021

INTRODUCTION

Recent data indicate that a relatively large number of peripheral and tissue-based immunocytes are chronically infected with human immunodeficiency virus (HIV), persisting as stationary cell intermediates from which HIV may be induced. By means of DNA amplification techniques such as the polymerase chain reaction (PCR), the frequency of infected peripheral $CD4^+$ T lymphocytes in AIDS patients was shown to be at least 1%,[1] while in asymptomatic HIV-seropositive persons, it ranges from 0.04% to 1.3%.[2] Apart from the classic target for HIV infection in peripheral blood, T cells bearing the high-affinity viral receptor $CD4^+$, minor cell subpopulations also appear to be susceptible. However, the nature of the primary reservoir(s) for such infection *in vivo* is yet unclear. Circulating monocytes do not appear to subserve this purpose. For example, one group reported HIV proviral DNA in only two of fourteen peripheral monocyte samples from HIV-seropositive individuals,[1] while another found HIV sequences in all of 27 $CD4^+$ T-cell samples, but in only two of 20 monocyte samples evaluated.[3] Yet this lineage may be an important source of infectious virus in other body compartments. In cerebrospinal fluid, a large percentage of macrophages appear to be HIV-infected, although the ratio of unintegrated to integrated provirus is 10-fold higher when compared with $CD4^+$ peripheral T cells.[4]

This is not simply an academic issue. Intermittent activation of HIV expression in chronically infected cells by direct or indirect involvement of a variety of microbial, antigenic, and humoral cofactors may play a role in determining the rate of development of HIV-related disease.[5] Indeed, the relentless progression of

---

[a] Address for correspondence: Cornell University Medical College, 411 East 69th Street, New York, New York 10021.

immunologic dysfunction (and consequent clinical symptoms) characteristic of HIV infection appears to be related to the complex nature of viral gene regulation and its dependence on interactions with cellular targets, networks susceptible to modulation by myriad cofactors. The possibility that blocking the activation of chronically infected cells might maintain the integrated provirus in a quiescent state, preventing lytic infection and active viral replication, makes this avenue of investigation of particular pertinence in the design of novel therapeutics.

The central role of the T lymphocyte in AIDS is covered by other papers in this volume. This review will focus on several distinct cell lineages in peripheral blood and lymphoid tissue—the dendritic cell, follicular dendritic cell, monocyte, and B lymphocyte—as potential reservoirs for HIV replication or carriage.

DENDRITIC CELL

The dendritic cell (DC) is a loosely adherent, nonphagocytic bone marrow–derived lymphoid cell with distinct morphological features (FIG. 1). Its cytoplasm is arranged in pseudopods of varying form and number, resulting in a variety of shapes, from bipolar elongate cells to elaborate stellate or dendritic ones. The cytoplasm contains many spherical, phase-dense mitochondria and prominent vacuoles. The nucleus is large, contorted in shape, and refractile. DCs represent less than 1% of the normal population of splenic white pulp and a smaller fraction of peripheral leukocytes. They are MHC class II+, lack Fc receptors, are sensitive to steroids and τ-irradiation and, at least in man, bear C3 receptors. Unlike macro-

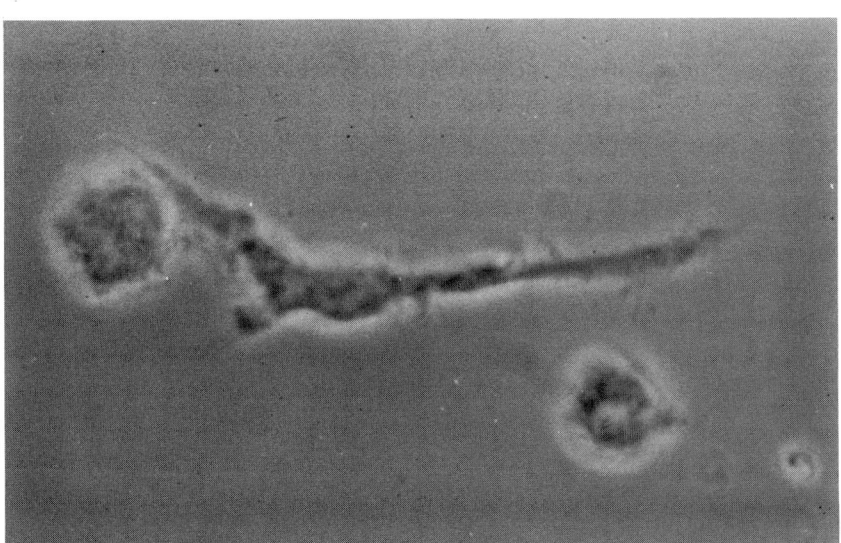

FIGURE 1. A human peripheral blood dendritic cell in culture, situated between two B lymphocytes. Note the prolonged, neuron-like processes.

phages, which are present at birth, DCs make a delayed appearance, recognized in the mouse at two to four weeks of age. They are nonproliferating and have a rapid turnover *in situ,* with a half-life of three to five days. Although they represent an extremely small fraction of circulating or tissue-based hematopoietic elements, they are found in all tissues except brain and are potent stimulators of both allogeneic and autologous mixed lymphocyte culture (MLC) responses. They also serve as accessory cells for T-cell proliferative responses to mitogen and antigen, development of cytolytic T cells, and oxidative mitogenesis.

One group[6] has described morphologically distinct subsets of dendritic cell, as recognized by immunoelectron microscopy, with those of type 1 having an irregular surface with numerous projections and distinct cytoplasmic vacuoles and type 2, a paler nucleus with only a thin rim of dense heterochromatin, large expanses of cytoplasm devoid of organelles, and few processes. This distinction may be important in adjudicating the controversy over whether DCs serve as active sites for HIV entry, replication, and latent infection, or are simply passive carriers of virus. Indeed, while Langerhans' cells of the dermis, peripheral DCs, lymphoid follicular dendritic cells, and lymphoid interdigitating dendritic cells share morphologic features, reflected in the confusing similarity of nomenclature, there are conflicting views as to their precise lineage[7] and their susceptibility to HIV infection.

Dr. Knight's group first described apparent infection of DCs by HIV, observing classical lentiviral budding from the plasma membrane within five days after viral exposure.[8] *In situ* hybridization revealed HIV transcripts in 3 to 21% of purified DCs in culture.[9] *In vivo* infection was documented by isolating peripheral DCs from HIV-seropositive persons at different clinical stages.[10] Infection paralleled qualitative, though not quantitative, DC abnormalities. A decrement in cells expressing high-density MHC-II alloantigen, as well as a decreased capacity to serve as stimulators in autologous and heterologous MLC, was shown.[10] In addition, after *in vitro* exposure to HIV, dendritic cells suppressed T-cell responses to mitogen.[11]

These data were corroborated by additional studies from Dr. Haseltine's group.[12] DCs supported the active replication of all isolates of HIV-1 tested, including T- and monocyte-trophic strains, yielding markedly higher titers of virus than parallel cultures of primary T lymphocytes, $CD4^+$ T cells, or monocytes. Replication occurred without evident cytopathic effects. These properties momentarily placed the DC in a position central to HIV pathogenesis, as it could conceivably represent a source for continuous spread of virus to $CD4^+$ T cells brought into close continuity with DC during antigen presentation. In addition, the presence of such accessory cells in skin and mucous membranes might facilitate HIV infection across what were previously thought to be impenetrable barriers.

This scenario was directly contradicted by several other reports. In one study, DC were isolated from 25 HIV-positive persons at various clinical stages. No evidence either for a prefential loss of peripheral DC, nor for a functional defect, assessed by stimulatory capacity for allogeneic $CD4^+$ T cells in a MLC, was found.[13] In addition, DC could fully initiate expansion of allogeneic $CD4^+$ T-lymphocyte clones, without cytopathicity for the proliferating cells.[13] In terms of viral load, limiting dilution and PCR analysis revealed HIV provirus in 0.1 to 0.2%

of $CD4^+$ lymphocytes from AIDS patients, but in only 1 in 50,000 cells from the DC-enriched fraction, a level consistent with potential T-cell contamination of this subset.

The basis for these discrepancies may be partially resolved by morphologic distinctions among "DCs".[6] By *in situ* hybridization, HIV DNA and RNA were found solely within two morphologic types of "dendritic cell," those with large expanses of cytoplasm devoid of organelles and with few processes, and those resembling the interdigitating cells of the afferent lymphatics, but not in the classic "type 1" DC. The lack of HIV infection in the latter population was confirmed and expanded by a second report.[14] After exposure to HIV-1 *in vitro*, dendritic cells continue to present antigens and superantigens, normally forming clusters with $CD4^+$ T cells, that are then driven to replicate. Infection of the DC could not be detected, even though the aggregated T cells formed syncytia and released mature virions. It was hypothesized that membrane trapping of HIV by DC facilitates T-cell lysis, and therefore loss of circulating antigen-specific $CD4^+$ T cells.[14]

The dendritic cell does appear to be much more efficient than antigen-presenting cells of monocyte/macrophage lineage in facilitating HIV infection of T lymphocytes *in vitro*.[14] An analogous mechanism may operate in the germinal centers of lymphoid organs, as well as other regions enriched for DC, such as intestinal mucosa and bronchial passages. These characteristics should broaden the concept of an HIV "reservoir" and highlight the importance of accessory cells in the immune dysfunction seen in HIV disease. For example, HIV participates in a superantigen-mediated facilitation of viral replication in certain $CD4^+$ T cells, without leading to gross deletion of these $V\beta$-selected T cells *in vivo*.[15] While neither macrophages nor DC are required for the presentation of superantigens *in vitro*, the latter render T cells that are undergoing a superantigen–T cell receptor $V\beta$ interaction anergic.[16] The DC, in presenting HIV epitope(s) as a superantigen, may therefore have a critical role in inducing T-cell anergy, rather than facilitating T-cell depletion.

The DC may also be of therapeutic utility in AIDS. Dendritic cells are potent stimulators of primary immune responses to contact sensitizers and alloantigens. They could serve as stimulators for the *in vitro* priming of $CD8^+$ cytolytic T-cell clones against HIV envelope antigens, for use in passive cellular immunotherapy.[17]

FOLLICULAR DENDRITIC CELLS

Controversy over active replication versus virion adherence for the DC extends to other cell types with similar morphology. Interdigitating cells (IDC), peripheral dendritic cells, and epidermal Langerhans' cells all derive from bone marrow progenitors, but the location, function, and phenotype of these cells are divergent; and their infectibility by, as well as expression and transmission of HIV may vary widely. In addition, the follicular dendritic cell (FDC), also known as the reticular DC, may not even be of hematopoietic origin, but may instead be related to marrow stromal cells, a type of myofibroblast.[18]

FDC are located only in primary and secondary lymphoid follicles,[18] forming long cellular extensions providing extensive networks among B lymphocytes.

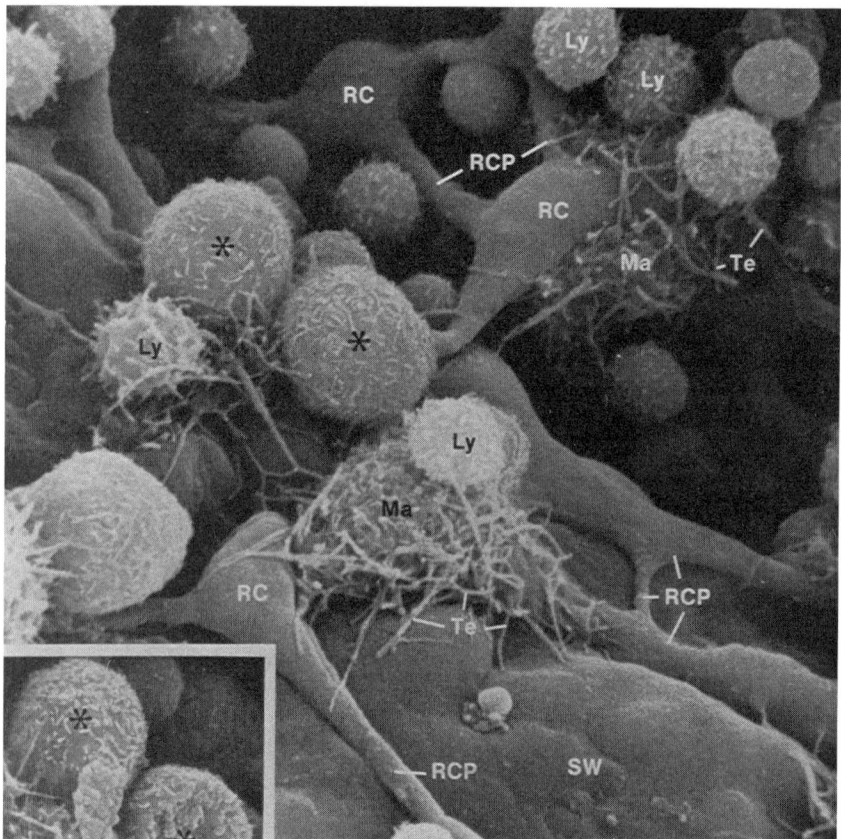

FIGURE 2. A scanning electron micrograph of a human lymph node sinus. Follicular dendritic cells (RC), with long processes (RCP) are shown within a trabecular meshwork with macrophages (Ma), macrophage tendril processes (Te), and lymphocytes (Ly). Large granular lymphocytes, near the sinus wall (SW), are marked with an asterisk. (Reproduced from Kessel, R. G. & R. H. Kardon. 1979. Tissues and Organs: A Text-Atlas of Scanning Electron Microscopy: 57. W. H. Freeman. San Francisco.)

They are nonphagocytic but efficient at capturing and retaining membrane complexes of antigen, antibody, and complement by virtue of Fc and C3 receptors (FIG. 2). FDCs influence B lymphocyte function by facilitating interactions with antigen–antibody complexes and cell matrix molecules.[18] Trapped immune complexes, with exposed antigenic determinants, are retained over long periods of time, a process critical to the regulation of antibody titers and initiation and maintenance of B-cell memory, through continuous restimulation of antigen-specific B cells.

Early in the history of HIV disease, it was clear that FDC were involved in various pathologic stages of the generalized lymphadenopathy syndrome (LAS), a hallmark of initial HIV disease.[19] Soon after an acute seroconversion reaction to HIV infection, there is a marked increase in FDC number, concordant with proliferation of B lymphoid elements. With clinical progression, both cell types decline in number, paralleling decreases in CD4+ T cells. Concurrently, the architecture of the lymph node undergoes tremendous disruption (FIG. 3). Germinal center involution and loss of FDCs are accompanied by replacement with CD8+ T lymphocytes and monocytes and the deposition of a fibrin-like matrix, resulting in a "burned out" fibrotic node.[20] This provides a visual portrait underlying the immune dysfunction characteristic of AIDS, as such destruction quite clearly results in a severely altered lymphoid microenvironment.[19,21]

The pathophysiology of this FDC disturbance is yet unclear. HIV RNA is consistently found only "in" CD4+/CD45RO+ T cells and FDCs, but for the latter the pattern of nucleic acid deposition is suggestive of surface immune complex trapping, rather than true infection.[22] HIV adheres to FDCs *in vitro* by mechanisms independent of CD4, as ostensible infection—more probably viral carriage—is unaffected by monoclonal antibodies against CD4.[23] Indeed, the ability to detect proviral DNA and RNA in FDC by PCR or *in situ* hybridization markedly declines after extensive protease treatment of tissue samples.[24] Yet, in the absence of evident HIV replication, it is still unknown how FDCs decline in number as HIV disease progresses. It may involve autocytolytic or autoantibody phenomena.[21]

In terms of HIV pathogenesis, it is likely that as soon as antibody production and germinal center activation begins, HIV–antibody complexes are trapped on FDCs in lymphoid germinal centers, assisting in the prompt removal of circulating virus characteristic of the first two months following infection. Those viral complexes not destroyed by monocytes should be free to interact with other cells trafficking through the germinal center, including CD4+ T lymphocytes, which constitute 5 to 25% of germinal center cellular components.[20] These observations have led to the suggestion that initiation of effective anti-viral therapy early after HIV infection may be critical, delaying establishment of a significant viral burden in lymphoid tissues, further extending the period before establishment of immune deficiency.

LANGERHANS' CELLS

Langerhans' cells (LCs) are MHC-II+ (HLA-DR+/DQ+), CD1+, CD4+ leukocytes with dendritic morphology. They function as the primary epidermal antigen-presenting cell. LC are the only components of the normal epidermis that express surface ATPase, a marker that may be used to identify and enumerate LCs.[25] Unlike dendritic cells, LCs arguably belong to the monocyte–macrophage lineage, although they exhibit 50-fold higher quantities of membrane MHC-II than do monocytes.[26] In contrast to the controversy surrounding DCs, Langerhans' cells are active replicators of HIV, capable of undergoing direct HIV infection *in vitro*.[27] Moderate to severe LC damage has been noted in skin and mucosal biopsies from AIDS patients, with budding virions from their surface membranes.[25] These cells are also functionally altered, with reduced MHC-II expression and ATPase activity.[28]

LCs may have a role in viral transmission. LCs are found in abundance in oral, vaginal, and cervical epithelium, including ectocervical squamous epithelium and

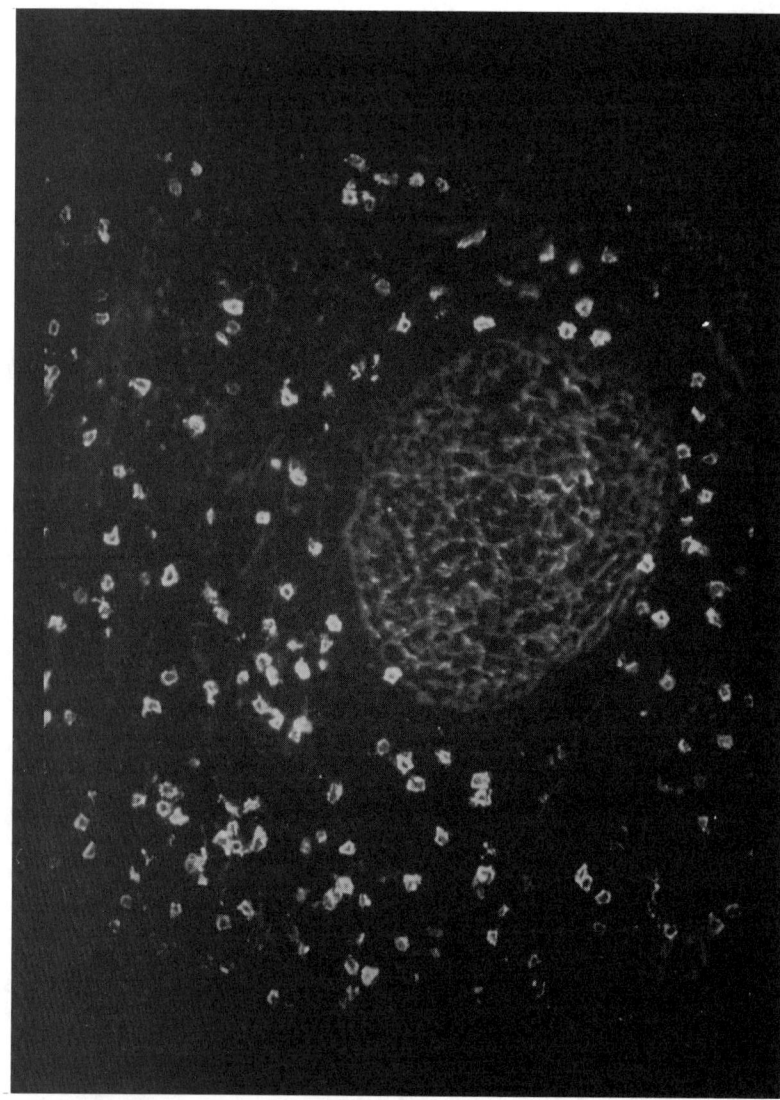

FIGURE 3A. Lymph node disruption in HIV disease. In a normal node (*above*), CD4$^+$ and CD8$^+$ T cells (white peripheral cells) populate the paracortex surrounding the spherical germinal center. B cells and follicular dendritic cells (white cells forming the central reticular pattern) form a regular network in the germinal center.

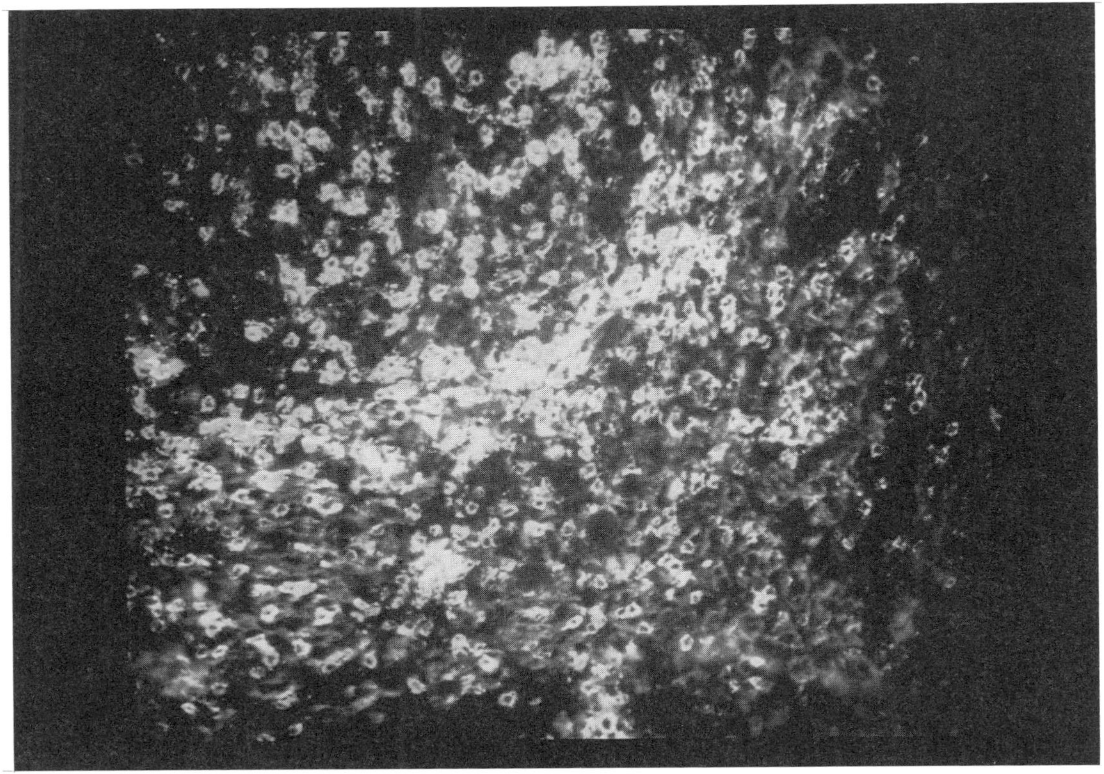

FIGURE 3B. Hyperplastic lymph node from an HIV+ person. T cells invade the germinal center, disrupting its regular architecture. Photographs reproduced in black and white from color figures in Laurence.[19]

the transformation zone represented by endocervical columnar epithelium, albeit rectal epithelium appears devoid of this cell type.[29] In the vaginal mucosa there may be as many as 10 to 50 Langerhans' cells for every 200 basal epithelial cells.[29] The prominent epidermal and mucosal locations of the LC led to the hypothesis, reminiscent of the DC discussion, that transmission of HIV across intact mucosa might occur via direct infection of LCs.[30] It should be noted that no epidemiologic, animal, or even clinical anecdotal evidence supports this contention.

B LYMPHOCYTES

HIV infection is also associated with a progressive decrease in circulating $CD19^+$, $CD20^+$, $CD21^+$ B cells, paralleling the decline in absolute numbers of $CD4^+$ lymphocytes with advancing clinical stage.[31] Intrinsic B-cell functional defects may also precede alterations in T helper cell activity. Infection of transformed B-cell lines has been documented, a process susceptible to blockade by anti-CD4 monoclonal antibodies, even in those cells lacking detectable membrane CD4 but expressing CD4 mRNA.[32] We[33] and others[34] have also demonstrated direct HIV infection of nonimmortalized peripheral human B cells *in vitro*. These results are consistent with the identification of HIV provirus in B cell-enriched subpopulations of peripheral blood from >40% of HIV-1 seropositive individuals in one recent study[35] (TABLE 1). They suggest that the types of cell capable of serving as reservoirs for HIV infection *in vivo* should include those of B lymphocyte lineage.

Our group has recently developed a model for chronic infection in human B cells, parallel to those available for cells of $CD4^+$ T and monocyte lineages.[36,37] The ability of HIV replication to be induced from one chronically infected B-cell oligoclone, B-HIV1,[38] is illustrated in TABLE 2. The protein kinase activator phorbol ester (PMA), but not a congener, 4β-phorbol, incapable of activating diacyelglycerol and PK, markedly upregulates HIV. This effect appears to be protein kinase specific, inhibitable in a dose-dependent manner by the PK inhibitor H7 and specific PKC inhibitors such as staurosporine (TABLE 2).

As FDCs are present in highest concentration in the B-cell-rich germinal centers of lymphoid follicles, they may serve as a ready conduit of virus to the B lympho-

TABLE 1. Frequency of Cells Containing HIV-1 DNA in Subpopulations of Peripheral Blood Leukocytes by PCR[a]

Patients	T cells	Adherent Monocytes	B Cell/Dendritic Cells
Asymptomatic	0.001	0	0
Asymptomatic	0.0001	0	0.0001
ARC	0.001	0	0.0001
ARC	0.001	0	0
ARC	0.001	0	0
AIDS	0.01	0	0.0001
AIDS	0.001	0	0.001
AIDS	0.0001	0	0
AIDS	0.001	0	0

[a] Data taken from Poznansky *et al.*[35]

TABLE 2. Effect of Protein Kinase Activator and Inhibitors on Induction of HIV-1 from B-HIV1 Cells[a]

Inducing Agent	Concentration (ng/ml)	Inhibitor	Concentration (μM)	[p24] Core Ag (pg/ml)	Inhibition (%)
—	—	—	—	620 ± 160	—
PMA	5	—	—	3405 ± 285	—
4B-phorbol	5	—	—	960	—
4B-phorbol	50	—	—	950	—
PMA	5	H7	10	2450	34.3
PMA	5	H7	50	1750	59.4
PMA	5	H7	75	1040	84.9
PMA	5	H7	100	670	98.2
PMA	5	Staurosporine	0.0001	480	100

[a] Cells were plated at 7.5×10^4/microwell in 0.2 ml of culture medium (RPMI-1640 + 10% FCS) together with the appropriate concentration of inhibitor for 2 hr, followed by addition of inducing agent with or without inhibitor. Supernatants were harvested 120 hr later and HIV p24 Ag concentration measured. (Data taken from Laurence et al.[38])

cyte. Cognate interactions among B, T, and antigen-presenting cells during an immune response may also serve as a source of HIV transmission to B lymphocytes. This is an underinvestigated area of HIV biology; additional studies are required in primary and transformed B-cell lines at various stages of differentiation.

MONOCYTE/MACROPHAGE

The mononuclear phagocytes encompass circulating peripheral blood monocytes, promonocytes, precursor cells from the bone marrow and possibly other organs, and fixed tissue macrophages or histiocytes. These latter cells include connective tissue histiocytes, the Kupffer's cells of liver, microglial cells, and alveolar macrophages. These cells have receptors for Fc and complement, are MHC-II$^+$, and constitute 3 to 8% of circulating leukocytes. The marginal pool, primarily those adhering to endothelial cell surfaces, is three to four times as great. The half-life of monocytes varies from 12 to 100 hours, while mature macrophages may survive for many months in tissues. There is increasing evidence that functionally and structurally heterogeneous subsets of monocytes exist. Variations in size, degree of aerobic glycolosis, Fc receptor avidity, phagocytic properties, expression of CD antigens, and quantity of membrane MHC-II have been correlated with immunoregulatory activity and tumoricidal or antigen- and superantigen-processing capabilities. In addition, certain subsets secrete soluble factors, including interleukin 1, arginase, prostaglandins, lymphocytotoxins, and τ-interferon. Like the dendritic cell, macrophages also serve as stimulators in the allogeneic and possibly autologous MLC, although in the latter reaction the DC is extraordinarily more potent.

It is beyond the intention of this article to review the extensive literature on HIV infection of the monocyte/macrophage; several excellent monographs have recently appeared.[39] It is important to note, however, that this lineage does not appear to be an important reservoir of HIV in peripheral blood (TABLE 1), despite earlier reports to the contrary. Macrophages, however, are infected with high frequency in the brain, spinal cord, lymphatic tissue, and lung, and this may parallel organ-specific manifestations of HIV disease. For example, *in situ* hybridization for HIV mRNA in brain tissue of HIV-seropositive individuals demonstrates productively infected macrophages in specific regions, representing some 15% of white matter.[40] In addition, subcortical structures, including the caudate and putamen of the basal ganglia, may also be involved, with generalized demylinization and secondary astroglial reaction. In contrast, the frequency of HIV transcripts in liver, skin, bone marrow, and blood is quite low, with monocytes and tissue macrophages rarely infected. *In vitro* infection of primary monocytes or monocytoid cell lines is usually not cytopathic, virions typically budding into vacuoles.

Like the other accessory cell components discussed here, HIV may be transmitted from monocyte/macrophage reservoirs during antigen presentation.[41] A second issue, frequently raised in discussions of both passive immunization with pooled human immunoglobulin of high neutralizing titer against HIV, and in the development of active immunization protocols, is the possibility of facilitating HIV infection of Fc receptor-positive monocytes via a process known as antibody-dependent enhancement. While ADE appears to occur *in vitro*,[42] with one possible exception[43] it has not been found clinically relevant in either animal models or phase-I clinical trials.

REFERENCES

1. SCHNITTMAN, S. M., M. C. PSALLIDOPOULOS, H. C. LANE, *et al.* 1989. The reservoir for HIV-1 in human peripheral blood is a T cell that maintains expression of CD4. Science **244**: 305–307.
2. PSALLIDOPOULOS, M.C., S. M. SCHNITTMAN, L. M. THOMPSON III, *et al.* 1989. Integrated proviral human immunodeficiency virus type 1 is present in CD4+ peripheral blood lymphocytes in healthy seropositive individuals. J. Virol. **63**: 4626–4644.
3. SPEAR, G. T., O. CHIN-YIH, H. A. KESSLER, J. C. MOORE, G. SCHOCHETMAN & A. L. LANDAY. 1990. Analysis of lymphocytes, monocytes, and neutrophils from human immunodeficiency virus (HIV) infected persons for HIV DNA. J. Infect. Dis. **162**: 1239–1244.
4. PANG, S., Y. KOYANAGI, S. MILES, C. WILEY, H. V. VINTERS & I. S. Y. CHEN. 1990. High levels of unintegrated HIV-1 DNA in brain tissue of AIDS dementia patients. Nature **343**: 85–89.
5. LAURENCE, J. 1990. Molecular interactions among herpesviruses and human immunodeficiency viruses. J. Infect. Dis. **162**: 338–346.
6. PATTERSON, S., J. GROSS, P. BEDFORD & S. C. KNIGHT. 1991. Morphology and phenotype of dendritic cells from peripheral blood and their productive and nonproductive infection with human immunodeficiency virus type 1. Immunology **72**: 361–367.
7. AUSTYN, J. M. 1987. Lymph node dendritic cells. Immunology **62**: 161–166.
8. PATTERSON, S. & S. C. KNIGHT. 1987. Susceptibility of human peripheral blood dendritic cells to infection by human immunodeficiency virus. J. Gen. Virol. **68**: 1177–1181.
9. MACATONIA, S. E., R. LAU, S. PATTERSON, A. J. PINCHING & S. C. KNIGHT. 1990. Dendritic cell infection, depletion, and dysfunction in HIV infected individuals. Immunology **71**: 38–45.

10. EALES, L-J., J. FARRANT, M. HELBERT & A. J. PINCHING. 1988. Peripheral blood dendritic cells in persons with AIDS and AIDS related complex: Loss of high-density class II antigen expression and function. Clin. Exp. Immunol. **71**: 423–427.
11. MACATONIA, S. E., S. PATTERSON & S. C. KNIGHT. 1989. Suppression of immune responses by dendritic cells infected with HIV. Immunology **67**: 285–289.
12. LANGHOFF, E., E. F. TERWILLIGER, H. J. BOS, K. H. KALLAND, M. C. POZNANSKY, O. M. L. BACON & W. A. HASELTINE. 1991. Replication of human immunodeficiency virus type 1 in primary dendritic cell cultures. Proc. Natl. Acad. Sci. USA **88**: 7998–8002.
13. CAMERON, P. U., H. FORSUM, H. TEPPLER, A. GRANELLI-PIPERNO & R. M. STEINMAN. 1992. During HIV-1 infection most blood dendritic cells are not productively infected and can induce allogeneic $CD4^+$ T cells clonal expansion. Clin. Exp. Immunol. **88**: 226–236.
14. CAMERON, P. U., P. S. FREUDENTHAL, J. M. BARKER, S. GEZELTER, K. INABA, & R. M. STEINMAN. 1992. Dendritic cells exposed to human immunodeficiency virus type-1 transmit a vigorous cytopathic infection to $CD4^+$ T cells. Science **257**: 383–387.
15. LAURENCE, J., A. S. HODTSEV & D. N. POSNETT. 1992. Superantigen implicated in dependence of HIV-1 replication in T cells on TCR Vβ expression. Nature **358**: 255–259.
16. ACHA-ORBEA, H. & E. PALMER. 1991. MLS—a retrovirus exploits the immune system. Immunol. Today **12**: 356–361.
17. MACATONIA, S. E., S. PATTERSON & S. C. KNIGHT. 1991. Primary proliferative and cytotoxic T-cell responses to HIV induced *in vitro* by human dendritic cells. Immunology **74**: 399–406.
18. SCHRIEVER, F. & L. M. NADLER. 1992. The central role of follicular dendritic cells in lymphoid tissues. Adv. Immunol. **51**: 243–260.
19. LAURENCE, J. 1985. The immune system in AIDS. Sci. Am. **253(6)**: 84–93.
20. FOX, C. H. & M. COTTLER-FOX. 1992. The pathobiology of HIV infection. Immunol. Today **13**: 353–356.
21. LAMAN, J. D., E. CLAASSEN, N. VAN ROOIJEN & W. J. A. BOERSMA. 1989. Immune complexes on follicular dendritic cells as a target for cytolytic cells in AIDS. AIDS **3**: 543–544.
22. SPIEGEL, H., H. HERBST, G. B. NIEDOBITEK, H-D. FOSS & H. STEIN. 1992. Follicular dendritic cells are a major reservoir for human immunodeficiency virus type 1 in lymphoid tissues facilitating infection of $CD4^+$ T-helper cells. Am. J. Pathol. **140**: 15–22.
23. STAAHMER, I., J. P. ZIMMER, M. ERNST, *et al.* 1991. Isolation of normal human follicular dendritic cells in CD4-independent *in vitro* infection by human immunodeficiency virus (HIV-1). Eur. J. Immunol. **27**: 1873–1878.
24. PANTALEO, G., C. GRAZIOSI, J. F. DEMAREST, *et al.* 1993. HIV infection is active and progressive in lymphoid tissue during the clinically latent stage of disease. Nature **362**: 355–358.
25. RAPPERSBERGER, K., S. GARTNER, P. SCHENK, *et al.* 1988. Langerhans' cells are in actual site of HIV-1 replication. Intervirology **29**: 185–194.
26. BJERCKE, S., G. GAUDERNACK & L. R. BRAATHEN. 1985. Enriched Langerhans' cells express more HLA-DR determinants than blood-derived adherent cells, monocytes, and dendritic cells. Scand. J. Immunol. **21**: 489–492.
27. BRAATHEN, L. R., G. RAMIREZ, R. O. F. KUNZE & H. GELDERBLOM. 1987. Langerhans' cells as primary target cells for HIV infection. Lancet **2**: 1094.
28. BELSITO, D. V., M. R. SANCHEZ, R. L. BAER, F. VALENTINE & G. J. THORBECKE. 1984. Reduced Langerhans' cell Ia antigen and ATPase activity in patients with the acquired immunodeficiency syndrome. N. Engl. J. Med. **310**: 1279–1282.
29. TOUCHETTE, N. 1991. AIDS research and mucosal immune studies begin to gel. J. NIH Res. **3**: 65–70.
30. LEHNER, T., L. HUSSAIN, J. WILSON & M. CHAPMAN. 1991. Mucosal transmission of HIV. Nature **353**: 709.
31. REDDY, M. M., R. R. GOETZ, J. M. GORMAN, M. H. GRIECO, L. CHESS & S. LEDERMAN.

1991. Human immunodeficiency virus type-1 infection of homosexual men is accompanied by a decrease in circulating B cells. J. AIDS **4:** 428–435.
32. MALKOVSKY, M., K. PHILPOTT, A. G. DALGLEISH, A. L. MELLOR, S. PATTERSON, A. D. B. WEBSTER, A. J. EDWARDS & P. G. MADDON. 1988. Infection of B lymphocytes by the human immunodeficiency virus and their susceptibility to cytotoxic cells. Eur. J. Immunol. **18:** 1315–1321.
33. LAURENCE, J. & S. M. ASTRIN. 1991. Immunodeficiency virus induction of malignant transformation in human B cells. Proc. Natl. Acad. Sci. USA **88:** 7635–7639.
34. HENDERSON, E. E., J-Y. YANG, R-D. ZHANG & M. BEALER. 1991. Altered HIV expression and EBV-induced transformation in co-infected PBL's and PBL subpopulations. Virology **182:** 186–192.
35. POZNANSKY, M. C., B. WALKER, W. A. HASELTINE, J. SODROSKI & E. LANGHOFF. 1991. A rapid method for quantitating the frequency of peripheral blood cells containing HIV1-DNA. J. AIDS **4:** 368–373.
36. FOLKS, T. M., D. POWELL, M. LIGHTFOOT, et al. 1986. Biological and biochemical characterization of a clone LAU-3-cell surviving infection with the acquired immune deficiency syndrome retrovirus. J. Exp. Med. **164:** 280–291.
37. FOLKS, T. M., J. JUSTEMENT, A. KINTER, et al. 1988. Characterization of a promonocyte clone chronically infected with HIV and inducable by 13-Phorbol-12-myristate acetate. J. Immunol. **140:** 117–122.
38. LAURENCE, J., B. GRIMISON, C. RODRIGUEZ-ALFAGEME & S. M. ASTRIN. 1993. A model system for regulation of chronic HIV-1 infection of B lymphocytes. Virology, in press.
39. KALTER, D. C., H. E. GENDELMAN & M. S. MELTZER. 1991. Monocytes, dendritic cells, and Langerhans' cells in human immunodeficiency virus infection. Dermatol. Clin. **9:** 415–428.
40. KOENIG, S., et al. 1986. Detection of AIDS virus and macrophages in brain tissue from AIDS patients with encephalothapy. Science **233:** 1089–1093.
41. MANN, D. L., S. GARTNER, F. LE SANE, H. BUCHOW & M. POPOVIC. 1990. HIV-1 transmission and function of virus-infected monocytes/macrophages. J. Immunol. **144:** 2152–2158.
42. LAURENCE, J., A. SAUNDERS, E. EARLY & J. E. SALMON. 1990. Human immunodeficiency virus infection of monocytes: Relationship to Fc-gamma receptors and antibody-dependent viral enhancement. Immunology **70:** 338–343.
43. HOMSY, J., M. MEYER & J. A. LEUY. 1990. Serum enhancement of human immunodeficiency virus (HIV) infection correlates with disease in HIV-infected individuals. J. Virol. **64:** 1437–1440.

HIV-1 Reverse Transcriptase

A Diversity Generator and Quasispecies Regulator

JOSÉ L. MUÑOZ,[a] WADE P. PARKS,[a]
STEVEN M. WOLINSKY,[b] BETTE T. M. KORBER,[c]
AND CECELIA HUTTO[d]

[a] *Department of Pediatrics*
New York University School of Medicine
New York, New York 10016

[b] *Department of Medicine*
Northwestern University Medical School
Chicago, Illinois 60611

[c] *Los Alamos National Laboratory*
Los Alamos, New Mexico 87545

[d] *Department of Pediatrics*
University of Miami School of Medicine
Miami, Florida 33136

Many striking characteristics of HIV-1 have emerged from its study over the past decade. From a molecular point of view, the most unusual features are the multiple accessory genes and the extreme divergence of HIV-1 nucleotide sequences. Perinatal HIV-1 infection offers advantages to the study of HIV-1 genetic variation, one being that the approximate timing of transmission from mother to child is known. The maternal–infant interface may serve as a well-defined model of HIV-1 transmission that can be used to test hypotheses about sequence variation in a biologically relevant context. Thus, the use of sequence variation can provide important insights into the pathogenesis of HIV-1 infection, protective immunity to the virus, and perinatal HIV-1 transmission.

A relevant example of the value of sequence variation studies has emerged from the nucleotide mapping of high-level resistance to dideoxynucleotides such as AZT and ddI used to treat HIV-1 infected individuals. Resistance to nucleoside antimetabolites are localized in specific nucleotide changes in the *pol* gene. Larder and associates have identified that tyr-215 mutants are the most important mutations in AZT-resistant HIV-1 populations.[1] Resistance to ddI, another dideoxynucleoside, crosses with the ddC but not with AZT. Mapping resistance to nonnucleoside reverse transcriptase inhibitors reveals yet another predominant mutation not directly related to either AZT or ddI resistance mutations. Utilizing this knowledge of nonoverlapping nucleoside variation in the presence of antiviral selection, Chow et al.[2] have proposed convergent combination chemotherapy that uses three antipolymerase drugs, AZT, ddI, and a nonnucleoside inhibitor. Mutations that make the reverse transcriptase resistant to each of the three drugs are incompatible with each other. When the reverse transcriptase was genetically manipulated to contain the four mutations necessary for resistance, the virus was unable to replicate. Thus, knowledge of nucleotide variation in the presence of a known selection pressure such as chemotherapy can be used to constrain the diversifying potential of HIV-1.

The target of the most effective anti-HIV-1 chemotherapy is also the source of HIV-1 nucleotide variation, namely, the reverse transcriptase. Many factors affect the fidelity of DNA synthesis from an RNA template including the inherent instability of the single-stranded RNA combined with the absence of an error-correcting mechanism in the enzyme. Many estimates of fidelity rates or error rates of nucleotide incorporation indicate that the HIV-1 RT is no more error prone than influenza or other viral RNA replicases.[3] Even so, the ability to generate diversity is related in part[e] to *both* error and replication rate. Given the very high levels of HIV-1 replication and its error rate, vast diversity is generated by the HIV-1 replication process. The *pol* gene itself is a target of mutation and thus also demonstrates variation.

Relatively few studies of variation in HIV-1 RT function have been reported. However, given the antibiotic resistance data, pol nucleotide variation would be predicted to be as great as any other HIV-1 gene. Variation in rates of viral replication can be expected even before host factors are considered. Given different HIV-1 *pol* gene variation, different rates of replication, and selection pressures, the definition of *the* HIV-1 virus in a given patient becomes problematic, as was first appreciated by Saag et al.[4]

Eigen coined the term quasispecies for RNA populations[5] that replicate with high replication rates; it was first applied to HIV-1 by Meyerhans et al.[6] Eigen's definition of a quasispecies is that of a "mutant clan or swarm that is ordered about one or a degenerate set of selected master sequences, containing weighted contributions from all the mutants in a population." The term quasispecies was chosen to emphasize that for these populations of sequences, selection acts on the whole ensemble, not just on individual sequences, the entire population behaves *like a species*—*it* is the organism. To characterize partially HIV-1 populations, a consensus sequence is often used, particularly in studies of the V3 loop, an immunodominant *env* gp120 epitope cluster.[7] The consensus sequence is simply a compilation of the most common nucleotide present in each position. A second, often overlooked aspect of describing a quasispecies is the analysis of the distribution of variants. By calculating the nucleotide differences between all possible

---

[e] Other factors include the efficacy of reproduction of each variant relative to the population's average and efficiency (selection value) and the length of the nucleotide sequences.

sequence pairs in a set of variants, a distribution can be determined that provides a measure of the diversity in the set. From a statistical standpoint, the consensus sequence is the sequence less different from all the sequences in the set. The mean internucleotide distance provides a measure of how much the sequences in the set deviate from the consensus.

A comparison of a variant distribution of HIV-1 sequences directly amplified from peripheral blood leukocytes from three HIV-1 infected mothers and their infected children is shown in FIGURE 1.[7] The distribution is shown by comparing each sequence of the *env* gp120 V3 region with every other sequence. As can be noted, each mother's sequence distribution was more divergent than the sequence distribution noted with the infant's sequences, which showed a very narrow distribution. The mean difference between each pair of maternal sequences was 4.79%; for the infants it was 2.87%. A similar shift was seen for the V4–V5 sequences. In addition, the consensus sequence in the infant was different from the mother's in two out of three cases, the infant sequence reflecting a minor variant in the

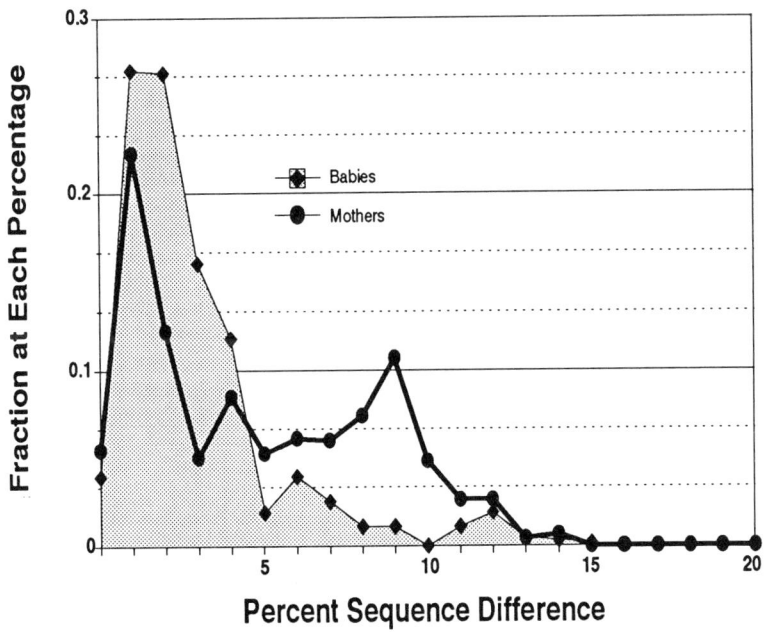

FIGURE 1. Shift in HIV-1 quasispecies diversity associated with perinatal transmission. All sequences from the V3 region of gp120 for each infant are first aligned. To construct the histogram, the percent difference between all possible sequence pairs is calculated. Each point represents the number of pairwise comparisons corresponding to each percent difference. Similar analysis was performed for the maternal sequences. The analysis shows the infants' sequences clustered at less than 5% difference. The mother's sequences are biphasic. They contain a homogeneous component like the infant's, but in addition contain a divergent component that stretches out beyond 10%. The overall diversity of the infants' sequences is thus much less.

mother. Perinatal transmission of HIV-1 thus involves a shift in the fine structure of the quasispecies. There are several possible explanations for this observed shift in quasispecies diversity and structure.

Narrow HIV-1 quasispecies distributions have been noted in other settings, including early after infection in adults[8] and in the late stages of infection[9] as well as with *in vitro* passage.[10] Nowak and May's[11] mathematical model of HIV-1 infection predicts that rapid replication alone would narrow the diversity of the virus. Thus, they argue that negative selective factors such as the immune response put pressure on the virus to diversify. If so, broadening of viral quasispecies sequence diversity may be a major factor in the pathogenesis of chronic persistent viral infections such as HIV-1. In the case of the maternal-infant pairs, we could argue that upon transmission to the infant, the maternal HIV-1 quasispecies found itself in a milieu lacking a critical immune effector mechanism—in this setting, a rapidly replicating, relatively homogeneous variant expands and becomes the predominant population.

Another possibility is that HIV-1 transmission from mother to child is the equivalent of a genetic bottleneck. In higher organisms, genetic bottlenecks result from extended periods of reduced population size that in turn lead to severe reductions in allelic polymorphism.[12] In RNA viruses, genetic bottleneck effects are commonly seen when the viruses are passaged by clone-to-clone transfers, or with very low multiplicities of infection.[13] These passages result in severe constrictions of the population diversity, and they can also lead to enhanced biological differences among the surviving viral subpopulations, eliminating any need to invoke specific selection forces.[14] In the case of perinatal HIV-1 transmission, a bottleneck effect could arise from both maternal and fetal factors.

On the maternal side, the placenta probably provides an effective barrier to transmission. We know that over two-thirds of infants born to HIV-1 positive mothers are *not* infected.[15] The simplest hypothesis for perinatal transmission is that it occurs by transfer of a small infectious inoculum at or near the time of delivery, thus providing a situation analogous to the passage of viruses *in vitro* at low multiplicities of infection. The bottleneck would thus narrow the quasispecies distribution, and only a very small portion of the maternal sequences would be transmitted. Initially, the distribution of these "selected" sequences would show a narrower distribution than the maternal sequences.

The transmission bottleneck may be on the infant side. Even if a very large inoculum of maternal viruses is transmitted to the infant, only a limited subset may be able to replicate in the infant environment. We know that HIV-1 requires activated T cells in order to replicate,[16] and that there is very little T-cell activation in the fetal environment, as evidenced by their very low numbers of HLA-DR-positive and CD45RA-positive T cells.[17] This restrictive environment would thus produce a genetic bottleneck on the fetal side. Whether any of these mechanisms or others are operative and to what degree will require further study. Before leaving the subject of bottlenecks, the strategy of convergent combination chemotherapy discussed earlier may also be seen as creating a severe bottleneck; a virus population may pass through but lack the diversity necessary to reestablish itself.

More detailed analysis of nucleotide changes in HIV-1 quasispecies provides another perspective on the pathogenesis of HIV-1 infection. Analysis of nucleotide substitutions indicates whether changes are positively or negatively selected for or are evolutionarily neutral. Nucleotide changes in the first or second position in a codon will likely result in an amino acid change and are termed nonsynonymous (N). Changes in the codon's third position may not change an amino acid and are thus termed synonymous (S). The ratios of synonymous to nonsynonymous (P_s/P_n) are expected to be near 1.0 if there is no selective pressure or if the change is evolutionarily neutral. If there are functional constraints as in the viral structural proteins encoded by *gag*, the P_s/P_n ratio is 5 to 7.[18] This high ratio is consistent with what is called purifying selection.

Conversely, if there is positive selection for change, there will be accelerated amino acid changes, P_n will be higher than P_s, and the P_s/P_n ratio will be significantly less than 1.0. Hughes and Nei in their analysis of antigen recognition sequences of MHC class I and II loci showed P_s/P_n ratios of less than 0.2.[19] This analysis was made possible by knowledge of the three-dimensional (3D) structure of the MHC, which allowed the analysis to be restricted to those regions of the Class I MHC molecule known to directly interact with peptide antigens.[20] Comparable analysis of HIV-1 is not possible because the 3D structure of HIV-1 *env* and *gag* products is not known. However, ratios calculated for HIV-1 V3 and V4–5 regions of transmitting mother–infant pairs are shown in TABLE 1. The fact that the ratios are so close to unity would at first suggest that these changes are neutral. In fact, the observed ratios are lower than what is seen even in genes known to be under strong selective pressures. We thus believe that averaging over such a wide region may actually mask a few residues that are under very high selective pressure but against a background of relatively conserved areas. We do not know what the selective pressure is, but if selection is on an immune basis, it could result from pressure exerted by either the B- or T-cell repertoire.

Before this can be determined, however, a better understanding of the immune response to HIV-1 will be needed. First, the immunodominant epitope of both B- and T-cell responses must be known in both linear and conformational terms. Second, the immune repertoire of individual patients must be more completely defined in order to relate viral nucleotide changes to host immune responses. Both the B- and T-cell responses are likely to display significant host-specific characteristics. The T-cell response is HLA-restricted, while the B-cell response is tightly linked to individual allotypes. Satisfying these diverse experimental requirements is possible and is necessary to test the specific hypotheses relating nucleotide changes to selective pressures.

TABLE 1. Ratios of Synonymous to Nonsynonymous Substitutions in Maternal and Infant Sequence Sets

	V3			V4–V5		
	1[a]	2	3	1	2	3
Mother	0.6	1.9	0.9	0.7	1.1	0.8
Infant	1.3	0.2	1.1	2.0	1.7	2.2

[a] Numbers indicate mother–infant pairs.

REFERENCES

1. LARDER, B. A. & S. D. KEMP. 1989. Multiple mutations in HIV-1 reverse transcriptase confer high-level resistance to zidovudine (AZT). Science **296:** 1155–1158.
2. CHOW, Y. K., M. S. HIRSCH, P. P. MERRILL, et al. 1993. Use of evolutionary limitations of HIV-1 multidrug resistance to optimized therapy. Nature **361:** 650–659.
3. DOUGHERTY, J. P. & H. M. TEMIN. 1988. Determination of the rate of base pair substitution and insertion mutations in retrovirus replications. J. Virol. **62:** 2817–2822.
4. SAAG, M. S., B. H. HAHN, J. GIBBONS, E. PARKS, W. P. PARKS & G. M. SHAW. 1988. Extensive variation of human immunodeficiency virus type-1 in vivo. Nature **334:** 440–444.
5. EIGEN, M., W. GARDINER, P. SCHUSTER & R. WINKLER-OSWATITSCH. 1981. The origin of genetic information. Sci. Am. **244:** 88–119.
6. MEYERHANS, A., R. CHEYNIER, J. ALBERT, et al. 1989. Temporal fluctuations in HIV quasispecies in vivo are not reflected by sequential HIV isolations. 1989. Cell **58:** 901–910.
7. WOLINSKY, S., J. L. MUÑOZ, S. C. HUTTO, et al. 1992. Selective transmission of human immunodeficiency virus type-1 variants from mothers to infants. Science **255:** 1134–1136.
8. MCNEARNY, T., Z. HARNICKOVA, R. MARKHAM, et al. 1992. Relationship of human immunodeficiency virus type 1 sequence heterogeneity to stage of disease. Proc. Natl. Acad. Sci. USA **89:** 10247–10251.
9. NOWAK, M. A., R. M. ANDERSON, A. R. MCLEAN, et al. 1991. Antigenic diversity thresholds and the development of AIDS. Science **259:** 963–969.
10. KUSUMI, K., B. CONWAY, S. CUNNINGHAM, et al. 1992. Human immunodeficiency virus type 1 envelope gene structure and diversity in vivo and after cocultivation in vitro. J. Virol. **66:** 875–885.
11. NOWAK, M. A., R. M. MAY & R. M. ANDERSON. 1990. The evolutionary dynamics of HIV-1 quasispecies and the development of immunodeficiency disease. AIDS **4:** 1095–1103.
12. MCCOMMAS, S. A. & E. H. BYANT. 1990. Loss of electrophoretic variation in serially bottlenecked populations. Heredity **64:** 315–320.
13. CLAKE, D. K., E. A. DUARTE, A. MOYA & S. F. ELENA. 1993. Genetic bottleneck effects and population passages cause profound fitness differences in RNA viruses. J. Virol. **67(1):** 222–228.
14. SANCHEZ-PALOMERO, S., J. M. ROJAS, M. A. MARTINEZ & E. M. FENYO. 1993. Dilute passage promotes expression of genetic and phenotypic variants of human immunodeficiency virus type 1 in cell culture. J. Virol **67:** 2938–2943.
15. HUTTO, S. C., W. P. PARKS, S. LAI, J. L. MUNOZ, et al. 1990. A hospital-based study of perinatal HIV-1 infection. J. Pediatr. **118:** 347–353.
16. ZACK, J. D., S. J. ARRIGO, S. R. WEITSMAN, et al. 1990. HIV-1 entry into quiescent primary lymphocytes: Molecular analysis reveals a labile lateral viral structure. Cell **61:** 213–222.
17. RABIAN-HERZOG, C., S. LESAGE & E. GLUCKMAN. 1992. Characterization of lymphocyte subpopulations in cord blood. Bone Marrow Transplantation (**Suppl. 1**): 64–67.
18. LEIGH BROWN, A. & P. MONAGHAN. 1988. Evolution of the structural proteins of human immunodeficiency virus: Selective constraints on nucleotide substitutions. AIDS Res. Hum. Retrovir. **9:** 339–407.
19. HUGHES, D. L. & M. NEI. 1988. Pattern of nucleotide substitution at major histocompatibility complex class I loci reveals overdominated selection. Nature **335:** 367–370.
20. BJORKMAN, P. J., M. A. SAPER, B. SAMARAOUI, et al. 1987. Structure of the human class I histocompatability antigen, HLA-A2. Nature **329:** 506–512.

Pathology of Pediatric AIDS

Overview, Update, and Future Direction

VIJAY V. JOSHI

Department of Pathology and Laboratory Medicine
East Carolina University School of Medicine
Greenville, North Carolina 27858-4354

INTRODUCTION

Human immunodeficiency virus (HIV) infection in children is a multisystem disease. A variety of pathologic lesions of infectious, degenerative, proliferative, and vascular types are seen in various tissues and organs in these children.[1] Pathologic studies have played an important role in the recognition of occurrence of acquired immunodeficiency syndrome (AIDS) in children when it was first suspected and subsequently in extending the clinical spectrum and in the study of its natural history.[1-4] On the basis of our experience in analyzing autopsy material from over 25 cases and biopsy material from various tissues in over 50 cases, we have suggested a classification of the various pathologic lesions. Currently, the emphasis of pathologic studies is on the study of perinatal lesions, particularly the structural abnormalities in the placentas of HIV-infected women and of neoplastic disorders in children with AIDS. The purpose of this article is to give a brief overview of the various pathologic lesions; give updated data on neoplastic disorders, other lesions, and perinatal lesions, and indicate the future direction of the pathologic study of pediatric AIDS including what we have called "pathologic surveillance."[5]

OVERVIEW

Scheme of Pathogenesis of Pathologic Lesions in Pediatric AIDS

The lesions can be classified according to known or proposed pathogenesis into three categories (TABLE 1). The primary lesions are due to HIV infection of tissues or organs. Associated lesions are those that are related to direct or indirect

TABLE 1.

I. **Primary Lesions of HIV Infection**
   A. Lymphoreticular system
      1. Thymus
      2. Lymph nodes
   B. Brain
II. **Association Lesions Due to Direct or Indirect Sequela(e) of HIV Infection**
   A. Lesions associated with immunodeficiency
      1. Opportunistic infections
      2. Repeated pathogenic bacterial infections
   B. Lesions associated with Epstein–Barr virus
      1. Pulmonary lymphoid hyperplasia/lymphoid interstitial pneumonitis (PLH/LIP) complex
      2. Nodal and extranodal lymphoid hyperplasia
      3. Lymphoproliferative disorder
      4. Malignant lymphoma
   C. Lesions associated with chronic debilitating disease process
      1. Inanition (failure to thrive) and its sequelae (villous atrophy of small intestine, developmental arrest of testes, atrophy of organs, etc.)
   D. Lesions associated with iatrogenic injury related to:
      1. Total parenteral nutrition
      2. Mechanical ventilation and oxygen therapy
      3. Other
III. **Lesions of Undetermined Pathogenesis**
   A. Arteriopathy
   B. Cardiomyopathy
   C. Nephropathy
   D. Neoplastic disorders
   E. Thrombocytopenia

sequelae of HIV infection or its treatment. The third category is of lesions of undetermined pathogenesis. We feel that such a classification of the lesions would lead to better understanding of the multisystem disease process of HIV infection and its numerous sequelae. It should be noted that in some of the lesions in TABLE 1 more than one mechanism may be involved. Tentative as the classification may be, the available data are reasonably supportive of its basic framework. Modifications and additions can be made as more data related to pathogenesis become available. The inclusion of encephalopathy in the category of primary HIV lesions is on the basis of the evidence available in the literature which shows that HIV is present in macrophages and multinucleated giant cells in the brain[6,7] and possibly in the parenchymal cells of CNS.[8,9] To the category of primary lesions, HIV enteropathy may be added. This condition, described in adults with AIDS and characterized by diarrhea and malabsorption in the absence of known demonstrable specific gastrointestinal infections, appears to be related to HIV.[10] HIV antigens and RNA have been demonstrated in the mononuclear cells, lymphocytes, enterocytes, and enterochromaffin cells in the biopsy specimens of duodenum and rectum by immunoperoxidase and *in-situ* hybridization techniques.[10,11] These results, which cannot be considered conclusive at this time, have not been confirmed in the biopsy material from children, although HIV-infected children with persistent diarrhea have been shown by polymerase chain reaction to shed HIV nucleic acid in the stool.[12] On histologic examination, the duodenal biopsy shows mucosal atrophy, normal crypt depth, reduced mitotic activity, and increased number of lymphocytes in the epithelium and in the lamina propria. These findings are nonspecific and were initially considered by us to be representative of an associated lesion related to chronic inanition due to AIDS and its complications.[1] It appears that investigation of intestinal mucosal biopsy specimens from children with AIDS who have diarrhea should be undertaken for demonstration of HIV itself or its antigens.

UPDATE

Arteriopathy and Nephropathy

In recent years, observations have been made that may have implications in pathogenesis of the lesions included in the third category (TABLE 1) such as arteriopathy, nephropathy, neoplastic disorders, and cardiomyopathy. Thus, Kure *et al.*[13] have demonstrated HIV antigens by immunocytochemical methods in aneurysmal cerebral arteries of a child with AIDS. AIDS-associated arteriopathy was considered a pathologic curiosity or an unusual terminal sequela seen at autopsy in children with AIDS. The occurrence of stroke associated with arteriopathy of meningocerebral arteries with or without aneurysm formation has clearly demonstrated the clinical relevance of arteriopathy. Cohen *et al.*[14] have demonstrated HIV antigens and nucleic acids in tubular and glomerular epithelial cells in nephropathy in adults with AIDS.

Malignant Lymphomas

A majority of the AIDS-associated lymphomas in adults show multiple rearrangements of immunoglobulin heavy- and light-chain genes, suggesting that these are multiclonal B-cell neoplasms.[15] Rearrangements of the C-myc gene are also present. The pattern of the C-myc gene rearrangements is similar to that seen in sporadic Burkitt's lymphoma, that is, recombination of truncated C-myc gene with a switch region of immunoglobulin heavy-chain focus. It is possible that these rearrangements play a role in the pathogenesis of lymphomas by disrupting the normal control of C-myc gene expression (? upregulation of C-myc gene with consequent increased cell proliferation). Epstein-Barr virus (EBV) DNA is present in about one-third of AIDS-associated B-cell lymphomas in adults and in CNS lymphomas in children.[15,16] Further studies of these pathogenetic mechanisms of AIDS-associated lymphomas by investigators of the National Cancer Institute (NCI)-sponsored Pediatric AIDS Lymphoma Network (PALN) are in progress at this time (see below).

Cardiomyopathy

The pathogenesis of AIDS-associated cardiomyopathy is not precisely known. Infection, immunologic factors, anemia, and nutritional deficiency have been implicated.[17] Focal myocarditis is one of the pathologic lesions seen in cardiomyopathy. Increased titers of anti-heart antibodies have been demonstrated in AIDS patients with myocarditis.[18] The immunopathologic findings of the presence of T lymphocytes and absence of B cells, monocytes, and natural killer cells have been considered indicative of a cell-mediated autoimmune injury to the myocardium.[19]

HIV has been cultured from the endomyocardial biopsy of a 32-year-old man with AIDS-associated congestive cardiomyopathy.[20] Although culturing of HIV by itself does not prove conclusively its etiologic role in cardiomyopathy, the observation is certainly worthy of further investigation. Among the nutritional deficiencies related to cardiomyopathy, selenium deficiency is an important factor as it relates to Keshan disease, which is characterized by cardiomyopathy and is endemic in mountainous areas of China. Selenium deficiency has also been associated with cardiomyopathy in patients with long-term total parenteral nutrition. Dworkin et al.[21] have documented low selenium levels in the cardiac tissue removed at autopsy (0.327 ± 0.082 µg/g dry weight as compared with 0.534 ± 0.184 µg/g dry weight in control hearts; $p < 0.01$) from eight patients with AIDS.

Perinatal Pathology

Maternal Genital Tract

Pomerantz et al.[22] studied cervical tissue from HIV-infected women. They found chronic cervicitis characterized by mononuclear cell infiltration and lymphoid aggregates in the mucosa and/or submucosa. HIV was isolated from these biopsy specimens, and HIV antigens were demonstrated in the mononuclear cells, endothelial cells, and lymphocytes. HIV has also been isolated from vaginal and cervical secretions of HIV-infected women.[23]

Placenta

Jauniaux and co-workers[24] studied 49 placentas, seven fetuses, and two stillbirths from central African and European HIV-positive women with or without fully developed AIDS. No villitis was noted in the placenta, but irrespective of gestational age, the villi were coarse, cellular, and hypovascularized. There was a high incidence of chorioamnionitis (43%). Ultrastructural studies revealed isolated retrovirus-like particles with some morphologic similarities to HIV (100 nM in size, dense central or eccentric core) in the syncytiotrophoblast, fibroblasts, and endothelial cells of villous capillaries and free membranes in 5 of the 13 of the placentas. The authors pointed out that the viral particles seen in their cases also resembled the type-c viral particles described in the syncytiotrophoblast of normal human term placenta. More recently, Chandwani et al.[25] have demonstrated HIV p24 antigen and nucleic acids in the trophoblast by the immunoperoxidase method and in situ hybridization in 2 of 20 (10%) term placentas from HIV-infected mothers

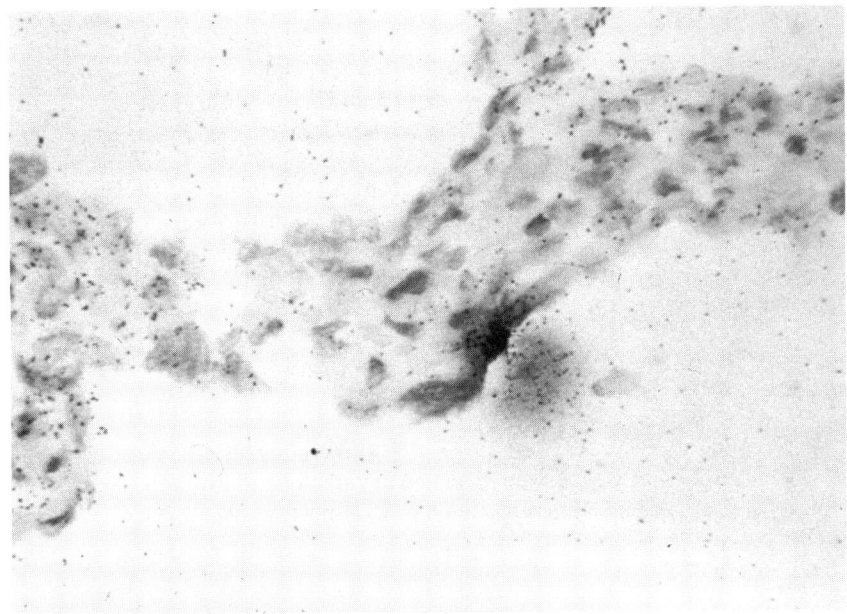

FIGURE 1. Immunoperoxidase stain for p24 and *in situ* hybridization for RNA of human immunodeficiency virus that shows a positive reaction for both in the trophoblastic cell of a placental villus. (Reproduced from Chandwani et al.[25] with permission from the *Journal of Infectious Disease*, © 1991 by the University of Chicago. All rights reserved.)

(FIG. 1). Chorioamnionitis was seen in 60% of the 43 placentas examined histologically. Martin et al.[26] found positive staining for p24 with the immunoperoxidase method in the Hofbauer cells, vascular endothelium, and intermediate trophoblast in four of nine (44%) placentas from HIV-positive women. Receptors for HIV, that is, CD4, are present on the trophoblastic and stromal cells of the chorionic villi and endothelial cells of the placental blood vessels.[27] HIV infection of first-trimester placental tissue has been shown in the organ culture.[27] In contrast to these positive findings, Peuchmaur et al.[28] failed to find HIV proteins by the immunohistochemical method or nucleic acids by *in situ* hybridization in any of the 75 placentas from HIV-positive women.

In one report, HIV was cultured from the placenta from an asymptomatic, HIV-positive mother.[29] The details of how contamination with maternal blood was avoided at the time of obtaining placental material to use were not given, and the authors commented that the positive culture was probably the result of positive maternal blood culture.

Amniotic Fluid

HIV has been cultured from and HIV antigens have been demonstrated in the amniotic fluid and amniotic cells.[30]

Fetal Tissues

Sprecher et al.[31] and Jovaisas et al.[32] found HIV reverse-transcriptase activity and antigens present in various organs (thymus, brain, lung, and spleen) from a 15- and a 20-week fetus. These findings have been confirmed by Lyman et al.,[33] Papiernik et al.,[34] and Gourgnaud et al.[35] In situ hybridization, immunofluorescence, and polymerase chain reaction (PCR) techniques were used by these investigators. Viral DNA could be demonstrated in fetal tissues (thymus and spleen) in about 75% of the cases even when attempts at viral cultures from these tissues were unsuccessful.[35] Attempts at culturing HIV cord blood from fetuses of HIV-positive mothers have been unsuccessful.[36]

Pathologic Features of HIV-Positive Fetal Tissues

Most of the reports discussed above[24,32,33] show either an absence of any pathologic findings or an absence of any mention of pathologic study of the fetal tissues. Focal lymphocytic depletion, infiltration by CD4-positive macrophages, increased density of epithelial cells, and thickening of lobular septa were found in the HIV-positive fetal thymuses by Papiernik et al.[34]

Mechanism and Timing of Fetal Infection

The results described above indicate that there are HIV receptors on the cells in the normal placentas (trophoblast, endothelium, stromal cells), and these cells are infectable by HIV. The frequency of HIV "infection" of the placenta varied from 0 to 44% in the different series.[24,25,28,35] The presence of HIV in the fetal tissues has been shown after 15 weeks of gestation. Fetal specimens from earlier gestations have not been tested. The brain and CD4 lymphocytes in the thymus and the spleen have been the primary sites of localization of HIV in the fetus. Cells expressing CD4 marker are detected in the thymus by 11 weeks' gestation.[37] Therefore, infection of fetal tissues is unlikely before 11 weeks' gestation.

Besides the infection of the placenta followed by that of the fetal tissues, other mechanisms of HIV transmission to the fetus include passive transfer during the maternal viremic phase, passage of infected CD4 lymphocytes from the mother, and active transport of HIV-immunoglobulin G complex.[28] It should be noted that in none of the known fetal infections (CMV, toxoplasmosis, syphilis, rubella, etc.) does passive transfer without infection of the placenta occur.

The low frequency of the localization of the virus in the placenta and the fetal tissues in some of the series[24,25,33,34] may be due to the low frequency of intrauterine transplacental maternofetal transmission of HIV in early pregnancy or to the low sensitivity of the techniques other than PCR. The presence of HIV in the secretions and tissues of the maternal genital tract and the exposure of the fetus to the maternal blood during delivery would support the intrapartum transmission of HIV. The failure of localization of HIV by in situ hybridization and PCR in 10 of 12 fetuses of HIV-positive mothers reported recently by Ehrnst et al.[38] supports perinatal (i.e., at the time of delivery) HIV transmission as the more frequent mode.

The placental barrier may be effective in preventing viral transmission—but concurrent placental inflammation may compromise the integrity of the placental barrier.[39] Thus, the presence of other placental infections such as chorioamnionitis (which is commonly present in placentas from HIV-positive mothers) or syphilis may enhance the perinatal transmission of HIV. It is of interest to note that maternal–fetal transmission of HIV has been observed in a chimpanzee.[40]

Importance of Timing of HIV Maternal–Fetal Transmission

The transmission can occur (1) transplacentally during intrauterine life (2) at the time of delivery, and (3) in the postpartum period (mainly via breast-feeding). The timing is of importance for embryological considerations. The morphogenesis of various organs takes place between the fourth and eighth to ninth week of gestation, which is referred to as the embryonic period. Exposure to noxious influences (infection, nutritional deficiency, drugs, etc.) during the embryonic period may interfere with normal development of the organs.

The time sequence of the development of the thymus and HIV transmission is of interest from this point of view. As indicated above, HIV has been localized in the fetal thymus in isolated cases and morphologic abnormalities of the fetal thymus have been described.[31,34] Up until the eighth week of gestation, the thymic primordium is primarily epithelial. During the ninth week, hematopoietic stem cells and lymphoid cells appear in the thymus. The differentiation into cortex and medulla start at 14 weeks and is complete by 17 weeks of gestation.[41] The observations on the thymic involvement in HIV infection have been made after 15 weeks of gestation. It will be of great importance to study the thymus in the abortuses during the embryonic period. If indeed the thymic injury occurs during the period of morphogenesis, there may be defective thymic development. Pathologic features that resemble thymic dysplasia are seen in some of the children with AIDS. This lesion, labeled thymic dysinvolution, suggests that the thymic injury may have occurred during the embryonic period.[42] If HIV transmission occurs during the perinatal period, the thymic injury would be of an acquired type, that is, precocious involution, which is also seen in children with AIDS.[1]

The timing of HIV transmission and localization of HIV in different organs is also pertinent in the consideration of the pathologic lesions in the brain, lungs, and heart in children with AIDS. HIV has been localized in the fetal brain and lungs but not the heart.[31,32] Microcephaly in children with AIDS has been described by Marion *et al.*,[43] although their findings were not confirmed by others.[44] Vogel and coauthors[45] observed congenital heart disease (valvular stenosis or atresia and septal defects) in 5 of a total of 175 children with HIV infection (2.8% incidence vs. 0.8% in the general population; $p < 0.04$), thus raising the question whether congenital infection contributed to these cardiac abnormalities. The localization of HIV in the fetal lung may be of significance in the consideration of pathogenesis of pulmonary lymphoid lesions in children.[1]

Another important aspect of perinatal pathology is the possible toxic effects of embryonic and fetal exposure to zidovudine (AZT) given to the HIV-infected mothers. To the best of my knowledge, no data regarding possible embryonic toxicity in man has been published. Toltzis et al. have presented preliminary evidence of a direct toxic effect of AZT on developing mouse embryo.[46] AZT given to pregnant mice was associated with significantly higher fetal wastage (abortions and resorption of fetus; $p = 0.003$). The adult animals themselves did not show any toxic effects of AZT with respect to growth, appetite, activity, or ovarian histology. In vitro studies on fertilized oocytes demonstrated failure to develop to the blastocyst stage in increasing concentrations of AZT.

Neoplastic Disorders in Children with AIDS

Until 1990 we had seen seven cases of neoplastic disorders (non-Hodgkin's malignant lymphoma of the brain, polyclonal polymorphic B-cell lymphoproliferative disorder, Kaposi's sarcoma, and leiomyosarcomatosis of the gastrointestinal tract) in a total of 102 consecutive cases of pediatric AIDS at Children's Hospital of New Jersey.[47,48] Since then, two more cases of B-cell non-Hodgkin's lymphoma (NHL) (one of kidney and one of lung) and a case of presacral leiomyosarcoma have been observed.[49] Mueller et al.[50] have recently reviewed the various neoplastic disorders in children with AIDS reported in the literature and described three more cases of smooth muscle tumors. The precise incidence of neoplastic disorders in pediatric AIDS is not known. It appears to be less than that in adults with AIDS. Nevertheless, it should be noted that the incidence in HIV-infected children is much higher than in noninfected children. The total incidence of various types of neoplastic disorders was found to be 70,000 per million children with AIDS at Children's Hospital of New Jersey as compared with 124 per million noninfected children.[48] In the Italian multicenter study, the incidence was found to be 1804 per million HIV-infected children.[51] Soft-tissue sarcomas have an incidence of 8.4 per million children.[52] Leiomyosarcomas represent <2% of the soft-tissue sarcomas in children.[53] The incidence of leiomyosarcoma is 3500 per million in HIV-infected children compared to < 0.016 per million in noninfected children.[53] The specific types of tumors known to occur in children with HIV infection/AIDS are given in TABLE 2.[47-82] It will be noted that B-cell lymphoproliferative disorders and smooth muscle tumors are the commonest in these children. Because of the occurrence of numerous cases of most of these neoplastic disorders given in TABLE 2 in this selected population of children, it can be concluded that there is a true association between them and HIV infection. Those disorders (e.g., hepatoblastoma; TABLE 2) of which only single cases have been reported may have occurred coincidentally in these children. The pathology and possible pathogenesis of lymphoproliferative disorders, smooth muscle tumors, Kaposi's sarcoma, and HPV-associated lesions are briefly discussed below.

Spectrum of Lymphoproliferation

The lymphoproliferative lesions form a broad spectrum extending from benign reactive hyperplasia, the lymphoproliferative disorder intermediate between be-

TABLE 2. Neoplastic Disorders in Children with AIDS

Type of Disorder	No. of Cases	References	Comments
Non-Hodgkin's malignant lymphoma	27	16, 47, 49, 51, 54–64	Extranodal sites (particularly brain) are more common. All lymphomas in which cell markers were done were B cell type. Majority were Burkitt's lymphoma.
Neoplastic angioendotheliomatosis (NAE) of brain	1	65	NAE represents intravascular B cell lymphoma.
Hodgkin's lymphoma	1	66	Hodgkin's lymphoma may be incidental.
Acute lymphoblastic leukemia	5	51, 54, 66	These were of B cell type.
Polyclonal polymorphic B cell lymphoproliferative disorder (PBLD)	4	67	In two of these cases PBLD represented progression of pulmonary lymphoid lesions. There was multiorgan involvement.
Leiomyoma/leiomyosarcoma	11	47, 49, 50, 53, 68–70	Mostly visceral sites (gastrointestinal tract, lung, liver).
Kaposi's sarcoma (KS) of skin	6	51, 71–74	KS is much less common in children than in adults with AIDS.
Kaposi's sarcoma, lymph node(s)	5	72, 75–77	Many lymph node groups may be involved. Most of these tumors have occurred in Haitian children and African children.
Condyloma acuminatum with/without dysplasia	3	80–82	Perianal and uterine cervix were sites of these human papilloma virus associated lesions.
Fibrosarcoma of liver	1	78	Immunohistologic and ultrastructural studies to rule out smooth muscle origin of the tumor were not done.
Embryonal rhabdomyosarcoma	1	79	Gallbladder was the probable site of origin.
Hepatoblastoma	1	51	Tumors occurring in single isolated cases may represent a coincidental occurrence.
Total	66		

nign and malignant lymphoproliferation, and malignant lymphoma (TABLE 3).[83] These lesions involve various nodal and extranodal sites such as lungs, liver, brain, and gastrointestinal tract. Overlap between the various lesions may be present. Thus, pulmonary lymphoid hyperplasia (PLH) and lymphoid interstitial pneumonitis (LIP) coexist commonly and are considered to be a continuum; hence the term PLH/LIP complex. A comparable spectrum of lymphoproliferation is seen in patients with congenital immunodeficiency syndromes and with immunosuppressive therapy.[83] Since the original description of this PLH/LIP complex,[84–85] we have seen a case with atypical features.[86] Besides the typical features consisting

TABLE 3. Spectrum of Systemic Lymphoproliferative Lesions[a] in Children with AIDS

A. Hyperplasia involving
  1. Lymph nodes
  2. Peyer's patches of ileum
  3. Lymphoid nodules in the esophagus and colon
  4. Thymus (lymphoid follicles with germinal centers in the medulla)
  5. Pulmonary lymphoid hyperplasia (PLH)[a]
B. Lymphoplasmacytic infiltrates in
  1. Lungs (lymphoid interstitial pneumonitis—LIP)[a]
  2. Salivary glands
  3. Liver
C. Overlapping lesions[a]
  1. PLH/LIP complex involving lungs
D. Atypical PLH/LIP complex
E. Polyclonal polymorphic B-cell lymphoproliferative disorder (PBLD) involving
  1. Lungs
  2. Liver
  3. Spleen
  4. Kidneys
  5. Salivary glands
  6. Lymph nodes
  7. Muscle
  8. Periadrenal fat
F. Non-Hodgkin's malignant lymphoma (B cell) involving
  1. Brain and other extranodal sites (lung, gastrointestinal tract)
  2. Lymph nodes
G. Hodgkin's lymphoma
H. B-Cell acute lymphoblastic leukemia

---

[a] The lesions listed above may show overlap. Thus, PLH and LIP are characteristically present in the same patient, hence the term PLH/LIP complex.

of peribronchiolar lymphoid follicles with germinal centers and a lymphoplasmacytic polyclonal infiltration of the alveolar septa, the lung biopsy in that case showed foci of monomorphic infiltration by atypical lymphocytes. Occasional atypical mitotic figures were present (FIGS. 2 and 3). No definitive conclusions can be drawn on the basis of a single case. Nevertheless, it is possible that atypical PLH/LIP complex belongs to the spectrum of systemic lymphoproliferation. It is suggested that lung biopsies showing PLH/LIP complex in children with AIDS be carefully examined for focal atypical features described above, and if found, the child be followed for development of more florid systemic lymphoproliferation.

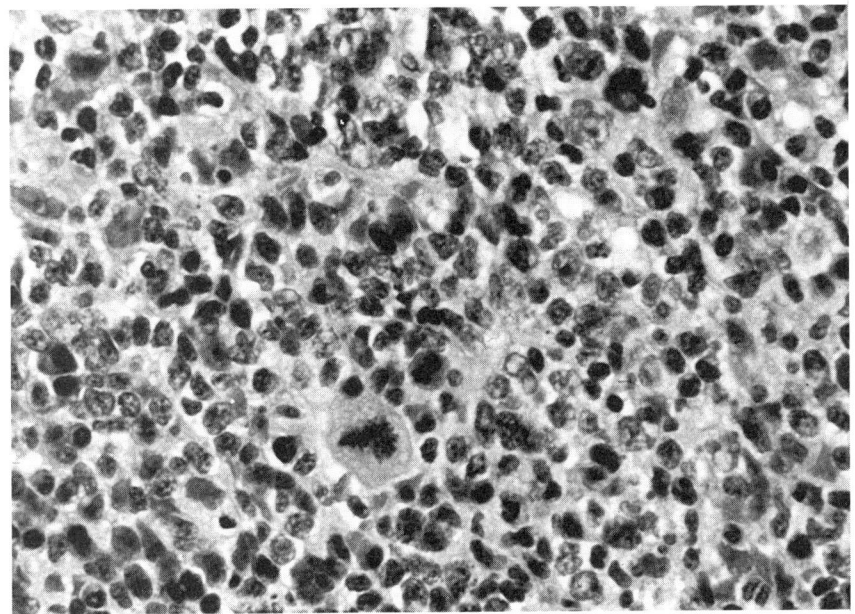

FIGURE 2. Lung biopsy from a case of atypical PLH/LIP complex showing monomorphic lymphoid infiltrate and an atypical mitotic figure.

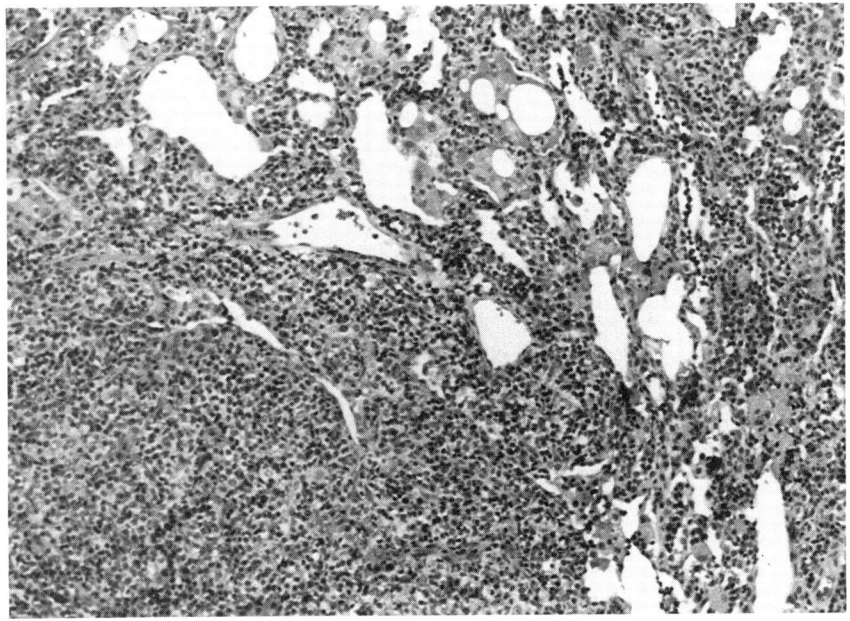

FIGURE 3. A low-power field from the lung biopsy from the case of atypical PLH/LIP complex illustrated in FIGURE 2 showing focus of typical features of PLH/LIP complex (lymphoid nodular aggregate with alveolar septal infiltration by polymorphic lymphoid cells).

Non-Hodgkin's Malignant Lymphoma

Of the various lesions in the spectrum described in TABLE 3, NHL is the most lethal. NHLs are more commonly extranodal, brain being one of the characteristic sites. All the NHLs reported so far have been of B-cell immunophenotype. Burkitt's lymphoma (NHL, small-cell noncleaved type) is the most common histologic type.

Pathogenesis of Lymphoproliferative Lesions

The probable role of Epstein–Barr virus and HIV in the pathogenesis of PLH/LIP complex, the polyclonal polymorphic B-cell lymphoproliferative disorder, and malignant lymphoma has been discussed previously.[87] HIV is known to produce primary pneumonia in rhesus monkeys. The histologic features consist predominantly of multinucleated giant cells and macrophages in the alveoli with a minimal interstitial lymphoid infiltration.[88] It is of interest to note that multinucleated giant cells and macrophages are also present in some of the cases of PLH/LIP complex.[84,85]

Smooth Muscle Tumors

It is essential that the smooth muscle origin of the tumor be established by immunohistological stain for muscle-specific action and/or by ultrastructural features consisting of external lamina, abundant pinocytotic vesicles, and intermediate filaments with dense bodies (FIGS. 4 and 5). Histoid reaction to *Mycobacterium avium-intracellulare* can produce a mass lesion consisting of fusiform to spindle-shaped cells and may be mistaken for a smooth muscle or other soft tissue-neoplasm. Acid-fast stain for demonstration of the bacilli should be done in these cases (FIG. 6).

Both leiomyoma and leiomyosarcomas have been described in children with AIDS (TABLE 2).[47–50,68–70] Most of the tumors arose in the viscera (TABLE 2). It appears that smooth muscle tumors (SMTs) are the second commonest neoplastic disorder in pediatric AIDS. SMTs have not been reported in adults with AIDS except for one case in a 23-year-old man.[54] Leiomyosarcoma has been reported in renal transplant patients given immunosuppressive therapy.[89,90]

Pathologic Diagnosis of Leiomyoma versus Leiomyosarcoma

Leiomyosarcomas are of low- and high-grade malignancy. The high-grade leiomyosarcomas have high mitotic activity with or without marked pleomorphism and can be readily differentiated from leiomyomas. Differentiation between leiomyoma and low-grade leiomyosarcoma, however, is problematical. Mitotic activity is used as a criterion for malignancy (FIG. 4). The extent of mitotic activity indicative of malignancy varies according to the site of origin. Thus for uterus and the retroperitoneum, five or more mitoses per 10 high-power fields (hpfs) are

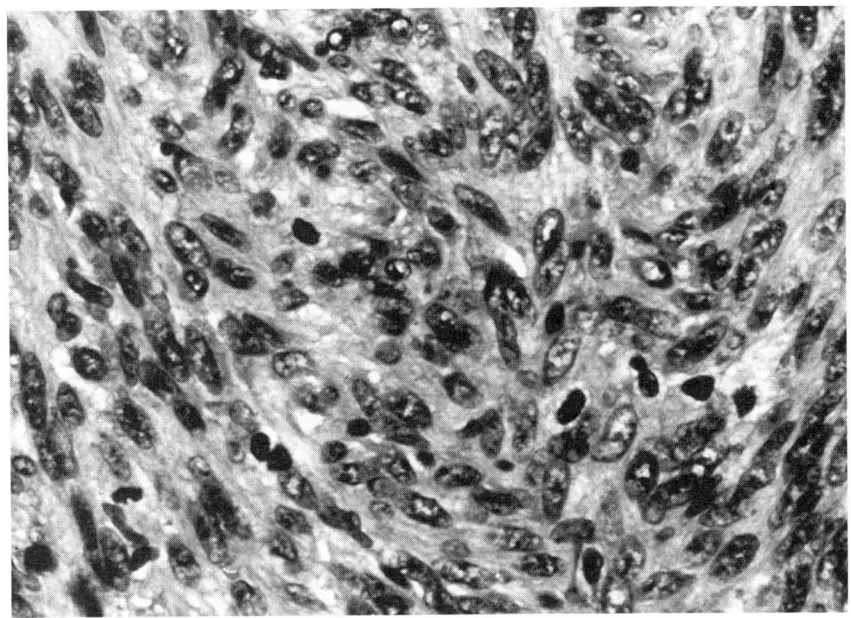

FIGURE 4. Leiomyosarcoma composed of fusiform to spindle-shaped cells with hyperchromatic nuclei. Note the mitotic figures.

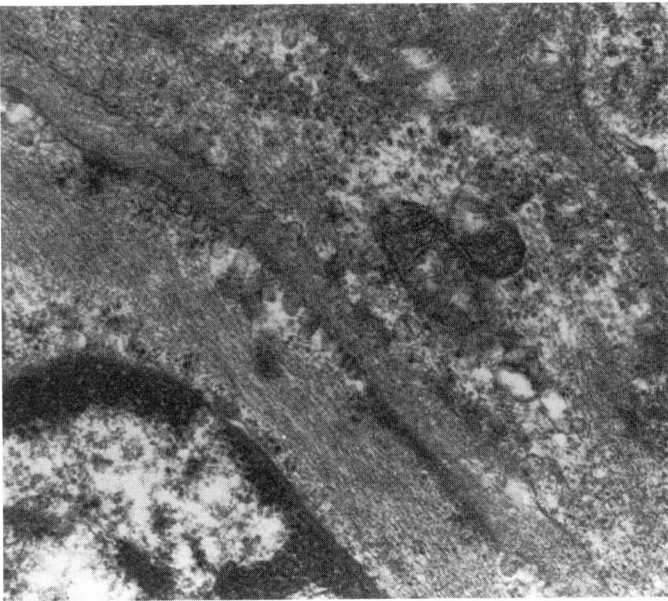

FIGURE 5. Electromicrograph of leiomyosarcoma showing pinocytotic vesicles and intermediate filaments with dense bodies.

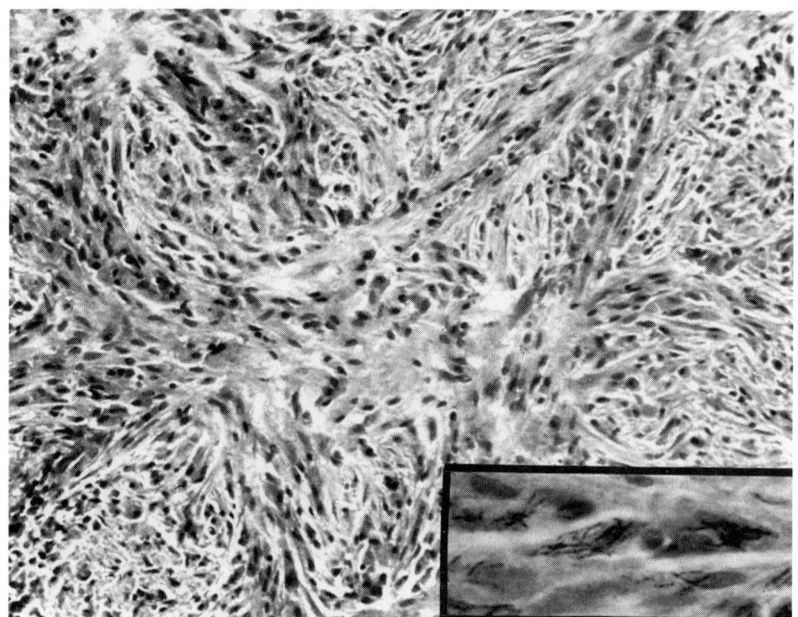

FIGURE 6. Histoid reaction in mycobacterium avium-intracellulase reaction showing fusiform to spindle-shaped histiocytes. Inset shows acid-fast bacilli within the histiocytes.

considered diagnostic of leiomyosarcoma.[91,92] In the gastrointestinal leiomyosarcomas, the criterion is two or more mitoses per 50 (hpfs). No formal cut-off point for mitotic activity has been established for hepatic or pulmonary leiomyosarcomas. Mitotic activity is best assessed by the method described by Hendrickson and Kempson.[93]

Pathogenesis of Smooth Muscle Tumors

Heterozygous and homozygous deletions of RB-1 gene are known to occur in leiomyosarcomas.[94] The RB-1 gene can be considered to be a prototype of a recessive gene, in which absence of both alleles or loss of their function results in oncogenesis. The factors that induce such structural alterations are not known. Another observation of interest in the pathogenesis of SMTs is the high level of expression of insulin-like growth factors (IGF I and II) in them.[95]

Kaposi's Sarcoma

The reported cases have occurred in two sites: the skin and lymph nodes. The lymphadenopathic form was seen mostly in children born to Haitian parents and

African children (TABLE 2) and probably represents the epidemic form of Kaposi's sarcoma unrelated to AIDS. The cutaneous form is a true indicator of disease related to AIDS.

Pathogenesis of Kaposi's Sarcoma

Two observations are pertinent to the pathogenesis: (1) The transactivating (tat) gene of HIV may contribute to the development of KS. The male germline mice in which the tat gene of HIV was introduced developed KS-like skin lesions.[96] It is noteworthy that there is a striking predominance of boys in childhood KS. (2) KS associated with AIDS in adults is seen predominantly in homosexual males. Most cases of pediatric AIDS are due to vertical transmission from the mother who has acquired HIV infection via i.v. drug use herself or via sex partners who are i.v. drug users. Thus, most of the children with AIDS are infected with the strain of HIV that infects i.v. drug users and not with the strain of HIV that infects homosexual males.

HPV-Related Genital Lesions

Only three cases of HPV-associated condylomatous lesions with or without dysplasia have been reported in children and adolescents with AIDS[80–82] (TABLE 2). In one of these cases (an 18-year-old woman), the uterine cervix was the site of the lesion. However, with increasing incidence of HIV infection in adolescents in recent years and the possibility of HIV transmission via sexual abuse in children,[97] HPV-related uterine cervical epithelial lesions are likely to become more prevalent. For example, by molecular biologic techniques HPV DNA has been demonstrated in the genital tract in 38% of urban female adolescents in New York.[98]

Pathologic Features of HPV-Related Lesions and Their Progression

These lesions comprise a spectrum extending from condyloma acuminatum with minimal, mild, moderate, or severe dysplasia to cervical intraepithelial neoplasia (CIN). The progression of the dysplastic lesions and CIN eventually to invasive carcinoma occurs over a period of many years. Therefore, HPV-related cervical neoplasia is unlikely to be seen in pediatric AIDS. Nevertheless, the precursor lesions as described above are likely to be more prevalent in adolescent females with HIV infection and should be looked for and treated promptly, if diagnosed, so that their progression to malignancy is prevented.

Diagnosis of HPV-Related Genital Lesions

These lesions may be flat or papillary. Colposcopic magnification with application of acetic acid is necessary for the diagnosis of flat condylomas. On application of acetic acid, the flat lesions stand out as white, slightly raised plaques. Cytologic examination and biopsy of the lesion establish the diagnosis. The morphologic hallmark of HPV-related genital lesions in the presence of koilocytotic atypia. (Koilos means hollow or empty.) Over 60 types of HPV have been delineated on the basis of DNA homology. Immunoperoxidase stains and *in situ* hybridization methods for detection of specific types of HPV (6/11 versus 16/18) are available and are widely used. The types 6/11 are more often associated with benign and low-grade dysplastic lesions and 16/18 with higher grade dysplastic and malignant lesions.

FUTURE DIRECTION OF PATHOLOGIC STUDY OF PEDIATRIC AIDS

Pathologic "Surveillance" of Pediatric AIDS

Although systematic and detailed pathologic study of every biopsy and autopsy in pediatric AIDS may not reveal any new features, rare cases may show atypical features of a previously described lesion, may shed light on the relationship between different lesions, or show a previously unreported lesion. Thus, for example, we have seen a case of atypical PLH/LIP as described above. In the past we have been able to formulate the relationship between PLH and LIP and between PLH/LIP complex and DIP.[1] Pathologic lesions such as arteriopathy, which were initially considered curiosities, have later been recognized to have clinical relevance as demonstrated by the detection of aneurysms of coronary and cerebral arteries[1,12] and by the occurrence of stroke in children.[99] We have called such ongoing pathologic study pathologic surveillance[5] and feel it should be continued in the future. Pathologic surveillance also enlarges the pathologic data base. For example, two of the three cases of SMTs described by Mueller *et al.*[50] were detected at autopsy as unexpected findings.

Pathologic Study of Placentas, Abortions, and Fetal Deaths

As indicated above in the section on perinatal pathology, there is a paucity of systematic pathologic study of perinatal material from abortions and fetal deaths. Multi-institutional cooperative studies for collection of an adequate number of cases should be conducted in the future. Some of the ongoing prospective national studies on HIV infection in women and children have incorporated abortions and fetal deaths.

Pathologic Study of Neoplastic Disorders

Horowitz and Pizzo[100] recommended establishing a central registry of all neoplastic disorders in children with AIDS. A prospective multi-institutional, multidisciplinary study of neoplastic disorders with emphasis on malignant lymphomas in children with AIDS (Pediatric AIDS Lymphoma Network) is now in progress. A central registry of histologic slides of the neoplastic disorders has also been started as part of the study. We urge all the pediatricians taking care of children with AIDS to participate fully in PALN. Dr. Sharon B. Murphy, Director of Hematology/Oncology Division of the Children's Memorial Hospital in Chicago is the principal investigator of PALN. Her office will be able to provide all the information regarding registration of patients on Pediatric Oncology Group Protocol #9182 and the various types of samples (blood, tissue) to be sent as well as the methods of sending the samples. It is estimated that there will be 6,000 to 20,000 cases of pediatric AIDS in the next several years. The risk of developing NHL is considered to be about 5%. Thus, 300 to 1000 cases of NHL are expected to occur within the next several years.[54] The antiretroviral and anticancer treatments will be integrated in this prospective study.

CD8 Lymphocytosis in Adults

The lymphoreticular neoplastic disorders occurring in adults with AIDS have also been described in children with AIDS. However, the diffuse infiltrative CD8 lymphocytosis syndrome characterized by parotid gland enlargement, sicca symptoms, and LIP described by Itescu *et al.*[101] in adults has not been reported in children. The lymphoid infiltrates in PLH/LIP complex and PBLD consist predominantly of B cells. Predominance of CD8 lymphocytes among the T cells present in the bronchoalveolar lavage in children with PLH/LIP complex has been reported.[102] Detailed and systematic *in situ* and flow cytometric immunophenotyping of the lymphocytic infiltrates in various organs in the lymphoproliferative lesions still need to be done.

Miscellaneous Lesions

The pathology of HIV-associated myopathy (HIVM) and AZT myopathy has been described adequately in adults.[103] Inflammatory, degenerative, and mitochondrial myopathic changes can occur in these patients. There is only one case report of AZT myopathy in a child with HIV infection.[104] In one of our cases, we have seen involvement of the muscle in the lymphoproliferative disorder (PBLD), which may be mistaken for inflammatory HIVM. There is one case report of possible HIV-related giant cell hepatitis in a child with AIDS.[105] The child died of CMV infection four months after the biopsy, and autopsy permission was not granted. Kahn *et al.* have described giant cell transformation of hepatocytes in three children with AIDS who did not have any other hepatic infection.[106] Pulmonary hypertension with plexiform arterial lesions has been reported in adults with LIP and AIDS.[107] We are not aware of any reports of pulmonary hypertension in pediatric AIDS. Pathologic study of bone marrow and liver for assessing possible toxicity of AZT and other anti-HIV drugs in children with AIDS also needs to be done.[108] Pathologic studies of the muscle, liver, lungs, and bone marrow would provide data that would be useful in increasing the awareness of the presence of these lesions in children with AIDS and in improving the understanding of their pathogenesis.

Besides systematic description of histologic features, these studies should also include special procedures such as immunoperoxidase stains and *in situ* hybridization for components of HIV and other viruses. A tendency exists to implicate HIV in the pathogenesis of many of the lesions seen in patients with AIDS. Such speculation is best avoided unless there are appropriate controls, thorough evaluations for other pathogens, and substantial evidence for the implication.[109]

Causes of Death in Children with AIDS

Kline *et al.*[110] have recently analyzed their data on mortality in 21 cases of pediatric AIDS. Over 75% of their patients died of infections. *Pneumocystis carinii* was the cause of infection in half of these cases. In the remaining cases *Mycobacterium avium-intracellulare,* Histoplasma, Cryptococcus, Cytomegalovirus, and *Streptococci* were the causative organisms. Cardiomyopathy, renal failure, and gastrointestinal hemorrhage were responsible in one case each (4.7%). In addition to the infections, we have seen neoplastic disorder (malignant lymphoma, disseminated Kaposi's sarcoma, and leiomyosarcomatosis) as the cause of death in our experience.[111] The gastrointestinal (GI) hemorrhage seen terminally can be due to probable GI involvement by Kaposi's sarcoma or to idiopathic thrombocytopenia. Cardiomyopathy was responsible for death in some of our patients. Arteriopathy was the cause of death in one case. Systemic analysis of causes of death in children with AIDS need to be done.

Collection of Tissues for Special Studies

It is of great importance that samples (blood, tissue) are collected for appropriate molecular biologic and virologic studies related to HIV and other viruses and cell marker studies and are sent to appropriate laboratories if such studies cannot be performed in the local institutions. Appropriate investigations conducted on these samples would be helpful in understanding the pathogenesis of previously described lesions and of new lesions. The requirements of the protocols of various ongoing national multi-institutional studies on various aspects of pediatric AIDS would also be satisfied.

ACKNOWLEDGMENTS

The author thanks Dr. James Oleske, Dr. Ed Connor, and Dr. Fred DiCarlo for their cooperation and help in collecting the data for the manuscript and Ms. Pauline Hardee and Ms. Tricia Robbins for their expert assistance in the computer-aided preparation of the manuscript.

REFERENCES

1. JOSHI, V. V. 1991. Pathologic findings associated with HIV infection in children. *In* Pediatric AIDS—The Challenge of HIV Infection In Infants, Children and Adoles-

cents. P. A. Pizzo & W. Wilfert, Eds. Chapter 8: 113–119. Williams and Wilkins. Baltimore.
2. OLESKE, J., A. B. MINNEFOR, R. COOPER JR., K. THOMAS, A. D. CRUZ, H. AHDIEH, I. GUERRERO, V. V. JOSHI & F. DESPOSITO. 1983. JAMA **249:** 2345–2349.
3. RUBINSTEIN, A., M. SICKLICK, A. GRUPTA, L. BERNSTEIN, N. KLEIN, E. RUBINSTEN, I. SPIGLAND, L. FRUCHTER, N. LITMAN, H. LEE & M. HOLLANDER. 1983. JAMA **249:** 2350–2356.
4. JOSHI, V. V., J. M. OLESKE, A. B. MINNEFOR, R. SINGH, T. BOKHARI & R. H. RAPKIN. 1984. Pediatr. Pathol. **2:** 71–87.
5. JOSHI, V. V. 1990. Pathologic surveillance of pediatric HIV infection. Pediatr. AIDS HIV Inf. Fet. Adolesc. **1:** 9–10.
6. SHARER L., L. G. EPSTEIN, E. S. CHO, V. V. JOSHI, M. F. MEYENHOFER, L. F. RANKIN & C. K. PETITO. 1986. Hum. Pathol. **17:** 271–284.
7. VAZEUX R., C. LACROIX-CIAUDO, S. BLANCHE, M. C. CUMONT, D. HENIN, F. GRAY, L. BOCCON-GIBOD & M. TARDIEU. 1992. Am. J. Pathol. **140:** 137–144.
8. STOLER, M. H., T. A. ESKIN, S. BENN, R. C. ANGERER & L. M. ANGERER. 1986. JAMA **256:** 2360–2364.
9. LYMAN, W. D., Y. KRESS, K. KURE, W. K. RASHBAUM, A. RUBINSTEIN & R. SOEIRO. 1990. AIDS **4:** 917–920.
10. ULLRICH R., M. ZEITZ, W. HEISE, M. LAGE, G. HOFFKEN & E. O. RIECKEN. 1989. Ann. Intern. Med. **111:** 15–21.
11. NELSON, J. A., C. A. WILEY, C. REYNOLDS-KOHLER, C. E. REESE, W. MARGARETTEN & J. A. LEVY. 1988. Lancet **1:** 259–262.
12. YOLKEN, R. H., S. LI, J. PERMAN & R. VISCIDI. 1992. J. Inf. Dis. **164:** 61–66.
13. KURE, K., T. S. KIM, Y. D. PARK, W. D. LYMAN, G. LANTOS, S. LEE, S. CHO, A. L. BELMAN, K. M. WEIDENHEIM & D. W. DICKSON. 1989. Pediatr. Pathol. **9:** 655–667.
14. Cohen, H. A., N. C. Sun, P. Shapshak & D. T. Imagawa. 1989. Mod. Pathol. **2:** 125–128.
15. KNOWLES, D. M. & A. CHADBURN. 1990. Neoplasms associated with AIDS. *In* AIDS and Other Manifestations of HIV Infection. V. V. Joshi, Ed. Chapter **6:** 83–120. Igaku-Shoin. New York.
16. ANDIMAN, W. A., R. EASTMAN, K. MARTIN, A. RUBINSTEIN, S. PAHWA, R. EASTMAN, B. KATZ, J. PITT & G. MILLER. 1985. Lancet **2:** 1390–1393.
17. JOSHI, V. V., C. GADOL, E. CONNER, J. M. OLESKE, J. MENDELSOHN & J. MARIN-GARCIA. 1968. Hum. Pathol. **19:** 69–73.
18. HERSKOWITZ, A., A. A. AMARI & D. A. NEUMANN. 1989. Circulation **89**(Suppl II): 322a
19. BESCHORNER, W. E., K. BAUGHMAN, K. P. TURNICKY, G. M. HUTCHINS, S. A. ROWE, A. L. KAVANAUGH-MCHUGH, D. L. SURESCH & A. HERSKOWITZ. 1990. Am. J. Pathol. **137:** 1365–1371.
20. CALABRESE, L. H., M. R. PROFFITT, B. YEN-LIEBERMAN, R. E. HOBBS & N. B. RATLIFF. 1987. Ann. Intern. Med. **107:** 691–692.
21. DWORKIN, B. M., P. P. ANTONECCHIA, F. SMITH, L. WEISS, M. DRAVIDAN, D. RUBIN & W. S. ROSENTHAL. 1989. J. Parent. Nutr. **13:** 644–647.
22. POMERANTZ, R. J., S. M. DE-LA-MONTE, S. P. DONEGAN, T. R. ROTA, M. W. CRAVEN & M. S. HIRSCH. 1988. Ann. Intern. Med. **108:** 321–327.
23. WOFSY, C. B., J. B. COHEN & L. B. HAUER. 1986. Lancet **1:** 527–529.
24. JAUNIAUX, E., C. NESSMANN, M. C. IMBERT, S. MEURIS, F. PUISSANT & J. HUSTIN. 1988. Placenta **9:** 633–642.
25. CHANDWANI, S., M. A. GRECO, K. MITTAL, C. ANTOINE, K. KRASINSKI & W. BORKOWSKY. 1991. J. Inf. Dis. **163:** 1134–1138.
26. MARTIN, A. W., K. BRADY, S. I. SMITH, D. DECOSTE, D. V. PAGE, A. MALPICA, B. WOLF & R. S. NEIMAN. 1992. Hum. Pathol. **23:** 411–414.
27. MAURY, W., B. J. POTTS & A. B. ROBSON. 1989. J. Inf. Dis. **160:** 583–588.
28. PEUCHMAUR, M., J. F. DELFRAISSY, J. C. PONS, E. EMILIE, R. VAZEUX, C. ROUZIOX, Y. BROSSARD & E. PAPIERNIK. 1991. AIDS **5:** 741–745.

29. HILL, W. C., V. BOLTON & J. R. CARLSON. 1987. Am. J. Obstet. Gynecol. **157:** 10–11.
30. MUNDY, D. C., R. F. SCHINAZI, A. R. GERBER, A. J. NAHMIAS & H. W. RANDALL, JR. 1987. Lancet **2:** 459–460.
31. SPRECHER, S., S. SOUMENKOFF, F. PUISSANT & M. DEGUELDRE. 1986. Lancet **2:** 288.
32. JOVAISAS, E., M. A. KOCH, A. SCHAFER, M. STAUBER & D. LOWENTHAL. 1985. Lancet **1:** 1129.
33. LYMAN, W. D., Y. KRESS, K. KURE, W. K. RASHBAUM, A. RUBINSTEIN & R. SOEIRO. 1990. AIDS **4:** 917–920.
34. PAPIERNIK, M., Y. BROSSARD, N. MULLIEZ, J. ROUNE, C. BRECHOT, F. BARIN, A. GOUDEAU, J. F. BACH, C. GRISCELLI, R. HENRION & R. VAZEUX. 1992. Pediatrics **89:** 297–301.
35. GOURGNAUD, V., F. LAURE & A. BROSSARD. 1991. AIDS Res. Hum. Retrovir. **7:** 337–341.
36. DAFFOS, F., F. FORESTIER, A. MANDELBROT, G. PIALOUX, M. A. REY & F. BRUN-VEZINET. 1989. J. AIDS **2:** 205–207.
37. KAMPS, W. A. & M. D. COOPER. 1984. J. Clin. Immunol. **4:** 36–39.
38. EHRNST A., S. LINDGREN, M. DICTOR, B. JOHANSSON, A. SONNERBORG, J. CZAIKOWSKI, G. SUNDIN & A. B. BOHLIN. 1991. Lancet **338:** 203–207.
39. BORKOWSKY, W. & K. KRASINSKI. 1992. Pediatrics **90:** 133–136.
40. EICHBERG, J. W., D. R. LEE, J. S. ALLAN, K. E. COBB, L. H. BARBOSA, G. J. NEMO & A. M. PRINCE. 1988. N. Engl. J. Med. **319:** 722–723.
41. GAUDECKER, B. V. 1986. The development of human thymus microenvironment. *In* The Human Thymus: Histophysiology and Pathology. Chapter 1: 1–41. Springer Verlag. Berlin.
42. JOSHI, V. V., J. M. OLESKE & E. M. CONNOR. 1990. Perspect. Pediatr. Pathol. **10:** 155–165.
43. MARION, R. W., A. A. WIZNIA, R. G. HUTCHEON & R. RUBINSTEIN. 1987. Am. J. Dis. Child. **141:** 429–431.
44. QAZI, Q. H., T. M. SHEIKH, S. FIKRIG & H. MENIKOFF. 1988. J. Pediatr. **112:** 7–11.
45. VOGEL, R. L., E. T. ALBOLIRAS, G. D. MCSHERRY, R. LEVINE & J. R. ANTILLON. 1988. Circulation **78:** 11–17.
46. TOLTZIS, P., C. M. MARX, N. KLEINMAN, E. M. LEVINE & E. V. SCHMIDT. 1991. J. Inf. Dis. **163:** 1212–1218.
47. JOSHI, V. V., E. M. CONNOR & F. DICARLO. 1989. (Abstr TBP 259). V International Conference on AIDS. Montreal, Canada 330.
48. JOSHI, V. V., F. J. DICARLO & E. M. CONNOR. 1992. Pathologic studies in pediatric AIDS. Related neoplastic disorders. *In* Management of HIV Infection in Infants and Children. Chapter 23: 461–476. Mosby Year Book. St. Louis.
49. DICARLO, F. J., J. M. OLESKE & E. M. CONNOR. 1992. Personal communication.
50. MUELLER, B. V., K. M. BUTLER, M. C. HINGHAM, R. N. HUSSON, K. A. MONTRELLA, P. A. PIZZO, I. M. FEUERSTEINAK & K. MANJUNATH. 1992. Pediatrics **90:** 460–462.
51. ARICO, M., D. CASELLI, D. ARGENIO, P. D. ARGENIO, A. R. DEL MISTRO, M. DEMARTINO, S. LIVADIOTTI, N. SANTRO & A. TERRAGNA. 1991. Cancer **68:** 2473–2477.
52. YOUNG, J. L., JR. & R. W. MILLER. 1975. J. Pediatr. **86:** 254–258.
53. CHADWICK, E. G., E. J. CONNOR, C. G. HARRISON, V. V. JOSHI, H. ABU-FOSAKH, R. YOGEV, G. MCSHERRY, K. MCCLAIN & S. B. MURPHY. 1990. JAMA **263:** 3182–3184.
54. MURPHY, S. B. & B. POLLOCK. 1992. Personal communication.
55. EPSTEIN, L. G., F. J. DICARLO, V. V. JOSHI, E. M. CONNOR, J. M. OLESKE, D. KAY, M. R. KOENIGSBERGER & L. SHEARER. 1988. Pediatrics **82:** 355–363.
56. PAHWA, S., M. KAPLAN, S. FIKRIG, R. PAHWA, M. G. SARNGADHARAN, M. POPOVIC & R. C. GALLO. 1986. JAMA **255:** 2299–2305.
57. KAMANI, N., J. KENNEDY & J. BRANDSMA. 1988. J. Pediatr. **112.:** 241–244.
58. COCCHI, P., G. CALABRI, G. SALVI, R. NIERI & M. D. MARTINO. 1988. Pediatrics **82:** 478–479.
59. MISTRO, A. D., A. LAVERDA, F. CALABRESE, M. D. MARTINO, G. CALABRI, P. COGO, P. COCCHI, E. D'ANDREA, A. D. ROSSI, C. GIAQUINTO, R. GIORDANO, R. M. NIERI,

G. Salvi, N. Pennelli & L. Chieco-Bianchi. 1990. Prim. Am. J. Clin. Pathol. **94:** 722–728.
60. Honda, N. S., N. C. J. Sun & D. C. Heiner. 1987. Am. J. Dis. Child. **141:** 398–399.
61. Goldstein, J., D. W. Dickson, A. Rubinstein, W. Woods, F. Mincer, A. L. Belman & L. Davis. 1990. Cancer **66:** 2503–2508.
62. Young, S. A. & D. W. Crocker. 1991. Pediatr. Pathol. **11:** 115–122.
63. Patton, D. F., J. W. Sisky & S. B. Murphy. 1988. J. Pediatr. **113:** 951.
64. Keohane, C., O. Robain, G. Ponsot & F. Gray. 1991. Irish J. Med. Sci. **160:** 179–182.
65. Dozic, S., V. Suvakovic, D. Ovetkovic, D. Jertoric & M. Skender. 1990. Clin. Neuropathol. **9:** 284–289.
66. Montalvo, F., R. Casanova & L. A. Clavell. 1990. J. Pediatr. **116:** 735–738.
67. Joshi, V. V., S. Kauffman, J. M. Oleske, S. Fikvig, T. Denny, C. Gadol & E. Lee. 1987. Cancer **59:** 1455–1462.
68. Sabatino, D., S. Martinez, R. Young, H. Balbi, P. Cininera & M. Frieri. 1991. Pediatr. Hematol. Oncol. **8:** 355–359.
69. McLoughlin, L. C., K. S. Nord, V. V. Joshi, F. J. DiCarlo & M. J. Kane. 1991. Cancer **67:** 2618–2621.
70. Ross, J. S., A. D. Rosarco, H. X. Bui, H. Sonbuti & O. Solis. 1992. Hum. Pathol. **23:** 69–72.
71. Connor, E., L. Boccon-Gibod, V. Joshi, J. Just, A. Grimfeld, S. Morrison, G. McSherry & J. Oleske. 1990. Arch. Dermatol. **126:** 791–793.
72. Bouqety, J. C., M. R. Siopathis, P. R. Ravisse, N. Lagarde, M. C. Georges-Courbot & A. J. Georges. 1989. Am. J. Trop. Med. Hyg. **40:** 323–325.
73. Gutierrez-Ortega, P., S. Hierro-Orozco, R. Sanchez-Cisneros & L. F. Montano. 1989. Arch. Dermatol. **125:** 432–433.
74. Malekadeh, M. H., J. A. Church, S. E. Siegel, W. G. Mitchell, L. Opal & E. Lieberman. 1987. Nephron **47:** 62–65.
75. Buck, B. E., G. B. Scott, M. Valdes-Dapena & W. P. Parks. 1983. J. Pediatr. **103:** 911–913.
76. Baum, L. G. & H. V. Winters. 1989. Pediatr. Pathol. **9:** 459–465.
77. Marquat, K. H., A. G. Mueller, P. Hartter, J. C. O. Oku & W. O. Ayuko. 1987. J. Trop. Med. Hyg. **90:** 93–94.
78. Ninane, J., D. Monlin, D. Latinne, M. D. Bruyere, J. M. Scheiff, J. Duchateau & G. Cornu. 1985. Eur. J. Pediatr. **144:** 385–390.
79. Scully, R. E., R. E. Mark & B. U. McNeely. 1986. N. Engl. J. Med. **314:** 629–640.
80. Larague, D. 1988. N. Engl. J. Med. **320:** 1220–1221.
81. Henry, M. J., M. W. Stanley, S. Cruihshank & L. Carson. 1988. Am. J. Obstet. Gynecol. **160:** 352–353.
82. Forman, A. B. & J. S. Prendiville. 1988. Arch. Dermatol. **124:** 1010–1011.
83. Joshi, V. V. 1990. Pediatr. AIDS HIV Inf. Fet. Adolesc. **1:** 44–48.
84. Joshi, V. V., J. M. Oleske, A. B. Minnefor, S. Saad, K. M. Klein, R. Singh, M. Zabala, C. Dadzie, M. Simpser & R. H. Rapkin. 1985. Hum. Pathol. **16:** 241–246.
85. Joshi, V. V. & J. M. Oleske. 1986. Hum. Pathol. **17:** 641–642.
86. Joshi, V. V. 1990. Unpublished data.
87. Joshi, V. V. 1991. Pediatr. Clin. N. Am. **38:** 97–120.
88. Letvin, N. L. & N. W. King. 1990. J. AIDS **3:** 1023–1040.
89. Walker, D., T. J. Gill & J. M. Corson. 1971. JAMA **2315:** 2084–2086.
90. Pritzker, K. P. H., S. N. Huang & K. G. Marshall. 1970. Can. Med. Assoc. J. **103:** 1362–1365.
91. Christopherson, W. M., E. D. Williamson & L. A. Gray. 1972. Cancer **29:** 1512–1517.
92. Enziger, F. M. & S. W. Weiss. 1988. Soft Tissue Tumors. 2nd edit. Chapter 15: 402–422. C. V. Mosby Co. St. Louis, MO.
93. Hendrickson, M. R. & R. L. Kempson. 1980. Surgical Pathology of Uterine Corpus: #471. WB Saunders. Philadelphia, PA.
94. Stratton, M. R., S. Williams, C. Fisher, A. Ball, G. Westburg, B. A. Guster-

95. SON, C. D. M. FLETCHER, J. C. KNIGHT, Y. K. FUND, B. R. REEVES & C. S. COOPER. 1989. Br. J. Cancer **60:** 202–205.
95. GLOUDEMANS, T., I. PRINSEN, J. A. M. VAN UNNIK, C. J. M. LIPS, W. D. OTTER & J. S. SUSSENBACH. 1990. Cancer Res. **50:** 6689–6695.
96. VOGEL, J., S. H. HINRICHS, R. K. REYNOLDS, P. A. LUCIW & G. JAY. 1988. Nature **335:** 606–610.
97. GUTMAN, L. T., K. K. ST. CLAIRE, C. WEEDY, M. E. HERMAN-GIDDENS, B. A. LANE, J. G. HIMEYER & R. E. MCKINNY. 1991. Am. J. Dis. Child. **145:** 137–141.
98. SHAFER, M. A. B. & A. B. MOSCICK. 1987. Chapters 4–6. *In* Rudolph's Pediatrics. 19th edit. A. M. Rudolph, Ed.: 71–81. Appleton & Lange. Norwalk, CT.
99. PARK, Y. D., A. L. BELMAN, T. S. KIM, K. KURE, J. F. LLENA, G. LANTOS, L. BERNSTEIN & D. W. DICKSON. 1990. Ann. Neurol. **28:** 303–311.
100. HOROWITZ, M. E & P. A. PIZZO. 1990. J. Pediatr. **116:** 730–731.
101. ITESCU, S., L. J. BRANCATO, J. BUNBAUM, P. K. GREGERSEN, C. C. RIZK, T. S. CROXSON, G E. SOLOMON & R. WINCHESTER. 1990. Ann. Intern. Med. **112:** 3–10.
102. BOCCON-GIBOD, L., J. P. SACRE & J. JUST. 1986. Pediatr. Pathol. **5:** 328.
103. DALAKAS, M. C. & G. H. PEZESHKAPOUR. 1988. Ann. Neurol. **235:** 38–48.
104. WALTER, E. B., R. P. DRUCKER, R. E. MCKINNEY & C. M. WILFERT. 1991. J. Pediatr. **119:** 152–155.
105. WITZLEBEN, C. L., G. S. MARSHALL, W. WENNER, D. A. POCCOLI & S. D. BARBOUR. 1988. Hum. Pathol. **19:** 603–605.
106. KAHN, E., M. A. GRECO, F. DAUM, M. MAGID, R. MORECKI, V. MANOVSKI & V. ANDERSON. 1991. Hum. Pathol. **22:** 1111–1119.
107. POLOS, P. G., D. WOLFE, R. A. HARLEY, D. C. STRANGE & S. A. SAHN. 1992. Chest **101:** 474–478.
108. PIZZO, P. A., J. EDDY, J. FALLOON, *et al.* 1988. N. Engl. J. Med. **319:** 889.
109. BARTLETT, J. G., P. G. BELIFSOS & C. L. SEARS. 1992. Clin. Inf. Dis. **15:** 726–735.
110. KLINE, M. W., B. BOHANNON, C. A. KOZINETZ, H. M. ROSENBLATT & W. T. SHEARER. 1992. Pediatr. Inf. Dis. J. **11:** 676–677.
111. JOSHI, V. V., E. M. CONNOR, F. DICARLO & J. M. OLESKE. 1992. Unpublished data.

Central Nervous System Pathology in Pediatric AIDS[a]

DENNIS W. DICKSON,[b,c] JOSEFINA F. LLENA,[d]
STEPHEN J. NELSON,[e] AND KAREN M. WEIDENHEIM[b]

[b] Department of Pathology (Neuropathology)
Albert Einstein College of Medicine
Bronx, New York 10461

[d] Department of Pathology (Neuropathology)
Montefiore Medical Center
Bronx, New York 10467

[e] Department of Pathology (Neuropathology)
University of Miami
Broward County Medical Examiner
Fort Lauderdale, Florida

INTRODUCTION

Involvement of the nervous system in the acquired immunodeficiency syndrome (AIDS) was noted in several reports shortly after the recognition of AIDS as a clinical syndrome.[1-6] Despite many subsequent clinical and pathological studies, there is still no clear understanding of the mechanisms of HIV-1 neurotropism or many of the neurological manifestations of HIV-1 infection. It is recognized, however, that some of the neurological findings in AIDS are not unique to AIDS, but rather are a consequence of the immunocompromised state of the host, including opportunistic infections and CNS lymphoma. Other neurological findings are related to systemic disease processes that are not clearly related to immunodeficiency, such as cerebral hemorrhages due to coagulopathies and encephalopathies due to metabolic disorders. Of possibly more significance are the CNS manifestations that may be directly attributable to HIV-1 infection of the brain.

Although many of the neuropathological findings in infants and children with HIV-1 infection are similar to those in adults with HIV-1 infection, there are some

---

[a] This work was supported by National Institute of Mental Health Grant MH47667.

[c] Address for correspondence: Dennis W. Dickson, M.D., Department of Pathology (Neuropathology), Albert Einstein College of Medicine, 1300 Morris Park Ave., Bronx, NY 10461.

differences, partly related to the fact that HIV-1 infection occurs in the setting of neurodevelopment in infants and children. The purpose of this overview is to describe the neuropathology of pediatric AIDS in a select autopsy population, with particular attention to differences between findings in pediatric and adult AIDS.

MATERIALS AND METHODS

Autopsy Cases

This report is based on the pathological evaluation of brains and/or spinal cords from 45 autopsies performed at Bronx Municipal Hospital Center, Montefiore Medical Center, and the J. D. Weiler Hospital of the Albert Einstein College of Medicine all in the Bronx, New York, or the Broward County Medical Examiner's Office in Fort Lauderdale, Florida. Some of the children participated in prospective studies of neurologic complications of pediatric AIDS.[7,8]

The 45 autopsies included evaluation of both brain and spinal cord in 18 cases, only brain in 24 cases, and only spinal cord in three cases. There were 26 boys and 19 girls. The average age at death was 36.5 ± 5.5 months with 13 cases ≤ 1 year of age and 22 cases >1 year of age at the time of death.

Clinical Features

The criteria for the diagnosis of AIDS were those of the Center for Disease Control, as revised in 1987.[9] None of the children were presymptomatic. The most common risk factor for AIDS was intravenous drug abuse in one or both parents. The most frequent neurologic finding was AIDS encephalopathy, characterized by cognitive and motor deficits. Focal neurological deficits were detected in several children. The differential diagnosis of focal signs in pediatric AIDS has been previously discussed.[10] Detailed description of the clinical course is beyond the scope of this review and has been reviewed in previous publications.[7,8,11]

Pathologic Methods

All tissues were fixed in formaldehyde for 10 days to two weeks before sections were taken. Tissue blocks were embedded in paraffin and stained with a variety of special stains, including stains for myelin (Luxol fast blue) and axons (Bodian) in all cases. Immunocytochemistry to localize HIV-1 antigen used a mouse monoclonal antibody (Genetic Systems, Seattle, WA; 1:200 to 1:400) to the major transmembrane glycoprotein of HIV-1, gp41, as previously described.[12] Additional antibodies were used to characterize lymphomas, including common leukocyte antigen (CD45; 1:50), L26 (CD20; B lymphochytes; 1:200) and UCHL (CD45RO; T lymphocytes; 1:50; all from DAKOPATTS, Santa Barbara, CA). A mouse monoclonal antibody to human glial fibrillary acidic protein (GFAP, 1:50) or bovine S-100 (1:250, DAKOPATTS) were used to detect gliosis. A biotinylated lectin,

Ricinus communis agglutinin (RCA), was used to detect microglia, as previously described.[13] Staining in the absence of RCA served as the control for the lectin, and isotype-specific monoclonal antibodies to irrelevant proteins (neurofibrillary tangles) were used for negative controls for immunocytochemistry. Nonspecific staining was blocked with 5% nonimmune serum. An avidin–biotin complex (ABC) peroxidase method and diaminobenzidine were used as the detection system.

RESULTS

Pathology Considered to Be Due to HIV-1

Brain Pathology

The most common neuropathologic finding was an acquired microcephaly, first emphasized by Kozlowski *et al.*[14] In this autopsy series observed brain weights usually differed from the expected by less than 25%, but in two cases the brain weights were only half the expected weight. Accompanying the decreased brain weight was cortical atrophy and ventriculomegaly. In cases with severe atrophy, the tissue also had an increased consistency due to gliosis. The degree of cerebral atrophy was to some extent a function of the age of the child (Fig. 1). In children one year of age or less, brain weights often did not differ from that expected for the age (average brain weight ratio: 0.99 ± 0.21), and some brains were actually heavier than expected because of brain swelling from anoxic encephalopathy (two cases) or intraventricular hemorrhage (one case). For children more than one year of age, the observed brain weights showed a greater departure from the expected, and only two children had normal or greater brain weights than expected (average brain weight ratio: 0.81 ± 0.13). The difference between the brain weight ratios of children less than one year of age and those more than one year of age was statistically significant (two-tailed Student's *t*-test, df = 36, t = 3.49, $p < 0.001$).

Despite sometimes marked microcephaly, there was no evidence of either gross or microscopic brain malformation, including absence of even subtle neuronal migration abnormalities. Although it is likely that neuronal loss contributed to microcephaly in at least some cases,[15,16] neuronal cell counts with morphometric methods have not yet been performed. On the other hand, more obvious histological changes were detected. Among the most remarkable features that accompanied microcephaly was diffuse gliosis, especially affecting the cerebral white matter and the deep gray matter. Both GFAP and S-100 immunocytochemistry revealed the gliosis in white matter and the perivascular brain parenchyma, but S-100 was superior for demonstrating gliosis in the cortical and deep gray matter (Fig. 2). Gliosis was frequently accompanied by mineralization in the walls of small and medium-sized blood vessels and calcospherites in the neuropil.[17] Mineralization was detected in 81% of the brains. Using a 0 to 4+ scoring system, the severity of mineralization was estimated. As was true for microcephaly, mineralization increased with age (Fig. 3). The average score for children one year of age or less

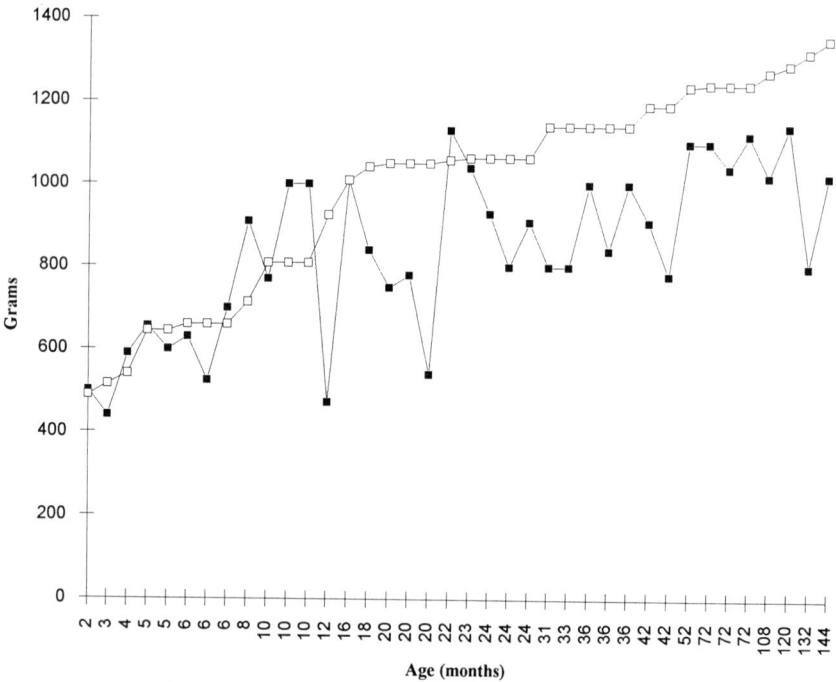

FIGURE 1. The brain weight obtained from fixed tissue for the pediatric AIDS cases (■) and the expected brain weight[42] (□) are plotted versus age. In general, there is greater departure from the expected brain weight the older the child.

was 0.85 ± 1.1, while it was 2.1 ± 0.18 for children greater than one year of age (two-tailed Student's t-test, df $= 40$, t $= -3.73$, $p < 0.001$).

Focal inflammatory cell infiltrates, usually perivascular, and microglial nodules with or without multinucleated cells were characteristic of HIV encephalitis[18] (FIG. 4). Although a few such foci were detected in the brain of a child as young as four months of age, they clearly increased in frequency with age. HIV encephalitis was detected in just over 60% of the brains. The severity of HIV encephalitis was estimated on a 0 to 4+ scale. There was a trend for inflammatory disease to increase with age, but the frequency and severity of inflammation was variable (FIG. 3). For children one year of age or less, the average score was 0.62 ± 0.96, while it was 1.5 ± 1.2 for children greater than one year of age (two-tailed Student's t-test, df $= 40$, t $= -2.27$, $p < 0.05$). The sum of the mineralization and inflammation scores, which reflects HIV-1-related disease processes, when plotted versus age, shows an age-related increase (FIG. 3).

Spinal Cord Pathology

In the 27 spinal cords examined, pathological changes were noted in 20 (74%); two cases had more than one disorder. The most common finding was corticospinal

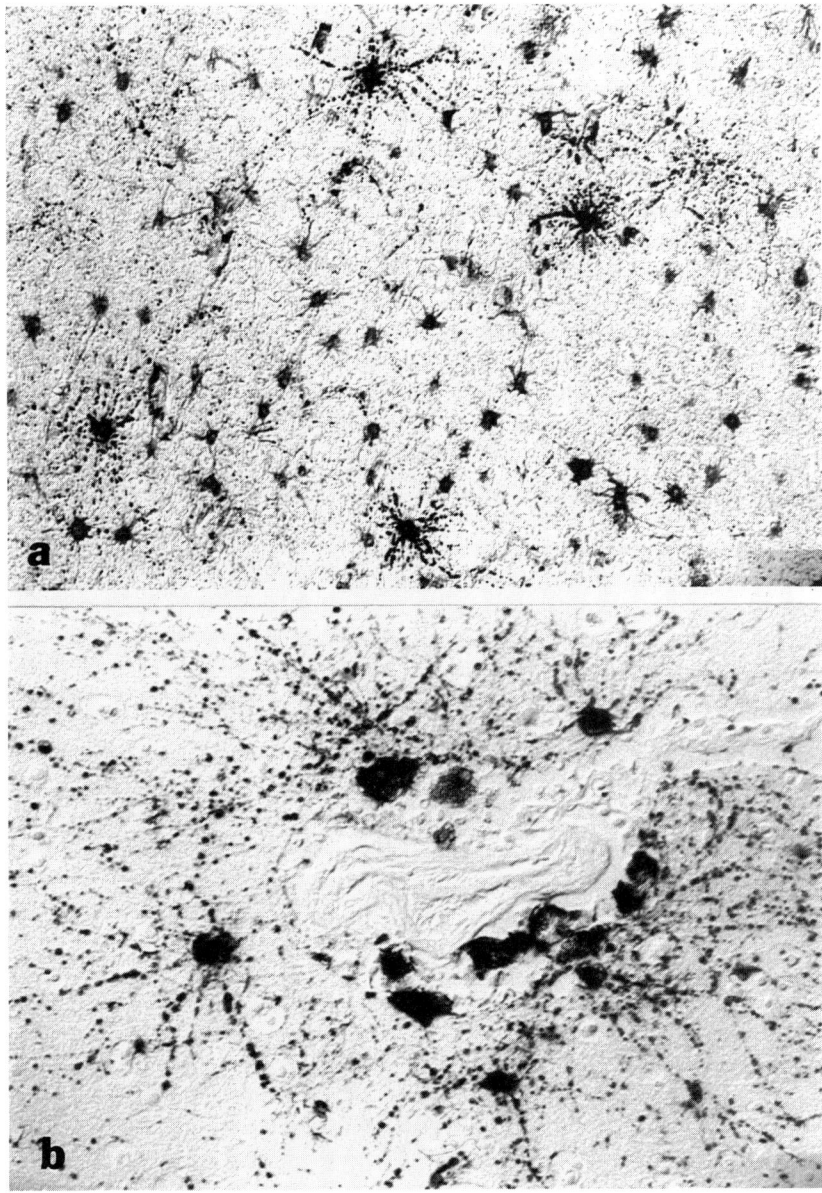

FIGURE 2. Immunocytochemistry with antibody to GFAP shows prominent gliosis in the white matter (a) and especially in the perivascular regions of the basal ganglia and deep gray matter (b).

tract (CST) degeneration,[19] which was most easily appreciated as pallor of myelin staining in the region of the lateral corticospinal tracts. CST degeneration was bilateral and symmetrical, and in some cases also affected, to variable degrees, the anterior, uncrossed CST. Six cases from children less than one year of age sometimes had pallor of the CST, which was interpreted as consistent with the degree of myelination expected for this age, since the lateral CST is not completely myelinated until around two years of age.[20] Only one of the children older than one year of age had a normal spinal cord.

Ten cases had disproportionate loss of myelin compared to axons in the CST and an axonal density in the CST comparable to the axonal density in the adjacent lateral funiculus as judged by Bodian's stain for neurofilament. These cases may represent delayed myelination (hypomyelination) or possibly selective injury to newly formed myelin mediated by soluble factors. These cases did not have detectable macrophages in the CST. Brainstem tracts that are last to normally myelinate (e.g., frontopontine fibers in the cerebral peduncle) were also deficient in myelin.

Nine cases had approximately equal degrees of axonal and myelin loss from the CST. The pathologic condition in these cases was suggestive of tractal degeneration secondary to lesions in the brain. Whether or not these changes can be superimposed on developmentally delayed myelination could not be determined. Axonal injury of the CST was asymmetrical in two cases and traceable to focal lesions in the internal capsule in both cases—one had an infarct and the other had CNS lymphoma.

Vacuolar myelopathy as described in spinal cords of adult AIDS[21] was not

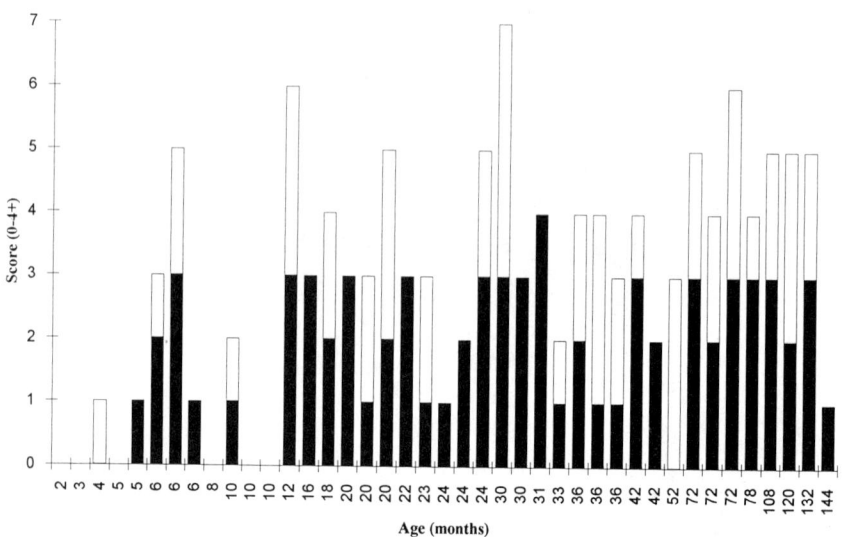

FIGURE 3. The major types of HIV-1-related CNS disorders in children, basal ganglia mineralization ■ and HIV encephalitis □, were scored on 0 to 4+ scale. The histogram demonstrates that both processes are more common in older children and the severity tends to increase with age.

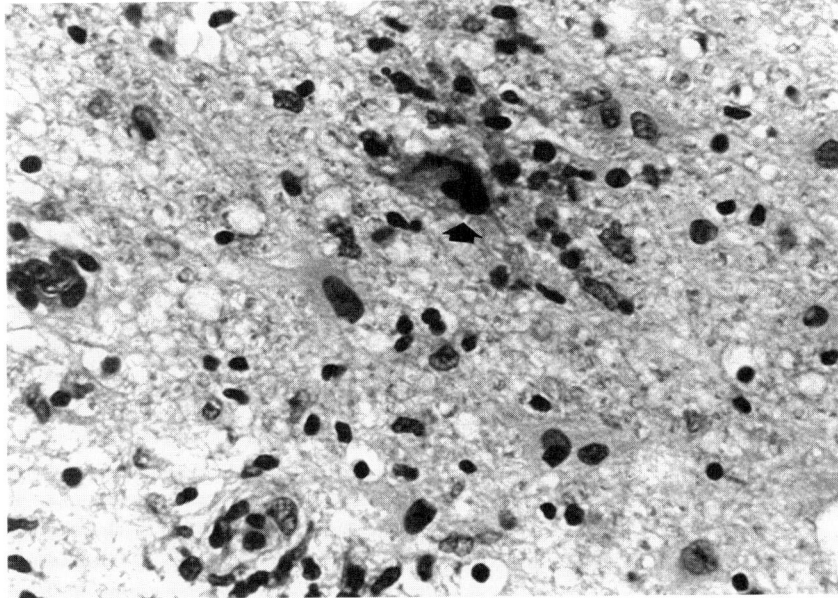

FIGURE 4. Multifocal inflammatory cell infiltrates with multinucleated cells *(arrow)* are hallmarks of HIV-1 encephalitis. The multinucleated cells are derived from microglia based on reactivity with RCA-lectin. In many cases of pediatric AIDS, even multinucleated cells were negative with HIV-1 gp41 immunocytochemistry[25] (not shown), which is different from the consistent staining of such cells in adults with HIV-1 encephalitis.

detected in any case. Two children (aged 72 and 96 months) had focal vacuolar change in the spinal cord. In one case it was localized to only a single focus in the posterior column, and the other case had more extensive vacuolation over several segments. As in adults with vacuolar myelopathy, the vacuolation was accompanied by macrophage infiltrates that could be best illustrated with RCA lectin histochemistry.

Other CNS Pathology in Pediatric AIDS

Cerebrovascular Disease

Lesions related to cerebrovascular disease were detected in 22 cases (52%). The most common disorder was anoxic-ischemic encephalopathy, characterized by homogenizing neuronal necrosis in the cerebral cortex, hippocampus, and basal ganglia. Anoxic encephalopathy alone or in combination with other ischemic or hemorrhagic lesions was detected in nine brains. Children with anoxic encephalopathy usually had cardiopulmonary disease that caused systemic hypoxemia and ischemia. Only one child had a catastrophic intracerebral hemorrhage associated with immune thrombocytopenia, but smaller petechial hemorrhages were not uncommon in several of the other brains. A child with multiple lymphomatous deposits had marked hemorrhage into the tumor bed of several of the nodules. Another child with lymphoma had severe radiation-induced brain damage. Multiple microinfarcts were detected in five brains, and three brains had focal cerebellar or hippocampal sclerosis. In one case several small blood vessels contained fibrin thrombi, possibly due to disseminated intravascular coagulation. Larger infarcts due to occlusion of penetrating meningocerebral arteries were detected in four children, including a neonate with thrombosis of meningeal arteries associated with purulent meningitis. Arteriopathy that was aneurysmal in one case[22] was found in three brains. Two children had histopathologic changes that were reminiscent of a subacute necrotizing encephalopathy. Neither child had received zidovudine (AZT).

Lymphoma

Lymphomatous perivascular and nodular infiltrates were detected in eight brains. In most cases the tumor cells were large and pleomorphic, and some had cytological features consistent with immunoblastic lymphoma. With immunocytochemical markers all tumors were composed of predominantly B cells with a variable admixture of presumably reactive small T lymphocytes. Small-cell neoplasms and other histological types of neoplasia were not detected. All but one case were considered to be primary CNS tumors. Two cases, in particular, were detected as incidental findings at autopsy and were focal lesions. The age range of the children with lymphoma was wide (6 to 120 months), but included lymphoma in a child as young as six months of age.

DISCUSSION

The CNS findings in children with AIDS share some similarities with the findings in adults with AIDS,[23] but there are also significant differences.[24] Although opportunistic infections, including toxoplasmosis, cytomegalovirus encephalitis, progressive multifocal leukoencephalopathy (papovavirus), and cryptococcal meningitis are common findings in the brains of adults, they are rare in infants and children with AIDS.[25] We have not detected toxoplasmosis at autopsy in children, but have recently seen toxoplasmosis in a brain biopsy from a cerebral abscess of a child with AIDS. There are now several reports in the literature describing CNS toxoplasmosis in children with AIDS.[26] In most of these settings, the infection is felt to be a primary infection, rather than a reactivation infection as occurs in adults.[27]

In this autopsy series, cytomegalovirus infection was the most common opportunistic infection. In a larger multicenter study, which includes cases from this series, CMV is also the most common infectious pathogen other than HIV.[14] Disseminated MAI is a relatively more common disease in children than adults with AIDS. We have detected macrophages containing acid fast bacilli consistent with MAI in the CNS of two children. In both cases the infected macrophages appeared to be either incidental perivascular macrophages or macrophages responding to another lesion, such as an infarct. These findings are natural demonstrations of recruitment of hematogenous macrophages in CNS disease processes and the turnover of perivascular macrophages.[28]

Lymphomas were the most common cause of CNS mass lesions in children with AIDS; in adults, toxoplasmosis is the most common cause of mass lesions.[27] All but one of the tumors were primary CNS lymphomas. Several occurred in the setting of a systemic immunoproliferative disease: a polyclonal B-cell proliferation affecting bronchial-, mucosal-, and gut-associated lymphoid tissue that is considered to be a disorder related to Epstein-Barr virus infection.[29] Several studies have now demonstrated that CNS lymphoma in AIDS is often linked to EBV infection.[30] Moreover, the fact that one child was only six months of age indicates that these tumors can evolve over a very short period of time. As in adult patients the prognosis of CNS lymphoma is grim, with survival measured in months. Radiotherapy may offer symptomatic improvement, however.[31]

Although cerebrovascular disease is a recognized complication in adults with AIDS,[3,32] it is not as pervasive as in children. The majority of the brains in this series (52%) had evidence of cerebrovascular disease. Strokes are, in fact, the most common cause of focal neurologic signs in pediatric AIDS.[33] Hemorrhages were most often incidental findings at autopsy associated with either encephalomalacia or subacute necrotizing encephalopathy. In two cases hemorrhages were associated with immune thrombocytopenia, and in one case the hemorrhage was catastrophic, resulting in the immediate death of the infant. Focal encephalomalacia were found in several cases in the form of multiple micro-infarcts, infarcts due to occlusion of large vessels and focal sclerosing lesions of cerebellum or hippocampus. In a minority of these cases, the infarcts were associated with arterial disease or emboli. In the remaining cases a definite cause of the infarcts could not be determined.

The most common cerebrovascular disorder was anoxic-ischemic encephalopathy that ranged from acute neuronal necrosis of vulnerable cell populations in the cortex, hippocampus, and cerebellum to extensive, cavitating laminar necrosis and leukoencephalopathy. Systemic cardiopulmonary disease processes, including lymphoid interstitial pneumonia and cardiomyopathy, were clinically evident in all cases. The pediatric brain, particularly one subjected to the additional insults associated with retroviral infection, may be unusually susceptible to anoxic-ischemic damage.

One child with CNS lymphoma received radiation therapy for her tumor. She sustained unusually severe and rapidly evolving radiation-related brain damage.[34] Analogous to the situation with respect to anoxic-ischemic injury, children with AIDS may be more susceptible to radiation-induced brain damage, because of pre-existing vascular and white matter disease. The nature of this hypothetical synergism is open to speculation, but recent studies have suggested that inflammatory cytokines or excitotoxic agents such as nitric oxide or quinolinic acid may produce additional stress on neuronal and glial function that is aggravated by hypoperfusion, hypoxemia, or ionizing radiation.

Two children had subacute necrotizing encephalopathies that were similar to those seen in mitochondrial cytopathies.[35] Both children had cardiomyopathy. Although cardiovascular disease may easily account for this disorder, its presence at least raises the possibility that AIDS may be associated with an acquired mitochondrial cytopathy. Such a process has been demonstrated in some patients treated with AZT,[36] but neither of the affected children described here had received AZT.

The most common histopathologic change in the brains of infants and children with AIDS was progressive calcification of the basal ganglia and deep cerebral white matter,[17] which was detected in 81% of the brains. As was true for other HIV-related lesions such as microcephaly and inflammation, calcification was more frequent and more severe in older children. In some cases, progressive calcification and brain atrophy was documented on serial CT scans. Histologically, the calcific deposits were usually in the walls of blood vessels of all sizes, including small capillaries and large arteries with well-formed elastic lamina. In the latter circumstance, calcification was most commonly detected in focal intimal lesions that were highly suggestive of dystrophic calcification occurring in a previous intimal injury. Although some immunocytochemical studies suggested that HIV can infect endothelial cells,[37] other studies have failed to document productive endothelial infections.[12,38,39] It is possible that the level of productive HIV-1 infection of endothelium is low or transient. On the other hand, vascular injury in AIDS may not be directly due to HIV, but may rather be an indirect manifestation of infection of perivascular macrophages or microglia, the cell types that have been most consistently shown to be infected.

Recognition of calcific vasopathy was perhaps the first indication that HIV-1 could injure endothelial cells. Three children in the current autopsy series had further evidence of vascular injury in the form of an arteriopathy characterized by fibrocellular intimal lesions. Immunocytochemical studies of these cases showed HIV-1 gp41 antigen in some of the cells in the wall of aneurysmal arteriopathy that have also undergone thrombosis. The other two cases were negative by immunocytochemical analysis. It is possible that the gp41-positive cells in aneurysmal arteriopathy may have been infected hematogenous cells involved in thrombus formation or organization. Further studies of additional cases will hopefully elucidate the pathogenesis of arteriopathies in AIDS. Of more practical significance is the recognition that cerebral arteriopathies do occur in pediatric AIDS and that they can lead to cerebral infarction.

The second most frequent finding in the brains of infants and children with AIDS was HIV encephalitis with multinucleated giant cells (60%). HIV encephalitis was characterized by inflammatory cell infiltrates around blood vessels and microglial nodules throughout the brain. The most severe damage was detected in older children, and lesser degrees were found in infants less than 12 months of age. Children with HIV encephalitis sometimes had immunocytochemical evidence of HIV infection, but more often HIV antigens were difficult to detect.[25] This has also recently been reported by Vaseux et al.[40] Even in fetuses that were positive for HIV by polymerase chain reaction, it has not been possible to detect HIV-1 antigens with immunocytochemistry.[25]

One of the most characteristic clinical features of pediatric AIDS encephalopathy is progressive long-tract signs. Although this has sometimes been attributed to cerebral white matter damage,[41] in this series the best pathological correlate has been corticospinal tract (CST) degeneration, which was detected in 74% of the spinal cords examined. In about half of the cases CST degeneration is characterized by a disproportionate loss of myelin compared to axons, suggestive of either delayed or hypomyelination or, alternatively, injury to newly formed myelin. In the other cases axonal loss is detected in addition to myelin loss. The latter cases more often had HIV encephalitis and leukoencephalopathy. In this group of patients, spinal cord degeneration may be secondary to cerebral degeneration. Although CST has been described in adults with AIDS, vacuolar myelopathy is the most frequent form of spinal cord involvement in adults. Two children had focal vacuolar change in the white matter of the spinal cord. The vacuolar change was less extensive than in adults with AIDS vacuolar myelopathy.

In summary, neurological disorders in children with AIDS differ from those in adults by progressive mineralization of the basal ganglia and cerebral white matter that has not been described in adults; the relatively increased frequency of cerebrovascular disease and lymphoma in children; and damage to myelin in the brain and spinal cord associated with extensive gliosis, highly variable degrees of inflammation, predilection for myelinated tracts that are last to myelinate, and a paucity of detectable HIV-1 antigens.

SUMMARY

Children with AIDS frequently have neurological manifestations due to complications of immunodeficiency or intrinsic effects of human immunodeficiency virus type 1 (HIV-1) on the central nervous system (CNS). The most common neurological disorders not directly related to HIV-1 infection include cerebrovascular disease and lymphoma. Global anoxic-ischemic and necrotizing encephalopathies are frequent, while CNS hemorrhages and arteriopathies are less frequent. Opportunistic CNS infections are uncommon, limited predominantly to monilial and cytomegaloviral encephalitides. Only a few cases of CNS toxoplasmosis have been reported in children. CNS lymphomas often occur in the setting of systemic polymorphous, polyclonal B-cell proliferations that have been associated with Epstein-Barr virus infection. Intrinsic effects of HIV-1 on the CNS include microcephaly, diffuse gliosis, basal ganglia mineralization, HIV encephalitis, and corticospinal tract degeneration. Although viral antigens can be detected in microglia and multinucleated cells in HIV encephalitis, most of the CNS effects of HIV-1 infection cannot be attributed to detectable levels of viral antigen, suggesting that the pediatric CNS is unusually susceptible to low-level HIV-1 infection or to systemic effects of HIV-1 infection, possibly mediated by soluble factors, including the inflammatory cytokines, interleukin-1β, and tumor necrosis factor-α, which have been shown to be increased in serum and cerebrospinal fluid of children with AIDS.

ACKNOWLEDGMENTS

Dikran Horoupian, M.D. and Anita Belman, M.D. were involved in neuropathological evaluations of some of the early autopsy cases in this series. Katsuhiro

Kure, M.D. performed many of the immunocytochemical analyses. Some of these studies would not have been possible without the clinical evaluations of Dr. Belman in Neurology and Drs. Arye Rubinstein and Larry Bernstein, among others, in Pediatrics. The efforts of all of these persons are gratefully acknowledged.

REFERENCES

1. SNIDER, W. D., D. M. SIMPSON, S. NIELSON, J. W. M. GOLD, C. E. METROKA & J. B. POSNER. 1983. Neurological complications of acquired immune deficiency syndrome: Analysis of 50 patients. Ann. Neurol. **14:** 403–418.
2. SHAW, G. M., M. E. HARPER, B. H. HAHN, G. EPSTEIN, D. C. GAJDUSEK, R. W. PRICE, B. A. NAVIA, C. K. PETITO, C. J. O'HARA, J. E. GROOPMAN, E.-S. CHO, J. M. OLESKE, F. WONG-STAAL & R. C. GALLO. 1985. HTLV-III infection in brains of children and adults with AIDS encephalopathy. Science **227:** 177–182.
3. LEVY, R. M., D. E. BREDESEN & M. L. ROSENBAUM. 1985. Neurological manifestations of the acquired immunodeficiency syndrome (AIDS): Experience at UCSF and review of the literature. J. Neurosurg. **62:** 475–495.
4. HO, D. D., T. R. ROTA, R. T. SCHOOLEY, J. C. KAPLAN, J. D. ALLAN, J. E. GROOPMAN, L. RESNICK, D. FELSENSTEIN, C. A. ANDREWS & M. S. HIRSCH. 1985. Isolation of HTLV-III from cerebrospinal fluid and neural tissues of patients with neurologic syndromes related to the acquired immunodeficiency syndrome. N. Engl. J. Med. **313:** 1493–1497.
5. STOLER, M. H., T. A. ESKIN, S. BENN, R. C. ANGERER & L. M. ANGERER. 1986. Human T-cell lymphotropic virus type III infection of the central nervous system: A preliminary *in situ* analysis. JAMA **256:** 2360–2364.
6. BELMAN, A. L., M. H. ULTMANN, D. S. HOROUPIAN, B. NOVICK, A. SPIRO, A. RUBINSTEIN, D. KURTZBERG & B. CONE-WESSON. 1985. Neurological complications in infants and children with acquired immune deficiency syndrome. Ann. Neurol. **18:** 560–566.
7. BELMAN, A. L., G. DIAMOND, D. W. DICKSON, D. S. HOROUPIAN, J. F. LLENA, G. LANTOS & A. RUBINSTEIN. 1988. Pediatric acquired immunodeficiency syndrome: Neurologic syndroms. Am. J. Dis. Child. **142:** 29–35.
8. ULTMANN, M., A. L. BELMAN & H. A. RUFF. 1985. Developmental abnormalities in infants and children with acquired immunodeficiency syndrome (AIDS) and AIDS-related complex. Dev. Med. Child. Neurol. **27:** 563–571.
9. CENTERS FOR DISEASE CONTROL. 1987. Classification system for human immunodeficiency virus (HIV) infection in children under 13 years of age. Morbid. Mortal. Wkly. Rep. **36:** 225–230.
10. DICKSON, D. W., J. F. LLENA, K. M. WEIDENHEIM, K. KURE, J. GOLDSTEIN, Y. D. PARK & A. L. BELMAN. 1990. Central nervous system pathology in children with AIDS and focal neurologic signs—stroke and lymphoma. *In* Brain in Pediatric AIDS. P. Kozlowski, D. A. Snider, P. M. Vietze & H. M. Wisniewski, Eds.: 147–157. Karger. Basel.
11. BELMAN, A. L. & D. W. DICKSON. 1992. Neurologic aspects. *In* Children and AIDS. M. L. Stuber, Ed.: 89–105. American Psychiatric Press. Washington, D.C.
12. KURE, K., W. D. LYMAN, K. M. WEIDENHEIM & D. W. DICKSON. 1990. Cellular localization of an HIV-1 epitope in subacute AIDS encephalopathy using an improved double-labeling immuno-histochemical method. Am. J. Pathol. **136:** 1085–1092.
13. DICKSON, D. W. 1986. Multinucleated giant cells in acquired immunodeficiency syndrome encephalopathy; origin from endogenous microglia? Arch. Pathol. Lab. Med. **110:** 967–968.
14. KOZLOWSKI, P. B., J. H. SHER, D. W. DICKSON, J. F. LLENA, L. SHARER, E.-S. CHO & M. D. KANZER. 1990. Central nervous system in pediatric HIV infection—a multicenter study. *In* Brain in Pediatric AIDS. P. Kozlowski, D. A. Snider, P. M. Vietze & H. M. Wisniewski, Eds.: 132–146. Karger. Basel.

15. WILEY, C. A., E. MASLIAH, M. MOREY, C. LEMERE, R. DETERESA, M. GRAFE, L. A. HANSEN & R. D. TERRY. 1991. Neocortical damage during HIV infection. Ann. Neurol. **29:** 651–657.
16. MASLIAH, E., N. GE, C. L. ACHIM, L. A. HANSEN & C. A. WILEY. 1991. Selective neuronal vulnerability in HIV encephalitis. J. Neuropathol. Exp. Neurol. **51:** 585–593.
17. BELMAN, A. L., G. LANTOS, D. S. HOROUPIAN, B. E. NOVICK, M. H. ULTMANN, D. W. DICKSON & A RUBINSTEIN. 1986. AIDS: Calcification of the basal ganglia in infants and children. Neurology **36:** 1192–1199.
18. BUDKA, H. 1986. Multinucleated giant cells in brain: A hallmark of the acquired immune deficiency syndrome (AIDS). Acta Neuropathol. (Berlin) **69:** 253–258.
19. DICKSON, D. W., A. L. BELMAN, T. S. KIM, D. S. HOROUPIAN & A. RUBINSTEIN. 1989. Spinal cord pathology in pediatric acquired immunodeficiency syndrome. Neurology **39:** 227–235.
20. BRODY, B. A., H. C. KINNEY, A. S. KLOMAN & F. H. GILLES. 1987. Sequence of central nervous system myelination in human infancy. 1. An autopsy study of myelination. J. Neuropathol. Exp. Neurol. **46:** 283–301.
21. PETITO, C. K., B. A. NAVIA, E.-S. CHO, B. D. JORDAN, D. C. GEORGE & R. W. PRICE. 1985. Vacuolar myelopathy pathologically resembling subacute combined degeneration in patients with acquired immunodeficiency syndrome. N. Engl. J. Med. **312:** 874–879.
22. KURE, K., Y. D. PARK, T. S. KIM, W. D. LYMAN, G. LANTOS, S. LEE, S. CHO, A. BELMAN, K. M. WEIDENHEIM & D. W. DICKSON. 1989. Immunohistochemical localization of an HIV epitope in cerebral aneurysmal arteriopathy in pediatric AIDS. Pediatr. Pathol. **9:** 655–667.
23. SHARER, L. R., L. G. EPSTEIN, E.-S. CHO, V. V. JOSHI, M. E. MEYENHOFER, L. E. RANKIN & C. K. PETITO. 1986. Pathologic features of AIDS encephalopathy in children: Evidence of LAT/HTLV-III infection of brain. Hum. Pathol. **17:** 271–284.
24. DICKSON, D. W., A. A. BELMAN, Y. D. PARK, C. WILEY, D S. HOROUPIAN, J. F. LLENA, K. KURE, W. D. LYMAN, R. MORECKI, S. MITSUDO & S. CHO. 1989. Central nervous system pathology in pediatric AIDS: An autopsy study. A.P.M.I.S. **97(Suppl. 8):** 40–57.
25. KURE, K., J. F. LLENA, W. D. LYMAN, R. SOEIRO, K. M. WEIDENHEIM & D. W. DICKSON. 1991. Human immunodeficiency virus-1 infection of the nervous system: An autopsy study of 268 adult, pediatric and fetal brains. Hum. Pathol. **22:** 700–710.
26. MITCHELL, C. D., S. S. ERLICH, M. T. MASTRUCCI, S. C. HUTTO, W. P. PARKS & G. B. SCOTT. 1990. Congenital toxoplasmosis occurring in infants perinatally infected with human immunodeficiency virus 1. Pediatr. Infect. Dis. J. **9:** 512–518.
27. NAVIA, B. A., C. K. PETITO, J. W. M. GOLD, E.-S. CHO, B. D. JORDAN & R. W. PRICE. 1986. Cerebral toxoplasmosis complicating the acquired immune deficiency syndrome: Clinical and neuropathological findings in 27 patients. Ann. Neurol. **19:** 224–238.
28. DICKSON, D. W., L. A. MATTIACE, K. KURE, K. D. HUTCHINS, W. D. LYMAN & C. F. BROSNAN. 1991. Biology of disease: Microglia in human disease, with an emphasis on the acquired immunodeficiency syndrome. Lab. Invest. **64:** 135–156.
29. JOSHI, V. V., S. KAUFMANN & J. M. OLESKE. 1987. Polyclonal polymorphic B-cell lymphoproliferative disorder with prominent pulmonary involvement in children with acquired immune deficiency syndrome. Cancer **59:** 1455–1462.
30. ROSENBERG, N. L., F. H. HOCHBERG, G. MILLER & B. K. KLEINSCHMIDT-DEMASTERS. 1986. Primary central nervous system lymphoma related to Epstein-Barr virus in a patient with acquired immune deficiency syndrome. Ann. Neurol. **20:** 98–102.
31. GOLDSTEIN, J., D. W. DICKSON, F. G. MOSER, A. D. HIRSCHFELD, K. FREEMAN, J. F. LLENA, B. KAPLAN & L. DAVIS. 1991. Primary central nervous system lymphoma in acquired immunodeficiency syndrome. A clinical and pathological study with results of treatment with radiation. Cancer **67:** 2756–2765.
32. MIZUSAWA, H., A. HIRANO, J. F. LLENA. 1988. Cerebrovascular lesions in acquired immune deficiency syndrome (AIDS). Acta Neuropathol. (Berl.) **76:** 451–457.

33. PARK, Y. D., A. L. BELMAN, T. S. KIM, K. KURE, J. F. LLENA, G. LANTOS, L. BERSTEIN & D. W. DICKSON. 1990. Stroke in pediatric acquired immunodeficiency syndrome (AIDS). Ann. Neurol. **28:** 553–560.
34. GOLDSTEIN, J., D. W. DICKSON, A. RUBINSTEIN, W. WOODS, F. MINCER, A. L. BELMAN & L. DAVIS. 1990. Primary central nervous system lymphoma in a pediatric patient with acquired immune deficiency syndrome: treatment with radiation therapy. Cancer **66:** 2503–2508.
35. DAVID, R. B., P. MAMUNES & W. I. ROSENBLUM. 1976. Necrotizing encephalomyelopathy of Leigh. *In* Metabolic and Deficiency Diseases of the Nervous System, Part II. Handbook of Clinical Neurology, vol. 28. P. J. Vinken, G. W. Bruyn & H. L. Klawans, Eds.: 349–363. North-Holland. New York.
36. MHIRI, C., M. BAUDRIMONT, G. BONNE, C. GENY, F. DEGOUL, C. MARSAC, E. ROULLET & R. GHERARDI. 1991. Zidovudine myopathy: A distinctive disorder associated with mitochondrial dysfunction. Ann. Neurol. **29:** 606–614.
37. WILEY, C. A., R. D. SCHRIER, J. A. NELSON, P. W LAMPERT & M. B. A. OLDSTONE. 1986. Cellular localization of human immunodeficiency virus infection within the brains of acquired immune deficiency syndrome patients. Proc. Natl. Acad. Sci. USA **83:** 7089–7093.
38. VAZEUX, R., N. BROUSSE, A. JARRY, D. HENIN, C. MARCHE, C. VEDRENNE, J. MIKOL, M. WOLFF, C. MICHON, W. ROZENBAUM, J.-E. BUREAU, L. MONTAGNIER & M. BRAHIC. 1987. AIDS subacute encephalitis: Identification of HIV-infected cells. Am. J. Pathol. **126:** 403–410.
39. GABUZDA, D. H., D. D. HO, S. M. DE LA MONTE, M. S. HIRSCH, T. R. ROTA & R. A. SOBEL. 1986. Immunohistochemical identification of HTLV-III antigen in brains of patients with AIDS. Ann. Neurol. **20:** 289–295.
40. VASEUX, R., C. LACROIX-CIAUDO, S. BLANCHE, M.-C. CUMONT, D. HENIN, F. GRAY, L. BOCCON-GIBOD & M. TARDIEU. Low levels of human immunodeficiency virus replication in the brain tissue of children with severe acquired immunodeficiency syndrome encephalopathy. Am. J. Pathol. **140:** 137–144.
41. EPSTEIN, L. G., L. G. SHARER, J. M. OLESKE, E. M. CONNOR, J. GOUDSMIT, L. BAGDON, M. ROBERT-GUROFF & M. R. KENIGSBERGER. 1986. Neurologic manifestations of human immunodeficiency virus infection in children. Pediatrics **78:** 678–687.
42. LUDWIG, L. 1972. Current Methods of Autopsy Practice.: 325. W. B. Saunders. Philadelphia.

Neurologic Syndromes

ANITA L. BELMAN[a]

*Departments of Neurology and Pediatrics
School of Medicine
State University of New York @ Stony Brook
Stony Brook, New York 11794*

INTRODUCTION

Central nervous system (CNS) involvement associated with pediatric HIV-1 infection can be divided into two major categories, as listed in TABLE 1. The first is HIV-1-associated CNS disease. This is CNS disease currently believed to be related to the retrovirus itself, due to either direct or indirect effects of HIV-1 on the CNS. The second major category consists of the CNS complications that are secondary to immunosuppression or are associated with distinct systemic AIDS-related conditions. CNS neoplasms, CNS infections caused by pathogens other than HIV-1, and cerebrovascular compromise and strokes are included in this division.

The focus of this article will be on HIV-1-associated CNS disease. Current information pertaining to neurological, neuropsychological, and neuroimaging aspects in infants and children will be summarized. Neuropathological features of HIV-1-associated CNS disease and secondary complications are covered by D. W. Dickson *et al.*

HIV-1-ASSOCIATED CNS DISEASE

Background

In the early years of the AIDS epidemic, CNS involvement was recognized as a frequent complication in infants and young children with AIDS/ARC. A "progressive encephalopathy" (PE) was described,[1-6] as was more stable neurologic impairment.[2,4] Neurological, neuropathological, and virologic investigations in both adults and children with HIV-1 infection and AIDS demonstrated that the

---

[a] Address for correspondence: Department of Neurology, HSC T12-020, School of Medicine, State University of New York @ Stony Brook, Stony Brook, New York 11794-8121.

TABLE 1. HIV-1 Infection and the CNS

1.	HIV-1 Associated CNS disease 　Direct 　Indirect
2.	Secondary complications 　CNS infections 　　Pathogens other than HIV-1 　　　Bacterial 　　　Viral 　　　Fungal 　　　Parasitic 　CNS neoplasms 　　Primary lymphoma 　　Metastatic lymphoma 　　Metastatic sarcoma 　Strokes 　　Intracerebral hemorrhage 　　Infarctions 　　　Hemorrhagic 　　　Ischemic

CNS was directly infected by HIV-1[7-18] (TABLE 2). "Progressive encephalopathy" in children and the adult counterpart, "AIDS dementia complex,"[19] were then causally linked to the retrovirus.

It is our current understanding that these syndrome complexes are related to HIV-1 CNS infection in basic and fundamental ways. Underlying pathophysiologic mechanisms, however, have not yet been elucidated.

Terminology

Because of the limitations in our understanding of general disease processes underlying HIV-1-associated CNS disease(s), terminology has been far from precise. A myriad of terms are found in the literature; for example, progressive en-

TABLE 2. HIV-1 Central Nervous System Infection[a]

Cerebrospinal Fluid Studies	Neuropathologic Studies
Isolation of HIV 　• Cocultivation techniques Detection of HIV-1 p24 　• Antigen-capture assay Anti-HIV-1 antibody 　• ELISA and Western Blot Intrathecal synthesis of anti-HIV-antibody	Detection of HIV-1 DNA/RNA 　• *In situ* hybridization 　• Southern blot Detection of HIV-1 proteins 　• Immunocytochemistry Visualization of viral particles 　• Electron-microscopy Increased levels of virus in brain 　• Southern blot

[a] Taken from Belman, A. L. 1992. Acquired immunodeficiency syndrome and the child's central nervous system. *In* Pediatric Neurology. J. Bodensteiner, Ed. Pediat. Clin. North Am. **39:** 691–713.

cephalopathy,[2-6] subacute progressive encephalopathy,[6] encephalopathy,[20-22] severe encephalopathy/moderate encephalopathy,[22] serious neurologic disease,[23] and more recently HIV-1-related or -associated CNS disease.[22,24] In fact at times these terms are used without accompanying descriptions of neurologic abnormalities. In a recent consensus report on nomenclature, it was suggested that the term "HIV-associated progressive encephalopathy of childhood" replace the various terms found in the literature.[25] The proposed nomenclature will be adhered to in this article, as will other clinically descriptive terms as described below. The term HIV-1-associated/related CNS disease will be used to refer to all of the clinical syndromes currently believed to be related to the direct or indirect effects of HIV-1 on the CNS. It is anticipated that in the future more precise definitions will evolve as clinical features are further delineated and correlated with underlying neuropathophysiologic processes.[1]

HIV-1-ASSOCIATED CNS DISEASE SYNDROMES OF CHILDHOOD

Pediatric HIV-1-related/associated CNS disease(s) may be thought of as a syndrome complex that has a characteristic constellation of cognitive, motor, and behavioral manifestations. Several patterns of CNS disease and progressive encephalopathy were recognized in the early years of the AIDS epidemic.[2] Continued longitudinal studies showed the *rate* of neurologic deterioration, *severity* of neurologic deficits, and *"domains"* of function most affected varied among patient subsets.[24] It is still unclear, however, if in some patients this reflects a continuum of disease processes, indicating different stages of disease progression. Alternatively, some patients' symptoms may reflect coexisting yet distinct underlying pathophysiologic processes that may be overlapping.[1] In other words, it is currently uncertain if there is one or several "etiopathological" causes for this syndrome complex (or these syndrome complexes). To this investigator, however, it seems most likely that different neuropathophysiological mechanisms account, at least in part, for the different clinical expressions of HIV-1-associated CNS disease(s) to be described below.

Clinical Features

The most frequent manifestations of HIV-1-related CNS disease(s) include acquired microcephaly, corticospinal tract signs (CST), cognitive impairment, and developmental delays.[2-6] Cerebellar signs and disorders of movement occur less frequently, and when movement disorders occur they are usually superimposed on spasticity[2-6] (TABLE 3).

On the basis of rapidity of progression and severity of neurologic deficits, several patterns of PE were recognized as children were followed longitudinally. Initially we described these patterns as (1) subacute progressive and (2) plateau, including (a) a plateau followed by further deterioration and (b) a plateau followed by improvement.[6] We introduced this clinically descriptive nomenclature to allow further characterization of syndrome clusters of features and signs.

TABLE 3. Manifestations of HIV-1 Related CNS Disease[a]

Cognitive impairment
Developmental delays
Corticospinal tract signs
Acquired microcephaly
Cerebellar signs
Ataxia
Tremor
Extrapyramidal tract signs
Rigidity
Opisthotonic
Dystonia
Tremor

[a] Data from Belman et al.[6] and Belman et al.[2]

During the past decade as we followed an increasingly larger cohort of infants and children with manifestations of HIV-1-related CNS disease, our initial observations regarding "neurologic/encephalopathic courses and diversity of disease patterns (see figures in Refs. 1 and 24) have been confirmed. In addition, there are clearly some patients that have a marked discrepancy between progression and severity of motor dysfunction compared with more stable, albeit impaired, higher cortical functions.[1,24] Conversely, some children have greater cognitive impairment than motor deficits. Thus, it is recognized that the classification scheme as presented below is problematic and will require modification and revision; nevertheless, it will be used herein under the heading of HIV-1-associated PE of childhood in the following section, since it still remains useful in describing clinical disease patterns.

HIV-1 ASSOCIATED PROGRESSIVE ENCEPHALOPATHY OF CHILDHOOD

Infants and Young Children

"Subacute Progressive"

This is the most severe and devastating syndrome. Characteristic features of "progressive encephalopathy" include (a) progressive motor dysfunction; (b) acquired microcephaly; and (c) "loss of milestones." Over time, deterioration occurs in cognitive, language, and/or adaptive development. Progressive CST signs often result in spastic quadriparesis with or without pseudobulbar signs, thus "loss of milestones" (previously acquired motor abilities).[5,6] Disorders of movement (rigidity, dystonic posturing, and/or extrapyramidal tremor) may also develop, but are less frequent.[6] Some children develop cerebellar signs as well. A characteristic facial appearance may be noted. These severely affected infants and young children often develop "mask-like" faces. They appear alert and wide-eyed, but have a paucity of spontaneous facial expression. However, full facial movements are seen when the child cries.[24] Serial head circumference measurements in infants and young children show acquired microcephaly (an indication of poor brain growth). At end stage the child may have markedly impaired higher cortical functions, may be mute, apathetic, and quadriparetic.[2-6]

Neurologic deterioration in this "subacute PE," is usually insidious. In some children there appears to be a slow decline. In others deterioration occurs more rapidly, over a period of weeks to one to two months. In still others the course may also be episodic with periods of deterioration interrupted by variable periods of relative neurologic stability (see figures in Refs. 2, 6, 24).

Serial psychometric testing in infants and young children (e.g., Bayley scales of infant development [BSID]) shows a decline in the mental developmental index (MDI). The mental developmental age (MDA) may stay the same for variable periods of time, but then may also decline with advancing disease.[1,6,24,27-30]

Plateau

Most children, however, have a more indolent neurologic course.[6] Cognitive impairment becomes evident as the *rate* of mental developmental progress declines. Over time, although the child may gain further cognitive, language, and socially adaptive skills, the *rate* of acquisition of these new skills is slow. It deviates from the norm. In some cases it deviates not only from the norm but also from the child's previous rate of early developmental progress.[6,24] Serial psychometric evaluations will show the MDI (or IQ) declining; however, the MDA may either remain the same over a period of months, or may gradually increase. (There is no loss of "milestones.") The MDA mirrors the "raw" scores. There may be an incremental rise over time; however, the slope of the curve is clearly deviant.[1,6,29,30]

Motor involvement is variable. Some infants and young children develop progressive CST signs as described above. They may have spastic diplegia, and progressive paraparesis, and some will progress to quadriparesis.[1,24] Other children remain hypotonic,[28] while still others have even less severe motor involvement. They may be hyperreflexic and/or clumsy.[1,6,24] Some may have a mildly spastic gait.[6,24] However, in some children these motor findings may remain stable for long periods of time. Poor brain growth may be documented by serial head circumference measurements and in some children may result in acquired microcephaly.[1-6,24]

Plateau Followed by Further Deterioration

With time as the disease advances, further neurologic deterioration may become manifest. The course then becomes similar to that of "subacute PE."[2,6]

Plateau Followed by "Improvement"

Some children with plateau show "improvement." They steadily acquire additional developmental skills. Their rate of acquisition of new skills accelerates compared to their previous performance.[6]

SCHOOL-AGED CHILDREN

HIV-1 associated CNS disease(s) and progressive encephalopathy has also been described in school-aged children. Because of the epidemiological nature of the disease, however, there is limited data from large series of older children. In our experience, early signs of CNS impairment in school-aged children may become manifest as loss of interest in school performance, social withdrawal, and/or increased emotional lability.[1,24,31,33] Other signs reported include attention deficits or worsening of previously documented attention-deficit disorders (ADD), psychomotor slowing, and in some cases, worsening of ADD combined with conduct disorders.[24,32-34] Motor involvement of varying severity may also develop as the disease progresses, as may movement disorders and cerebellar signs.[24,31,33]

Psychometric test results show a decline in IQ score (for example, see case three, Ref. 6). At end stage the child may have cognitive impairment and be apathetic and abulic.[24,31]

ADOLESCENTS

Little information is currently available concerning HIV-1 associated CNS disease in adolescents. It is unknown if the disease differs in early signs and progression from that of adults or children.

Longitudinal Studies in Progress

Cohen and co-workers studied a cohort of HIV-1 infected children who acquired infection via blood transfusions as neonates.[35] Overall IQ test scores at baseline did not differ between the cohort and the HIV-1 seronegative control groups. Nevertheless, the investigators reported small but consistently significant differences in motor speed, visual scanning, and cognitive flexibility. This is in agreement with Diamond and colleagues' earlier studies of vertically HIV-1 infected children.[36] Other clinicians have noted that expressive language and difficulties with attention were the most affected domains of mental function.[30,33,34,38,40,41] Attentional problems have been reported as an early manifestation of the AIDS-dementia complex in adults. Although it would seem that this is also the case in children, it has been somewhat more difficult to establish whether disorders of attention in HIV-1 infected children are attributable to HIV-1 related CNS disease. The prevalence of ADD in children is relatively high, especially in children with *in utero* exposure to drugs and those born prematurely (reviewed in Refs. 1, 33). Thus, a large series of HIV-1 infected children (and controls) will need to be followed prospectively to address this question.

Longitudinal neuropsychological and neurological studies of children with transfusion-acquired HIV-1 infection (hemophilia and other blood dyscrasias) are in progress.[42-44] Baseline studies have revealed subtle impairments in motor, attentional, memory, and sensory-perceptual functioning relative to age norms. Equally frequent problems, however, were detected in the age-matched HIV-1 seronegative hemophiliac control patients.[43,44] Abnormalities have also been noted on neurological examinations in both the HIV-1 infected and noninfected groups (indicating that hemophilia and/or associated treatments may contribute to neurologic dysfunction).[42,43]

"STATIC/STABLE" ENCEPHALOPATHY

In the early years of the AIDS epidemic, we used the term "static" encephalopathy to describe the more stable neurologic course of a group of youngsters who had (a) developmental abnormalities (delays in acquisition of language and motor milestones), (b) cognitive and/or motor impairment, and (c) no *history* of "loss of milestones" or progressive neurologic deficits.[2,4,6] A pattern of continued but impaired development was seen as we followed the children in our longitudinal studies.[24,40,45,46] Developmental and intelligence quotients ranged from low average or borderline to retarded. These scores remained relatively stable during the study period. The children acquired new skills and abilities at a rate fairly consistent with their level of functioning at the initial evaluation, although slower than expected for age. This was in direct contrast to the deteriorating neurologic pattern described above.

Other investigators[33,41,47,48] have corroborated these findings in their cross-sectional clinical series. Nevertheless, it still remains unclear what role, if any, HIV-1 plays in the pathogenesis of this impairment. It is important to remember that infants and children with HIV-1 infection and AIDS often have other etiopathologic conditions that may affect the CNS and development (TABLES 4–6). Unfortunately, these occur with significant frequency in this population. Confounding uncontrolled factors (TABLES 4–6, and reviewed in Ref. 1)[1,24,33] have made interpretation and analysis difficult.

Preliminary data from our own prospective study show that some infants do manifest this course in the *absence* of *in utero* exposure to drugs, prematurity, perinatal complications, or other medical conditions that could explain the neurologic impairment.[29,30] These infants followed prospectively from birth have "cog-

TABLE 4. Medical and Psychosocial Conditions[a]

1. Metabolic and endocrinologic derangements
    HIV-1 systemic infections
    AIDS-related diseases
2. Medical conditions necessitating blood transfusion
    Hematologic, neoplastic, etc.
    Complications of therapy
3. Psychosocial stressors
    Changing caretakers, impoverished environments, frequent and painful medical treatments, etc.
4. Iatrogenic complications
    ? Possible metabolic or toxic complications of therapies for HIV-1 infection and/or AIDS-related diseases

[a] Taken from Belman.[76]

TABLE 5. Factors Related to Maternal Conditions[a]

Maternal illness:
  HIV-1 disease
  Infections with pathogens other than HIV-1
  HIV-1 associated noninfectious diseases
Inadequate maternal nutrition
Deficient maternal prenatal care
Maternal substance use:
  Cocaine/crack, heroin, alcohol, methadone, etc.

[a] Taken from Belman[1] with permission from *Pediatric Clinics of North America.*

TABLE 6. Neonatal Conditions[a]

Low Birth Weight	Perinatal Asphyxia	CNS Infection
Prematurity Small for dates	Hypoxic-ischemic encephalopathy Periventricular leukomalacia Intracranial hemorrhage	Common pathogens Opportunistic pathogens Other neonatal illnesses

[a] Taken from Belman[1] with permission from *Pediatric Clinics of North America.*

nitive impairment" and "delays" in acquisitioning of motor milestones and mental abilities. In addition, they did not "lose milestones." Moreover, they showed more "impairment" than controls. Thus, it seems likely that in at least some cases, HIV-1, in an as yet undetermined fashion, compromises the normal developmental process. However, further information awaits completion and analysis of large multicenter studies that are now in progress as well as studies of pathophysiologic mechanisms.

NEUROIMAGING FINDINGS

Neuroimaging findings are summarized in TABLE 7. Computed tomographic (CT) examinations of the head in infants and children with HIV-1 associated PE usually show variable degrees of cerebral atrophy and white matter (WM) abnormalities (rarefaction).[1-3,5,6,24] Some patients have bilateral symmetrical calcification of the basal ganglia (BG) and, less frequently, calcification of the frontal WM.[1-3,5,6,24,31] Serial studies often show progressive atrophy and WM changes, and, in some, progressive calcification of the BG.[2,6,29] Nevertheless, serial CT studies in a subset of children show *no* change, even though poor brain growth is demonstrated by serial head circumference measurements, and serial clinical examinations show "plateau" or marked delays in mental and motor function (with or without progressive motor findings).[2,6,24,49]

Magnetic resonance imaging (MRI), may reveal atrophy on T1 and T2-weighted images. T2-weighted images may show abnormal signal intensity in the WM and deep gray structures.[24,31]

MRI is the more sensitive technique for imaging WM abnormalities and maturational changes in myelination (delayed verses normal). CT is the more sensitive technique for detecting calcification. Cerebral atrophy is well demonstrated by both techniques.[1]

TABLE 7. Neuroimaging

CT
 Cerebral atrophy
  Present in majority of patients
  Serial studies often show progressive atrophy
 Calcification of basal ganglia
  ± Frontal white matter present in a subset of patients
  Serial studies may show progressive "calcification"
 White matter
  White matter changes (hypodensity)
  Serial studies often show progressive changes
MRI
 Cerebral atrophy
  Present in majority of patients
  Serial studies often show progressive atrophy
 Basal ganglia
  May show abnormally high signal (T2-weighted images) (at time when CT is "normal")
  May show abnormally low signal (T2-weighted images) (at time when CT shows calcification)
 White matter
  May show abnormally high signal (T2-weighted images)

CEREBROSPINAL FLUID STUDIES

CSF profiles are usually normal, although pleocytosis and elevation in protein content have been described.[5,6,48] In our experience these findings occur more frequently in children during later stages of HIV-1 associated PE and correlate well with neuroimaging abnormalities of marked WM rarefaction and progressive atrophy.

CSF studies in some neurologically asymptomatic as well as symptomatic patients have shown intrathecal production of anti-HIV-1 antibody, oligoclonal bands, detectible levels of HIV-1 antigen and cytokines.[5,8,18,22,50-52] These findings helped establish that the CNS was infected with HIV-1. They also indicated that at least in some patients, the CNS was invaded early in the course of the illness. However, the prognostic significance of these findings is unclear. It should be kept in mind that evidence of HIV-1 CNS infection is not synonymous with HIV-1 CNS disease. Questions regarding latency to clinical manifestations of HIV-1 related CNS disease still remain, as do questions regarding CSF findings and relationship to "stage" of HIV-1 CNS disease. Current understanding is limited by lack of data from prospective and longitudinal studies of a large cohort of patients.[24]

LOCALIZATION OF HIV-1, NEUROPATHOLOGIC FINDINGS, AND PATHOGENESIS

Localization

Neuropathological studies of brain have localized HIV-1 most frequently in bone marrow derived CNS cells of monocyte/macrophage lineage. These cells include macrophages, intrinsic microglia (the mononuclear phagocytic system of the brain), and multinucleated giant cells (formed by the fusion of these cell types).[53] Endothelial cell infection has also been reported, but not consistently (see Ref. 26, 53 for reviews).

In vitro studies have shown that HIV-1 can infect neuronal and glial cell lines (astrocytes, oligodendrocytes); however, there is minimal evidence from *in vitro* studies demonstrating productive infection in these cells.[53] It is noteworthy, though, that low levels of HIV-1 expression have recently been demonstrated in some pediatric cases.

Route of Entry

The route of HIV-1 CNS invasion is unclear. It is thought that the virus enters the brain from the blood, and most likely within infected mononuclear cells/or macrophages (Trojan horse). Direct CNS invasion by cell-free virus is also a possibility.[24,51] It remains unclear if the virus enters the brain via choroid plexus or across cerebral endothelial cells. However, the frequent finding of basal ganglia calcification suggests the latter. Findings that also suggest early CNS infection in some patients as well as the vulnerability of the immature vasculature to the direct or indirect effects of HIV.

Neuropathology

TABLE 8 summarizes neuropathological findings. (For a more comprehensive description and discussion see D. Dickson *et al.* in this volume.)

TABLE 8. Neuropathology

Brain
Gross
Variable degrees of cerebral atrophy:
Ventricular enlargement
Widening of sulci
Attenuation of deep cerebral white matter
Microscopic
HIV-1 encephalitis
Foci of inflammatory cells: microglia, macrophages, multinucleated giant cells
HIV-1 leukoencephalopathy
Myelin loss, reactive astroglosis, macrophages, multinucleated giant cells
Calcific vasculopathy
Basal ganglia, ± white matter mineralization in walls of blood vessels
Spinal Cord
Corticospinal tract "degeneration"
"Axonopathy type"
"Myelinopathy type"
Myelitis
Vacuolar myelopathy

Pathogenesis

Although it seems likely that HIV-1 associated or mediated CNS disease(s) is related in fundamental ways to HIV-1 CNS infection, pathogenetic mechanisms are uncertain. Both direct and indirect mechanisms have been proposed (see Janssen et al.[25]) and are the focus of ongoing research efforts.[54-67] These include, for example, the effects of cytokines released locally from infected macrophages impairing cellular functioning or modifying neurotransmitter function. These soluble factors might also contribute to the white matter pathology. Alternately, the white matter pathology may result from a local inflammatory response with damage caused by products such as proteases, arachidonic acid metabolites, and other products of activated macrophages (innocent bystander). The leukoencephalitis may, however, also result from immune-mediated processes.

Neuronal and glial function may possibly be altered by "toxic" viral proteins, products, or sequences that result in cytotoxicity or neuronal-altering effects, or which block neuroreceptors or neurotrophic factors.[26] Other postulated pathogenetic mechanisms involve immune-mediated neurotoxic or neuronal-altering effects of cytokines, including possible bidirectional interactions (mediated via cytokines) between glial cells and the activated lymphoid cells within the CNS, and/or interactions of astroglia and neurons (mediated via glial produced cytokines—the autocrine loop).[56-66]

Continuing research efforts are also focused on further defining the biologic properties of HIV-1 that determine neurotropism, neuroinvasiveness, and viral persistence. Immunopathologic mechanisms involved in HIV-1 encephalitis continue to be studied, and the possible viral effects on endothelial cells, including alterations of the blood–brain barrier, are under investigation.

It seems probable that the different clinical patterns ("encephalopathic courses") of HIV-1 associated CNS disease described above reflect (at least in part) different pathophysiologic processes. It also seems likely that the developmental stage of the nervous system when exposed to the direct or indirect effects of HIV-1 is a critical variable.

NEUROEPIDEMIOLOGY

The true incidence of HIV-1 related CNS disease is not known. Current knowledge comes from retrospective studies,[21] longitudinal clinical studies,[5,6,22] and preliminary data from prospective studies that are still in progress.[23] Early in the AIDS epidemic, studies were conducted in cohorts of children with severe symptomatic HIV-1 infection, AIDS, and ARC. Most of the children had AIDS (opportunistic infections).[5,6,8] More recently, children with less symptomatic infection (Centers for Disease Control [CDC] P-2 classification) were included in such studies.[22,23] Currently, children with asymptomatic and mildly symptomatic HIV-1 infection are also being identified and included in surveillance studies.[22] Although the cohorts have been dissimilar, review of the literature suggests that HIV-1 associated CNS disease parallels the progression and severity of immunodeficiency and systemic disease. Nevertheless, it is also clear that some patients do develop HIV-1 associated CNS disease syndromes in the absence of other major AIDS-defining diseases, severe immunodeficiency, and severely depressed CD4 cell counts.[29,68]

THERAPY

Therapeutic interventions with antiretroviral agents have been promising. Improvements in cognitive and behavioral function were documented in the initial clinical trials of the nucleoside analogue, AZT.[20-71] Unfortunately, however, not all children show neurologic "improvement" with orally administered antiretroviral agents, although "stabilization" has been reported.[71-73] Furthermore, some children who initially appeared to have a favorable response with time "relapsed" and manifested clinical and neuroimaging signs of HIV-1 associated CNS disease(s).[74]

Clinical trials in progress are investigating other antiretroviral agents, varying dosage regimens, combinations therapy, and immunomodulating therapies. New "targets" for therapy are under investigation, and new protocols are in development (TABLE 9).

TABLE 9. Current and Future Research

Prevention of maternal HIV-1 infection

Prevention of maternal–fetal transmission

Timing of congenital HIV-1 infection

Timing and route of HIV-1 CNS invasion

Pathophysiologic mechanisms of HIV-1 associated CNS disease
   Direct
   Indirect
   Developing nervous system[a]

Further delineation of HIV-1 associated CNS disease syndromes
   Neurological
   Neuropsychological
   Behavioral

Correlation with
   Neurophysiological
   Surrogate markers

Uniform measures of mental and motor function

Therapy
   Antiretroviral
   Immunomodulation
   "Other targets"
   Rehabilitation

[a] List not complete.

In parallel are rehabilitation programs, including infant stimulation programs, therapeutic nursery schools, and special educational classes, as well as physical and occupational therapy programs.

SUMMARY

It is now well recognized that HIV-1 associated CNS disease may complicate the course of HIV-1 infection and AIDS in infants and children. It is also well recognized that the neurologic dysfunction in these young patients adds significantly to the morbidity of the disease and is often a devastating complication.[24]

It is apparent that HIV-1 CNS infection in infants and young children is complicated by numerous developmental issues. The effects, direct and indirect, of HIV-1 on the developing nervous system must be considered. The effects of HIV-1 on the immature immune system must also be considered. Moreover, the possible effects of HIV-1 on the many complex interactions between these two systems during development will clearly also require investigation.[75] In order to care for these children and to design rational approaches for treatment and prevention, it is now critical to develop a better understanding of how HIV-1 affects the developing nervous system.[1]

REFERENCES

1. BELMAN, A. L. 1992. AIDS and the child's central nervous system. Ped. Neurol. Pediatr. Clin. N. Am. **39:** 691-714.
2. BELMAN, A. L., M. H. ULTMANN, D. HOROUPIAN, et al. 1985. Neurologic complications in infants and children with acquired immune deficiency syndrome. Ann. Neurol. **18:** 560-566.
3. EPSTEIN, L. G., L. R. SHARER, V. V. JOSHI, et al. 1985. Progressive encephalopathy in children with acquired immune deficiency syndrome. Ann. Neurol. **17:** 488-496.
4. ULTMANN, M. H., A. L. BELMAN, H. A. RUFF, B. E. NOVICK, B. CONE-WESSON, H. J. COHEN & A. RUBINSTEIN. 1985. "Developmental abnormalities in infants and children with acquired immune deficiency syndrome (AIDS) and AIDS-related complex. Dev. Med. Child Neurol. **27:** 563-571.
5. EPSTEIN, L. G., L. R. SHARER, J. M. OLESKE, et al. 1986. Neurologic manifestations of human immunodeficiency virus infection in children. Pediatrics **78:** 678-687.
6. BELMAN, A. L., G. DIAMOND, D. DICKSON, et al. 1988. Pediatric AIDS: Neurologic syndromes. Am. J. Dis. Child. **142:** 29-35.
7. HO, D. D., T. R. ROTA, R. T. SCHOOLEY, et al. 1985. Isolation of HTLV-III from CSF and neural tissues of patients with AIDS related neurologic syndromes. N. Engl. J. Med. **313:** 1493-1497.
8. HUTTO, C., G. SCOTT, E. PARKS, M. FISCHL, W. PARKS. 1989. Cerebrospinal fluid (CSF) studies in adults and pediatric HIV infections. III International Conference on AIDS, Washington, D.C. June 1-5. p. 38.
9. LEVY, J. A., J. SHIMABUKURO, H. HOLLANDER, et al. 1985. Isolation of AIDS associated retrovirus from cerebrospinal fluid and brain of patients with neurological symptoms. Lancet **2:** 586-588.
10. GOUDSMIT, J., E. C. WOLTERS, M. BAKKER, et al. 1986. Intrathecal synthesis of antibodies to HTLV-III in patients without AIDS or AIDS related complex. Br. Med. J. **292:** 1231-1234.
11. RESNICK, L., F. DIMARZO-VERONESE, J. SCHUPBACH, et al. 1985. Intra-blood–brain

barrier synthesis of HTLV-III specific IgG in patients with neurologic symptoms associated with AIDS or AIDS-related complex. N. Engl. J. Med. **313:** 1498–1504.
12. EPSTEIN, L. G., L. R. SHARER, S-E. CHO, *et al.* 1985. HTLV-III/LAV-like retrovirus particles in the brains of patients with AIDS encephalopathy. AIDS Res. **1:** 477–454.
13. WILEY, C. A., R. D. SCHRIER, A. S. NELSON, *et al.* 1986. Cellular localization of human immunodeficiency virus infection within the brains of acquired immune deficiency syndrome patients. Proc. Natl. Acad. Sci. USA **83:** 7089–7093.
14. GABUZDA, D. H., D. D. HO, DE LA MONTE, *et al.* 1986. Immunohistochemical identification of HTLV-III antigen in brain of patients with AIDS. Ann. Neurol. **20:** 289–295.
15. KOENIG, S., H. E. GENDELMAN, J. M. ORENSTEIN, *et al.* 1986. Detection of AIDS virus in macrophage in brain tissue from AIDS patients with encephalopathy. Science **233:** 109.
16. PUMAROLA-SUNE, T., B. A. NAVIA, D. CORDON-CARDO, *et al.* 1987. HIV antigen in the brains of patients with the AIDS dementia complex. Ann. Neurol. **21:** 490–496.
17. SHAW, G. M., M. E. HARPER, B. H. HAHN, *et al.* 1985. HTLV-III infection in brains of children and adults with AIDS encephalopathy. Science **227:** 177–181.
18. EPSTEIN, L. G., J. GOUDSMIT, D. A. PAUL, *et al.* 1987. Expression of human immunodeficiency virus in cerebrospinal fluid of children with progressive encephalopathy. Ann. Neurol. **21:** 397–401.
19. NAVIA, B. A., B. D. JORDON & R. W. PRICE. 1986. The AIDS dementia complex: I. Clinical features. Ann. Neurol. **19:** 517–524.
20. PIZZO, P. A., J. EDDY, F. M. BALIS, *et al.* 1988. Effect of continuous intravenous infusion of Zidovudine (AZT) in children with symptomatic HIV infection. N. Engl. J. Med. **319:** 889–896.
21. SCOTT, G. 1989. Survival in children with perinatally acquired human immunodeficiency virus type infection. N. Engl. J. Med. **3211:** 1791–1796.
22. BLANCHE, S., M. TARDIEU, A. M. DULIEGE, *et al.* 1990. Longitudinal study of 94 symptomatic infants with materno fetal HIV infection: Evidence for a bimodal expression of clinical and biological symptoms. AJDC **144:** 1210–1215.
23. European Collaborative Study: P. COGO, A. M. LAVERDA, A. E. ADES, *et al.* 1990. Neurologic signs in young children with human immunodeficiency virus infection. Ped. Inf. Dis. J. **9:** 402–406.
24. BELMAN, A. L. 1990. AIDS and pediatric neurology. *In* Pediatric Neurology. J. Bodensteiner, Ed. Neurol. Clinics **8:** 571–603.
25. R. S. JANSSEN, D. R. CORNBLATH, L. G. EPSTEIN, *et al.* 1991. American Academy of Neurology AIDS Task Force, nomenclature and research case definitions for neurologic manifestations of human immunodeficiency virus type I. Neurology **41:** 778–785.
26. JOHNSON, R. T., J. C. MCARTHUR & O. NARAYAN. 1988. The neurobiology of human immunodeficiency virus infections. FASEB J. **2:** 2970–2981.
27. BELMAN, A. L., T. CALVELLI, M. NOZYCE, *et al.* 1990. Neurologic and immunologic correlates in infants with vertically transmitted HIV infection. Neurology (Suppl. 1) **40:**409.
28. BELMAN, A. L., G. DIAMOND, Y. PARK, *et al.* 1989. Perinatal HIV infection: A prospective longitudinal study of the initial CNS signs. Neurology **39**(Suppl.): 278–279.
29. BELMAN, A. L., J. MARCUS, L. MUENZ, S. DURAKO & A. WILLOUGHBY. 1993. Neurologic status of infants born to HIV-I infected mothers and their controls: A prospective study from birth to 24 months of age. Neurology (Abstract) **43:** A347.
30. NOZYCE, M., J. HITTELMAN, L. MUENZ, S. DURAKO & A. WILLOUGHBY. Effect of perinatally acquired human immunodeficiency virus infection on neurodevelopment in children during the first two years of life.
31. BELMAN, A. L., G. LANTOS, D. HOROUPIAN, *et al.* 1986. AIDS: Calcification of the basal ganglia in infants and children. Neurology **36:** 1192–1199.
32. LIFSCHITZ, M., C. HANSON, G. WILSON, W. T. SHEARER. 1989. Behavioral changes in children with human immunodeficiency virus (HIV) infection. T.B.P. 175. V International Conference on AIDS. June 4–9. Montreal, Canada.
33. BROUWERS, E., A. L. BELMAN & L. EPSTEIN. 1990. Central nervous system involvement: Manifestations and evaluation. *In* Pediatric AIDS: The Challenge of HIV Infec-

tion in Infants, Children and Adolescents. P. A. Pizzo & C. M. Wilfert, Ed.: 318–335. Williams & Wilkins. Baltimore.
34. Moss, H., P. Wolters, J. Eddy, L. Wiener, P. Pizzo & P. Brouwers. 1989. The effects of encephalopathy and AZT treatment on the social and emotional behavior of pediatric AIDS patients. V International Conference on AIDS. June 4–9. Montreal, Canada.
35. Cohen, S. L., T. Mundy, B. Kaarassik, et al. 1991. Neuropsychological functioning in children with HIV-1 infected through neonatal blood transfusion. Pediatrics 88: 58–68.
36. Diamond, G. W., J. Kaufman, A. L. Belman, et al. 1987. Characterization of cognitive functioning in a subgroup of children with congenital HIV infection. Arch. Clin. Neuropsychol. 2: 1–16.
37. Condini, A., G. Axia, A. Viero, A. M. Laverda, et al. 1991. Study of language in HIV infected Italian children. (Abstract) Neuroscience of HIV-1 Infection. p. 25. Padova, Italy. Satellite Conference, VII International Conference on AIDS.
38. Wolters, P., et al. 1991. VIII International Conference on AIDS. June. Florence, Italy.
39. Nozyce, M., G. Diamond, A. Belman, et al. 1989. The course of neurodevelopmental functioning in the infants of IVDA and HIV-seropositive parents. M.B.O. 41. V International Conference on AIDS. June 4–9. Montreal, Canada.
40. Ultmann, M. H., G. Diamond, H. A. Ruff, A. L. Belman, et al. 1987. Developmental abnormalities in infants and children with acquired immune deficiency syndrome (AIDS): A follow-up study. Int. J. Neurosci. 32: 661–667.
41. Hittelman, J., S. Fikrig, H. Mendez, et al. 1989. Neurodevelopmental assessment of children with symptomatic HIV infection. T.B.P. 180. V International Conference on AIDS. June 4–9. Montreal, Canada.
42. Bale, J., B. Garg, A. Tilton, et al. 1991. Neurologic examination in hemophilic subjects: Relationship to human immunodeficiency virus serostatus. Ann. Neurol. 30: 508.
43. Papavasiliou, A., S. Aronis, E. Stamboulis, et al. 1991. Involvement of central and peripheral nervous system of HIV-infected hemophilic children. (Abstract) Neuroscience of HIV-1 Infection. p. 49. Padova, Italy. Satellite Conference, VII International Conference on AIDS.
44. Whitt, J. K., S. R. Hooper, M. B. Tennison, et al. 1991. Longitudinal patterns of neuropsychologic functioning in HIV-infected children with hemophilia. p. 66. (Abstract) Neuroscience of HIV-1 Infection. Padova, Italy. Satellite Conference, VII International Conference on AIDS.
45. Diamond, G. W., P. Gurdin, A. A. Wiznia, A. L. Belman, et al. 1990. Effects of congenital HIV infection on neurodevelopmental status of babies in foster care. Dev. Med. Child. Neurol. 32: 399–1005.
46. Diamond, G. W., P. Gurdin, A. Wiznia, A. Belman, A. Rubinstein & H. Cohen. 1991. Environmental and viral related factors in neurodevelopmental impairments of HIV seropositive children in foster care. p. 27. (Abstract) Neuroscience of HIV-1 Infection. Padova, Italy. Satellite Conference, VII International Conference on AIDS.
47. Kairam, R., S. Kugler, R. Zawadzki, V. Rojas, C. Mellins & R. Levenson. 1991. Range of neurological and psychological dysfunction in pediatric HIV infection. p. 41. (Abstract) Neuroscience of HIV-1 Infection. Padova, Italy. Satellite Conference, VII International Conference on AIDS.
48. Epstein, L. G., L. R. Sharer, J. Goudsmit. 1988. Neurological and neuropathological features of HIV in children. Ann. Neurol. 23(Suppl): S19–S23.
49. Wiley, C. A., A. L. Belman, D. Dickson, A. Rubinstein & J. A. Nelson. 1990. Human immunodeficiency virus within the brains of children with AIDS. Clin. Neuropathol. 1: 1–6.
50. Gallo, P., A. M. Laverda, A. DeRossi, et al. 1991. Immunological markers in the cerebrospinal fluid of HIV-1 infected children. ACTA Ped. Scand. 80: 659–666.
51. Laverda, A. M., P. Gallo, B. Tavolato, et al. 1991. Cerebrospinal fluid findings in neurologically symptomatic and asymptomatic HIV-1 infected children. p. 120. (Abstract) Neuroscience of HIV-1 Infection. Padova, Italy. Satellite Conference, VII International Conference on AIDS.

52. MINTZ, M., R. RAPAPORT, M. OLESKI, et al. 1989. Elevated serum levels of tumor necrosis factor are associated with progressive encephalopathy in children with acquired immunodeficiency syndrome. Am. J. Dis. Child. **14:** 771–774.
53. KURE, K., K. M. WEIDENHEIM, W. D. LYMAN & D. W. DICKSON. 1990 Morphology and distribution of HIV-1 qp 41 positive microglia in subacute AIDS encephalitis. ACTA Neuropathol. (Berlin) **80:** 393–400.
54. PRICE, R. W. 1992. The challenge of HIV and its effects on the central nervous system. J. Neurol. Sci. **113:** 126.
55. BUDKA, H. 1991. Neuropathology of human immunodeficiency virus infection. Brain Pathol. **1:** 163–175.
56. ACHIM, C. L., R. D. SCHRIER & C. A. WILEY. 1991. Immunopathogenesis of HIV encephalitis. Brain Pathol. **1:** 177–184.
57. WILEY, C. A. & H. BUDKA. 1991. HIV-induced CNS lesions. Brain Pathol. **1:** 153–154.
58. DICKSON, D. W. 1992. Microglia and macrophages in HIV-related CNS neuropathology. J. Neurol. Sci. **113:** 128.
59. BENVENISTE, E. 1992. Cytokine circuits in brain. Reprinted from J. Neurol. Sci. **113(2):** 127.
60. CHIODI, F. & E. M. FENYO. 1991. Neurotropism of human immunodeficiency virus. Brain Pathol. **1:** 185–191.
61. DA CUNHA, A. & L. VITKOVIC. 1992. Cytokine expression and control of pathogenesis in AIDS brain. J. Neurol. Sci. **113:** 130.
62. LI, Y., H. HUI, R. W. PRICE, G. M. SHAW & B. H. HALN. 1992. Molecular biology of HIV-1 in AIDS dementia complex. J. Neurol. Sci. **113:** 126.
63. LIPTON, S. A. 1991. HIV related neurotoxicity. Brain Pathol. **1:** 193–200.
64. O'BRIEN, W. A. 1992. Genetic and biologic basis of HIV "neurotropism." J. Neurol. Sci. **113:** 126.
65. OLDSTONE, M. 1992. The anatomy of viral persistence. J. Neurol. Sci. **113:** 127.
66. GENIS, P., M. JETT, E. W. BENNTON, et al. 1992. Cytokines and arachandonic metabolites produced during HIV infected macrophage-astroglia interactions: Implications for the neuropathogenesis of HIV disease. J. Exp. Med. **176:** 1703–1718.
67. BUTLER, K. M., R. N. HUSSON, R. M. BALIS, et al. 1990. Dideoxginosine in children with symptomatic human immunodeficiency virus infection. N. Engl. J. Med. **324:** 137–144.
68. CALVELLI, T. A., A. L. BELMAN, C. BUETI, M. GOLODNER & A. RUBINSTEIN. 1989. Divergence of onset of neurologic and immunologic impairment in infants born to HIV seropositive mothers. T.B.P. 184. V International Conference on AIDS. June 4–9. Montreal, Canada.
69. BROUWERS, P., H. MOSS, P. WOLTERS, et al. 1990. Effect of continuous-infusion zidovudine therapy on neuropsychologic functioning in children with symptomatic human immunodeficiency virus infection. J. Ped. **117:** 980–985.
70. DECARLI, C., L. FUGATE, J. FALLOON, et al. 1991. Brain growth and cognitive improvement in children with HIV induced encephalopathy after 6 months of continuous infusion therapy. J. AIDS **4:** 585–592.
71. PIZZO, P. A., K. BUTLER, F. BALIS, et al. 1990. Dideoxycytidine alone and in an alternating schedule with zidovudine in children with symptomatic human immunodeficiency virus infection. J. Ped. **117:** 799–808.
72. MCKINNEY, R. E., M. A. MAHA, E. M. CONNERS, et al. 1991. A multicenter trial of oral zidovudine in children with advanced HIV disease. N Engl. J. Med. **324:** 1018–1025.
73. NOZYCE, M., M. HOBERMAN, S. ARPADE, et al. 1992. The effects of oral AZT on neurodevelopmental, immunological, and clinical outcomes in vertically HIV infected children. Unpublished.
74. MINTZ, M. & L. G. EPSTEIN. 1992. Neurologic manifestations, clinical features and therapeutic approaches. Semin. Neurol. **12:** 51–56.
75. BELMAN, A. L. & D. W. DICKSON. 1992. Neurologic aspects. *In* Children with AIDS. M. L. Stuber, Ed.: 89–106. American Psychiatric Press. Washington, DC.
76. BELMAN, A. L. 1992. Central nervous system involvement in pediatric HIV-I infection, an overview. Int. Pediatr. **7:** 126–135.

Reliability of Neurologic Assessment in a Collaborative Study of HIV Infection in Children[a]

RAM KAIRAM,[b] JENNIE KLINE,[c] BRUCE LEVIN,[c]
DONALD BRAMBILLA,[d] DAVID COULTER,[e] KARL
KUBAN,[f] LESTER LANSKY,[g] PAUL MARSHALL,[h] JESUS
VELEZ-BORRAS,[i] AND EVELYN RODRIGUEZ[j]

INTRODUCTION

A growing number of studies of HIV infection, whether of disease progression or to evaluate treatments, require collaboration and combination of data from many sites. Proper conduct of these studies requires the use of reliable instruments to produce comparable data across sites. This paper summarizes the results of a study to assess the reliability of a structured neurologic examination administered by seven neuologists collaborating in a national study of vertically transmitted HIV infection in children. We consider the implications for analysis of already collected data and for measurement of hard neurologic signs in future collaborative studies.

HIV infection in children is associated with a progressive encephalopathy that is characterized by loss of developmental milestones, acquired microcephaly or brain atrophy, and pyramidal tract dysfunction. The latter is manifest in weakness and abnormalities in tone, and less frequently by ataxia and rigidity.[1,2] Involuntary movements such as tremors, peripheral neuropathy, and seizures are uncommon.

The more severe neurologic manifestations of infection occur in the end stages

---

[a] This work was supported in part by grants from the National Institutes of Health Women and Infant Transmission Study (NOI-AI-05072, 82506, 82507, 85005, 82505, and NO1-HD-82913.
[b] St. Luke's/Roosevelt Hospital Center and Columbia University, New York, New York 10025.
[c] New York State Psychiatric Institute and Columbia University, New York, New York.
[d] New England Research Institute, Watertown, Massachusetts.
[e] Boston University School of Medicine, Boston, Massachusetts.
[f] Children's Hospital, Harvard Medical School, Boston, Massachusetts.
[g] Children's Memorial Hospital, Chicago, Illinois.
[h] University of Massachusetts Medical Center, Worcester, Massachusetts.
[i] University of Puerto Rico Medical Sciences Campus, San Juan, Puerto Rico.
[j] National Institute of Allergy and Infectious Diseases, Bethesda, Maryland.

of disease. It is a reasonable assumption that such severe deterioration is readily apparent to a variety of clinicians, although neurologic and radiologic expertise may be needed to document the extent and types of abnormalities—for example, hypertonia, hyperreflexia, or cerebral atrophy. The same cannot be presumed for earlier and less severe signs of neurologic involvement. Indeed, work in the area of perinatal insult and neurologic sequelae such as cerebral palsy raises concerns about the criteria and comparability of diagnoses from different neurologists, at least during infancy, even when diagnosis is simply the categorization "normal," "abnormal," or "suspect."

It is in this context that the Neurologic Examination for Children (NEC)[3,4] is being developed to provide a valid and reliable measure of neurologic status in children with HIV infection. The term "validity" refers to "the degree to which a measurement measures what it purports to measure."[5] The term "reliability" refers to the reproducibility of similar examination results,[5] between examiners and over very short periods of time, when it is fair to assume stability in characteristics of the child.

One application of the NEC has been in the Women and Infant Transmission Study (WITS), a multicenter study to describe the natural history of pediatric HIV disease. More recently, the examination has been adopted for use in selected AIDS Clinical Trials Group protocols, with the hope that it will provide a valid and reliable measure of both beneficial and adverse neurologic changes following different treatments. This use presents a special challenge, because there is the need to achieve reliability across as many as 33 sites.

The goals of the NEC reliability study within the context of the WITS were:

1. To train the WITS neurologists in the administration and coding of the examination.
2. To evaluate the consistency or reliability of their measures.
3. To improve reliability, where needed, by training or revisions to the examination.

METHODS

The Neurologic Examination for Children

The NEC draws on the standard clinical neurologic examination described by Paine and Oppe,[6] thus achieving content validity.[5] Several steps were taken to achieve reliability.

First, the examination is *structured,* that is, it requires the uniform administration of items. Procedures are described in a manual, and, more recently, also demonstrated in a videotape.

Second, following principles of psychologic testing (e.g., the Bayley Scales of Infant Development[7]), examiners code the responses of the child, rather than clinical judgments about normality or severity. For example, observations of the head during the maneuver "pull-to-sitting" provide information about neck tone. The NEC distinguishes three responses based on the head and eye position, namely, (1) head aligned with the back for 90% or more of the pull, (2) head lag with eyes toward ceiling, and (3) head lag with eyes toward back of room. These relatively precise descriptions of the response contrast with judgmental alternatives such as coding "mild" or "severe" head lag, or the judgment "neck hypotonia."

Third, examiners are trained by observation and trial to carry out and code the examination according to a uniform protocol.

A fourth aspect that relates to reliability is that the examination is designed to yield composite scores in eleven domains by combining observations from several items. One criterion for retaining an individual item is whether it correlates as expected with other items thought to reflect the same domain (e.g. hypertonia). Evaluation of this type of reliability, that is, the internal consistency of composite scores, is planned.

Before the present study, reliability was assessed in terms of interrater agreement between the two neurologists who worked in the development of the NEC.[4] That study led to some revisions in the examination. The revised examination (NEC, version 4) was tested in the present study.

Training

Six pediatric neurologists were trained in the examination protocol. Training consisted of a 1½-day meeting in February of 1991 during which we discussed specific items, demonstrated the examination procedures, and had examiners practice both administration and coding. The training in administration was particularly important for the measurement of angles, which uses procedures not customary in clinical practice, and also for measurement of reflexes, since these are especially sensitive to technique. For training in coding, examiners coded while observing each other, reported their codes, and discussed disagreements. In addition, the neurologist most expert in the protocol (RK) carried out additional examinations with neurologists at their sites. In the fall of 1991 we carried out a two-day study to test the interrater agreement of all examiners (including RK).

SUBJECTS

The two-day reliability study drew on 35 children ranging in age from 5 to 34 months, with a mean age of 21 months (TABLE 1). Fourteen children were HIV positive, eight were HIV seroreverters, two were HIV negative; the remaining 11 children, drawn from a general pediatric clinic, were untested but presumed to be HIV negative. We deliberately selected a sample in which about half the children had been judged neurologically abnormal (by RK or another neurologist responsible for care) because accurate assessment of reliability requires that there be adequate variability in the responses of the children. The proportions of children with a neurologic abnormality were evenly distributed over the age range.

TABLE 1. Description of the Study Sample

Number of children	35
Age	
Mean (SD)	21.3 months (8.8)
Range	5–34 months
HIV serologic status	
Positive	14
Seroreverted	8
Negative	2
Not tested/tested result unknown	11
Neurologic status before study	
Normal	15
Abnormal	15
Not examined previously	5
Number of boys/girls	18/17

DESIGN

The NEC used in WITS has 74 neurologic items, plus an item on state during the examination, and diagnosis codes. For the sake of efficiency, these items were tested in two ways.

Test–Retest Design

Thirty-seven items that required "hands-on" manipulation of the child were evaluated in a test–retest design; these included most of the items to measure eye movements, tone, and reflexes. Thirty children were each examined independently by two of the seven neurologists. Pairing of neurologists and ordering of examinations was accomplished blind to both HIV and neurologic status. Assignments were randomized within blocks of five or six children, each of similar ages (range 10 months).

Group Examinations

The remaining 37 items were observational and did not require hands-on contact. Of these, 22 relate to standing, walking, and gait. Each of 26 children, including 21 who were also administered the hands-on items, were examined by one neurologist, with the remaining neurologists observing and coding. Examining neurologists were chosen such that none had performed a hands-on examination of the child being examined. The group examinations were carried out in a single room, with no discussion of items permitted, both during and after administration because that could bias estimates of agreement.

In both the test–retest and group examinations, the numbers of children examined per examiner varied because three neurologists were unable to attend for the entire two days. The statistical analysis takes account of the actual examiner/subject matchups.

Statistical Analysis

All but four items are categorical. For categorical items, reliability was assessed by two statistics, the percent agreement and the kappa coefficient.[8,9] The percent agreement is simply the number of children for whom both (or all) examiners agree divided by the number of children examined. One shortcoming of this measure is that it does not take account of the degree of agreement expected purely by chance. It is most misleading when there is very little variability between children.

The kappa coefficient takes account of the extent of agreement expected by chance. Kappa is an index bounded between plus and minus one with negative values indicating agreement less than expected by chance, 0 indicating agreement at exactly chance expectation, and positive values indicating above chance agreement, with 1 indicating perfect agreement. Chance expected agreement is derived from the (null) assumption that each examiner assigns ratings at random and without regard to variation in children's signs (although each examiner is allowed to maintain individual inclinations across rating categories). The main disadvantage of kappa is that it is sensitive to the variability of response to a particular item. For example, when a particular response is rare, even a single disagreement between examiners will produce a poor kappa (close to 0). Note that lack of variability occurs either because all or nearly all subjects are alike (in which case kappa will be poor even if examiners are nearly perfect in measurement), or because examiners almost always code one category (in which case kappa will be poor even if subjects are truly heterogeneous).

Our study design called for a slightly more elaborate estimation of kappa than is computed in simple designs where all examiners examine all children. Estimation procedures are contained in the APPENDIX; the footnote to TABLE 3 provides information on the lower 95% confidence bounds. For continuous items such as head circumference, we estimated reliability by the intraclass correlation coefficient (ICC).[10]

We interpret reliability coefficients taking into consideration the variability of items. In the NEC, the first coded response ordinarily represents the "normal" or developmentally advanced response. We defined variability as the proportion of children in which the consensus was that the child manifested Response 1 (or the most common response, for the few items in which Response 1 is not the most common). In the event of a draw (e.g., in the test–retest study when one examiner codes Response 1 and the other does not), the child was scored ½ towards response 1. We have grouped items in four categories of variability: *none; poor*, defined as 95% or more scored Response 1; *limited* with 85 to 95% scored response 1; and *good*, with 50% to 85% scored Response 1. In the test–retest study, *good* variability translates into at least five (of 30) children manifesting a response other than Response 1; in the group examination into at least four (of 26) children. It is only in this *good* category that variability is sufficient to make informed judgments about reliability of an item.

RESULTS

TABLE 2 summarizes the results of the reliability study. It provides counts of items organized by degree of variability in responses, kappa coefficients, and

TABLE 2. Variability and Reliability of NEC Items in WITS

Variability[a]	Kappa[b]	Agreement[b]	Number of Items Tested		
			Hands-on	Group	Total
Categorical items					
None	NC	Perfect	9	0	9
None	Poor	Excellent	0	8	8
None	Poor	Poor	0	1	1
Poor	Perfect	Perfect	1	0	1
Poor	Fair	Excellent	0	1	1
Poor	Poor	Excellent	8	3	11
Limited	Perfect	Perfect	1	0	1
Limited	Excellent	Excellent	1	4	5
Limited	Good	Excellent	0	1	1
Limited	Fair	Excellent/good	1	4	5
Limited	Fair	Fair	0	1	1
Limited	Poor	Excellent	4	0	4
Good	Perfect	Perfect	1	0	1
Good	Excellent	Excellent	1	5	6
Good	Good	Excellent/good	1	1	2
Good	Good	Fair	0	1	1
Good	Fair	Excellent/good	1	1	2
Good	Poor	Excellent/good	4	0	4
Good	Poor	Poor	0	1	1
Continuous items[c]					
Good	Excellent	—	1	0	1
Good	Fair	—	1	0	1
Good	Poor	—	2	0	2
Not assessed (30+ month items)				5	5
Sum			37	37	74

[a] Variability defined as percent of cases in which consensus was that child manifested Response 1 (or most common response). None = 1.0; Poor = [0.95–1.0); Limited = [0.85–0.95); Good = [0.50–0.85.). These definitions correspond to, respectively, binary variability, pq, at levels up to 0%, 5%, 50%, and 100% of maximum binary variability, $0.25 = 0.5 \times 0.5$.

[b] Agreement and kappa: Perfect (1.0); Excellent (0.75–0.99); Good (0.60–0.74); Fair (0.40–0.59); Poor (≤0.39); NC, not completed.

[c] Estimated by intraclass correlation coefficient.

percent agreement. In 18 items, or 24%, no child was judged to exhibit a response other than 1, although within the group setting, there were sporadic codings other than 1. In another 13 items variability was poor, with only one to two children exhibiting responses other than 1. And in a further 17 items, variability was limited, usually with three to four children exhibiting a response other than 1. These three classes of items total 48 or 65% of items tested. In these items variability is too low to consider our observations informative about reliability. Items falling in this majority include abnormal movements such as tremors, developmentally early responses such as "follows face," asymmetries in movement of limbs or face which are uncommon in HIV infection, abnormalities of gait such as scissoring, and severe signs of pyramidal dysfunction such as cortical fist (TABLE 3B–D).

Agreement between examiners was excellent or perfect in 42 of the 48 items with less than good variability (or 88%). Thus the data offer some evidence that examiners can identify children without the "abnormal" response. On the other hand, in 31 or 65% of these items, the corresponding kappa was below 0.60, suggesting that examiners disagree in their judgments.

For 21 items, comprising 28%, there was good variability between children with which to evaluate agreement of examiners (TABLE 3A). Eight items were tested in the test–retest examinations. Reliability, as measured by kappa, was

TABLE 3. Summary of WITS Reliability Study

	Kappa[a]		Agreement	
A. Items with Good Variability (0.50–0.85)	Best	Worst	Best	Worst
Test–retest study of 30 children				
Hip position on ventral suspension[b] (0.71)[c]	0.33		0.71	
Head position on ventral suspension (0.80)[c]	1.0		1.0	
Position of lower limbs when supported under arms (0.80)[d]	0.50		0.80	
Upgoing toe (0.84)	0.34		0.81	
Ankle jerk (0.80)[e]	−0.03		0.60	
Biceps reflex (0.73)[e]	0.09		0.60	
Seizures (0.80)	0.90		0.97	
Handedness (0.50)[e]	0.69		0.80	
Reflexes collapsing with or without limb displacement				
Ankle jerk collapsed	0		0.97	
Biceps reflex collapsed	NC[f]		1.0	
Knee jerk collapsed	NC		1.0	
Head circumference[g]	0.98		NC	
Adductor angle[g]	0.46		NC	
Popliteal angle[g]	0.38		NC	
Ankle angle[g]	−0.15		NC	
Group exam of 26 children				
Picks up Cheerio (0.77)	0.68	0.67	0.60	0.58
Picks up Cheerio collapsed	0.75	0.73	0.68	0.65
Crawls 9+ inches (0.83)	0.69	0.60	0.83	0.58
Pulls-to-stand (0.85)	0.51	0.43	0.92	0.42
Stands alone 3 sec[b] (0.65)	0.97	0.87	0.95	0.81
Stands alone 30 sec (0.60)	0.91	0.85	0.95	0.77
Three steps holding furniture[b] (0.71)	0.40	0.33	0.56	0.19
Three steps without support[b] (0.65)	0.97	0.88	0.96	0.85
Walks independently 6+ feet (0.65)	0.97	0.88	0.96	0.85
Gets up off floor to standing (0.60)	0.87	0.76	0.85	0.65

(*continued*)

TABLE 3 *Continued*. Summary of WITS Reliability Study

B. Items with Good Variability (0.85–0.95)	Kappa[a]		Agreement	
	Best	Worst	Best	Worst
Test–retest study of 30 children				
Upper eyelid covers pupil (0.95)	−0.05		0.90	
Slips with support under arms (0.91)[h]	−0.32		0.78	
Knee jerk (0.88)	0.20		0.83	
Crossed adductor response (0.88)	0.59		0.90	
Cortical fist (0.93)	0.28		0.90	
Rigidity of elbow (0.93)	0.82		0.96	
Rigidity of knee (0.95)	1.0		1.0	
Group exam of 26 children				
Sitting posture (0.88)	0.75	0.72	0.88	0.85
Sits 1+ minute (0.92)	0.90	0.83	0.96	0.88
Grasps red ring (0.92)	0.93	0.93	0.96	0.96
Upper limb symmetry during spontaneous movement (0.90)	0.42	0.39	0.72	0.69
Group exam of 17 children who walked[i]				
Toe walking (0.88)	0.52		0.71	
Broad-based gait (0.88)	0.52		0.71	
Stumbles while walking (0.91)	0.65		0.82	
Falls while walking (0.94)	0.78		0.88	
Stumbles while turning around (0.94)	0.43		0.59	
Falls while turning around (0.94)	0.50		0.65	

C. Items with Poor Variability (0.95–1.0)	Kappa[a]		Agreement	
	Best	Worst	Best	Worst
Test–retest study of 30 children				
Nystagmus (0.98)	0		0.97	
Head position after pull-to-sit (0.97)	1.0		1.0	
Head during pull-to-sit (0.98)	0		0.97	
Ankle clonus (0.97)	−0.02		0.93	
Athetosis—arms (0.98)	0		0.97	
Limb dystonia—arms (0.98)	0		0.97	
Limb dystonia—legs (0.98)	0		0.97	
Limb tremors—arms (0.98)	0		0.97	
Opisthotonus (0.97)	0		0.93	
Group exam of 26 children				
Lower limb symmetry during spontaneous movement (0.98)	0.27	0.24	0.84	0.81
Nasolabial fold symmetry (0.96)	0.28	0.25	0.84	0.81
Group exam of 17 children who walked[i]				
Dystonic arm posture (0.97)	0.28		0.82	
Decreased arm swing (0.94)	0.47		0.82	

TABLE 3 Continued. Summary of WITS Reliability Study

D. Items with No Variability in Response	Kappa[a]		Agreement	
	Best	Worst	Best	Worst
Test–retest study of 30 children				
Looks at person	NC		1.0	
Follows face	NC		1.0	
Horizontal eye movements	NC		1.0	
Athetosis—legs	NC		1.0	
Chorea—arms	NC		1.0	
Chorea—legs	NC		1.0	
Limb tremors—legs	NC		1.0	
Induced tremors—arms	NC		1.0	
Induced tremors—legs	NC		1.0	
Group exam of 26 children				
Neck extension in prone position (1.0)	0.36	0.22	0.89	0.65
Eye symmetry (1.0)	0.06	0.07	0.84	0.81
Angle of mouth symmetry (1.0)	0.17	0.14	0.92	0.88
Tandem stance 5+ seconds[b] (1.0)[e]	0.28	0.17	0.50	0.04
Group exam of 17 children who walked[i]				
Knee flexion (1.0)	0.12		0.76	
Knee hyperextension (1.0)	0.16		0.88	
Circumducting gait (1.0)	0.16		0.88	
Scissoring (1.0)	0.35		0.94	
Cortical arm posture (1.0)	0.16		0.88	

[a] For test–retest examination, the single estimates of kappa and agreement exclude children for whom one or both examiners coded not assessed/not in state. For group examination, two estimates are given. Worst estimates include all observations. Best estimates exclude single codings of not assessed/not in state for kappa and exclude all codings of not assessed/not in state for agreement. The lower 95% confidence bounds (not shown) were 0.60 or better for 11 of the 12 kappas of 0.80 or better; 0.4 or better for 4 kappas of 0.60–0.79; 0.20 or lower for all remaining kappas.
[b] Item will be deleted from NEC.
[c] 7 children assessed by both examiners.
[d] 10 children assessed by both examiners.
[e] Percent with a modal response other than response 1.
[f] NC, not computed.
[g] For continuous measures, reliability estimated by intraclass correlation coefficient.
[h] 9 children assessed by both examiners.
[i] For gait items, kappa and agreement estimated from all examinations. Results were not changed much by exclusion of children coded "not assessed/does not walk" except for "turning" items where five children were coded as "not assessed/does not walk" by 1–3 examiners.

good for two items based on report of the caretaker—seizure history and handedness. Kappa was perfect for "head position on ventral suspension," but poor in the companion item, "hip position on ventral suspension." Because this item is only administered to children under 20 pounds, these observations derive from only seven children. Despite these small numbers, we think that the poor performance on "hip position" may be real; children were tested with their diapers on, and this may interfere with assessment. The third item in this category, "position of legs when supported under arms" performed poorly; we have no easy explanation.

For reflexes, kappas indicate essentially chance agreement for both the ankle and biceps. The knee jerk, which had only limited variability, also showed a poor kappa of 0.20. Nearly all disagreements involved distinctions between two classes of response that are considered normal clinically—contraction without limb displacement and contraction with limb displacement. Potential sources of disagreements are several. First, the characteristic may not be stable; that is, the child may in fact have different responses on examinations several minutes apart. Second, examination techniques can produce discordances. We discovered this during development of the NEC, and thus specified particular procedures to improve reliability. However, we observed departures from these procedures during the reliability study. For example, with knee and ankle reflexes, not all examiners positioned the child across the side of the caretaker's thigh, as specified in the protocol. Third, judgments about whether displacement occurred might differ.

Nine items assessed in the group examination had good variability (TABLE 3A). The best and worst estimates reflect different treatment of codes indicating that the item was "not assessed." In some instance this code may represent the correct response, that is, the item was not administered. For example, not all examiners attempted to administer the crawling item to children who walked. In other instances, the "not assessed" code may indicate the observer could not see the child's response. The "worst" estimates include all examinations; the "best" estimates exclude single codings of "not assessed" on the assumption the examiner could not see the response, rather than disagreed with other examiners about whether the item was administered.

Seven of the nine items showed good to excellent reliability. The two items with kappas below 0.6 were "takes 3 steps holding onto furniture" and "pulls-to-stand." In both items, one source of inconsistency stemmed from coding when the item was not administered, as was usually the case with children who could walk independently. For "takes 3 steps holding onto furniture," however, we also had not achieved uniform administration.

For the four continuous items, we used the intraclass correlation coefficient to estimate reliability. As expected, reliability of head circumference measures is excellent. We did not fare as well on the angle measures, with ICCs ranging from 0.46 for the adductor angle to -0.15 for the ankle angle.

DISCUSSION

This reliability study has identified 11 items with good or better reliability, 10 items with fair or poor reliability, and 53 items with low variability, which precluded definitive assessment of reliability.

For the reliable items—mainly those related to power and head size—it appears safe to combine data across study sites. For items with poor reliability, there are two courses of action. For reflexes, where disagreements are not clinically significant, we can combine categories of "normal" response at analysis. For other items, including angle measures, disagreements are probably clinically important. To use already collected data, we need to identify those examiners with uniform administration and coding procedures. The most efficient way to do this is to videotape study examinations.

For items where the study sample was uninformative, we recommend that the criterion for combining data across sites be uniformity in administration and in coding. Administration techniques can be assessed by videotape. We can think of no simple way to assess coding of rare signs. One possibility is to assess coding from scoring a test videotape with an artificially high representation of such signs.

With respect to the future use of the NEC, our plans and recommendations are several.

First, we will make a few revisions to the examination. For reflexes, as in the analytic approach mentioned above, we will code the two clinically normal responses as one response. For power items, we will use the item "walks independently for 6 feet or more" to determine whether items such as "pulls-to-stand," that are achieved at an earlier developmental stage, should be administered. We anticipate this new ordering will eliminate ambiguities in procedures (and hence coding inconsistencies) for administration of developmentally inappropriate items. We will also delete two items (i.e., "stands alone for 3 seconds" and "3 steps without support") that appear to provide essentially the same information as their companion items (i.e., "stands alone for 30 seconds" and "walks independently for 6+ feet," respectively) and one item ("takes 3 steps holding onto furniture") where we did not achieve uniform administration.

Second, we would like to draw on data from selected study sites to assess reliability of the composite scores. This is the final step in the evaluation, since the NEC was designed with the idea of combining information from items to assess dimensions of tone, power, reflexes, and so forth. We would use videotaped examinations to identify sites with uniform administration and coding procedures.

Third, the training procedures for some items may need to be more intensive. Measures of angles fall in this category. These measures differ from other items in that they are not routine in clinical practice, and thus were not familiar to most examiners. The poor performance of these items is due, in large part, to our failure to achieve uniform measurement techniques between examiners. In our previous reliability study, with considerably better standardization and longer practice, ICC's were 0.69 for adductor, 0.79 for popliteal and 0.68 for ankle angle.[4] We consider these quantitative measures potentially more sensitive to subtle changes in tone than measures of function, which often simultaneously measure power. For this reason, we consider it worthwhile to undertake the added training needed to achieve reliable measurement.

Fourth, we recommend that careful consideration be given to characteristics of the examiners who use the NEC. We need examiners who are blind to the independent variable under study (e.g. HIV status) and who are committed to administering the NEC in the manner specified by protocol. Our recent experience in training nurse practitioners, pediatricians, and a developmental psychologist to administer the examination suggests that a variety of professionals, in addition to neurologists, can learn to administer the examination as intended. Serious commitment to the goal of uniform administration cannot fail to improve the ultimate worth of neurologic assessments in collaborative studies and the potential contribution to describing sequelae of infection and evaluating treatments.

ACKNOWLEDGMENTS

The authors thank Ann Kinney and Jane Carrington for help in fieldwork and data analysis and Dr. Ann Willoughby for helpful comments on the manuscript.

REFERENCES

1. BELMAN, A. L., G. DIAMOND, D. DICKSON, et al. 1988. Pediatric acquired immunodeficiency syndrome: Neurologic syndromes. Am. J. Dis. Child. **142:** 29–35.
2. EPSTEIN, L. G., L. R. SHARER, J. M. OLESKE, et al. 1986. Neurologic manifestations of HIV infection in children. Pediatrics **78:** 678–687.
3. KAIRAM, R., J. KLINE & C. CHIRIBOGA. 1991. Neurological Examination for Children, version 4.
4. CHIRIBOGA, C., R. KAIRAM & J. KLINE. 1993. Neurological examination for children: Reliability and utility in studies of HIV infection. Pediatr. AIDS HIV Infect. **4(3):**
5. LAST, J. M. 1988. A *Dictionary of Epidemiology, 2nd edit.* Oxford University Press, New York.
6. PAINE, R. & T. OPPE. 1966. Neurological Examination of Children. J. B. Lippincott. Philadelphia.
7. 1969. Bayley Scales of Infant Development. The Psychological Corporation. New York.
8. COHEN, J. 1960. A coefficient of agreement for nominal scales. Educ. Psychol. Meas. **20:** 37–46.
9. FLEISS, J. L. 1981. Statistical Methods for Rates and Proportions, 2nd edit.: 212–236. Wiley. New York.
10. SHROUT, P. E. & J. L. FLEISS. 1979. Intraclass correlations: Uses in assessing rater reliability. Psychol. Bull. **86(2):** 420–428.

Appendix

ESTIMATION OF KAPPA

Assume there are m examiners who independently score up to n subjects, placing a subject into one of c categories. The examiners are assumed to comprise a fixed set, not necessarily a random sample from a larger population of raters. Despite efforts to standardize procedures among examiners, in practice each may use different strategies for scoring. In particular, examiners may tend to classify subjects in different overall proportions across categories. The kappa statistic developed below allows for such propensities, and also the possibility that, by design or by accident, examiners may not observe every subject.

For $i = 1, \ldots, n$ and $j = 1, \ldots, m$, let $\delta_{ij} = 1$ indicate that subject i was scored by examiner j, otherwise set $\delta_{ij} = 0$. We refer to the set $\{\delta_{ij}\}$ as the examination schedule. Let $m_i = \sum_j \delta_{ij} = \delta_{i1} + \cdots + \delta_{im}$ denote the number of examiners scoring subject i, and let $n_j = \sum_i \delta_{ij} = \delta_{1j} + \cdots + \delta_{nj}$ denote the number of subjects scored by examiner j. The scores for any given item comprise a three-way array of zeros and ones, $\{Z_{ijk}\}$, where $Z_{ijk} = 1$ indicates that subject i was observed by examiner j and placed into category k ($k = 1, \ldots, c$). If $\delta_{ij} = 1$, we have $\sum_k Z_{ijk} = Z_{ij1} + \cdots + Z_{ijc} = 1$ because scoring categories are assumed to be mutually exclusive and exhaustive. If $\delta_{ij} = 0$, then we code each Z_{ijk} arbitrarily to zero. For a given examination schedule, let $X_{ik} = \sum_j \delta_{ij} Z_{ijk}$ denote the number of examiners classifying subject i into category k. Note that $\sum_k X_{ik} = m_i$ for any i.

Kappa is broadly defined as an index of the extent of agreement above the level of purely chance agreement. For a given measure of underlying true agreement in a population of subjects, say A_1, relative to some maximum level of agreement, say A_m, plus a definition of expected chance agreement, say A_0, kappa is defined to be

$$K = \frac{A_1 - A_0}{A_m - A_0} = 1 - \frac{A_m - A_1}{A_m - A_0} \tag{1}$$

assuming the nondegeneracy conditon $A_m > A_0$. (Kappa is undefined if $A_m = A_0$, which occurs when there is no variation in scoring.) In the data, observed agreement about any subject i among examiners is measured most simply by the number of pairs of examiners in agreement, which is $\frac{1}{2} \sum_k X_{ik}(X_{ik} - 1) = \frac{1}{2} \sum_k X_{ik}^2 - \frac{1}{2} m_i$. The total observed agreement is obtained by summing over subjects and is denoted by $a_1 = \frac{1}{2} \sum_i \sum_k X_{ik}(X_{ik} - 1) = \frac{1}{2} \sum_i \sum_k X_{ik}^2 - \frac{1}{2} \sum_i m_i$. Here and below, we use lower case symbols for sample quantities such as a_1. The total observed agreement a_1 is an obvious unbiased estimate of its expectation, which will be used to define the underlying true agreement, $A_1 = E_1\{\frac{1}{2} \sum_i \sum_k X_{ik}(X_{ik} - 1)\}$. The expectation E_1 is taken with respect to the distribution of subject characteristics and with respect to some probability model for the misclassification rates of the examiners, all conditional on the examination schedule $\{\delta_{ij}\}$.

Because at most $\frac{1}{2} m_i(m_i - 1)$ pairs of examiners can agree over subject i, we have $A_m \equiv a_m \equiv \frac{1}{2} \sum_i m_i(m_i - 1) = \frac{1}{2} \sum_i m_i^2 - \frac{1}{2} \sum_i m_i$. Thus $2(a_m - a_1) = \sum_i m_i^2 - \sum_i \sum_k X_{ik}^2 = \sum_i \sum_k X_{ik}(m_i - X_{ik})$, which is unbiased for its expectation, $2(A_m - A_1) = E_1\{\sum_i \sum_k X_{ik}(m_i - X_{ik})\}$. The statistic $d \equiv \sum_i \sum_k X_{ik}(m_i - X_{ik})$ is a pivotal measure of interrater disagreement. Once we have defined expected chance agreement, indicated by expectations E_0 with respect to some chance model, the definition of kappa becomes

$$K = 1 - \frac{E_1\{\sum_i \sum_k X_{ik}(m_i - X_{ik})\}}{E_0\{\sum_i \sum_k X_{ik}(m_i - X_{ik})\}} \tag{2}$$

Purely chance agreement would occur if examiners assigned classifications at random, for example, as a multinomial response with cell probabilities $(P_{j1}, \ldots, P_{jc})$ for examiner j, *irrespective* of subject characteristics. Given the m by c array of classification probabilities $\{P_{jk}\}$ in this model, we have $E_0 X_{ik} = \sum_j \delta_{ij} E_0 Z_{ijk} = \sum_j \delta_{ij} P_{jk} = m_i P_k(i)$, where we have defined $P_k(i) \equiv m_i^{-1} \sum_j \delta_{ij} P_{jk}$ to be the average probability of classification into category k over those examiners observing subject i. Note that $\sum_k P_k(i) = 1$. Also, $Var_0\{X_{ik}\} = \sum_j \delta_{ij}^2 Var_0\{Z_{ijk}\} = \sum_j \delta_{ij} P_{jk} Q_{jk}$, where $Q_{jk} = 1 - P_{jk}$. Thus the expected number of pairs of examiners in agreement for subject i is $\frac{1}{2} E_0\{\sum_k X_{ik}^2 - m_i\} = \frac{1}{2}\{\sum_k \sum_j \delta_{ij} P_{jk} Q_{jk} + \sum_k [m_i P_k(i)]^2 - m_i\}$. It follows that the total expected chance agreement under random classification is $A_0 = \frac{1}{2}\{\sum_j \sum_k n_j P_{jk} Q_{jk} + \sum_i m_i^2 \sum_k P_k(i)^2 - \sum_i m_i\}$, and that $E_0\{\sum_i \sum_k X_{ik}(m_i - X_{ik})\} = E_0\{d\} = 2(A_m - A_0) = \sum_i m_i^2 \{\sum_k P_k(i) Q_k(i)\} - \sum_j n_j \sum_k P_{jk} Q_{jk}$. Define the observed quantities $p_{jk} = n_j^{-1} \sum_i \delta_{ij} Z_{ijk} = 1 - q_{jk}$ and $p_k(i) = m_i^{-1} \sum_j \delta_{ij} p_{jk} = 1 - q_k(i)$. Then $E_0\{p_{jk}\} = P_{jk}$ and $E_0\{p_k(i)\} = P_k(i)$, so that an estimate of $E_0\{\sum_i \sum_k X_{ik}(m_i - X_{ik})\}$, which is consistent as n_j becomes large for each j, is

$$e_0 = 2(a_m - a_0) = \sum_i m_i^2 \{\sum_k p_k(i) q_k(i)\} - \sum_j n_j \sum_k p_{jk} q_{jk} \qquad (3)$$

Therefore we take as our point estimate of kappa

$$\kappa = 1 - d/e_0 = 1 - \frac{\sum_i \sum_k X_{ik}(m_i - X_{ik})}{\sum_i m_i^2 \{\sum_k p_k(i) q_k(i)\} - \sum_j n_j \sum_k p_{jk} q_{jk}} \qquad (4)$$

We observe that Eq. 4 reduces to the estimate of kappa given by Davies and Fleiss[2] in the case of equal m_i. It differs somewhat from the one-way ANOVA estimate in the binary case ($c = 2$), where groups comprise subjects with m_i replicate zero-one observations (unless the m_i are equal, in which case the estimates agree; see Fleiss[3] p. 227). The ANOVA estimate derives from a different probability model wherein examiners are selected at random from a pool for each subject, the analysis of which effectively assumes identical rater characteristics.

Next, consider estimation of confidence limits for kappa in Eq. 2. Here we focus on the one-sided lower confidence limits of the form K_L for which $K_L \leq K \leq 1$ has approximate coverage probability $100(1 - \alpha)\%$. Two main approaches are available. Using unconditional inference methods, we can jackknife the estimate Eq. 4 and use the resulting standard error $se(\kappa)$ together with normal or Student's t critical values c_α to set the conventional limit $\kappa - c_\alpha se(\kappa)$.[4,5] Alternatively, we may use conditional inference methods to construct confidence limits for kappa conditional on fixed values of $\{\delta_{ij}\}$ and $s_{jk} \equiv \sum_i \delta_{ij} Z_{ijk}$ for all $j = 1, \ldots, m$ and $k = 1, \ldots, c$. This fixes p_{jk} and renders Eq. 4 a simple linear function of the pivotal statistic d. We consider each method briefly.

(i) To jackknife Eq. 4, calculate the estimates $\kappa_{(-i)}$ for $i = 1, \ldots, n$, each time deleting subject i (and corresponding δ_{ij} for $j = 1, \ldots, m$). Form the pseudovalues $\kappa_{(i)} = n\kappa - (n - 1)\kappa_{(-i)}$. Then the jackknife estimate of kappa is $\kappa_J = n^{-1} \sum_i \kappa_{(i)}$ and the jackknife standard error is $se_J = n^{-1/2}\{(n - 1)^{-1} \sum_i (\kappa_{(i)} - \kappa_J)^2\}^{1/2}$ which is taken as both $se(\kappa)$ and $se(\kappa_J)$. Then with c_α as above, set $K_L = \kappa_J - c_\alpha se_J$. The jackknife reduces bias in the estimation of kappa, is easy to apply, and provides a unique estimate in contrast to simulation based resampling methods. The jackknife confidence intervals have reasonably accurate coverage probability, albeit slightly conservative compared with the conditional estimates obtained below.

(ii) In order to examine the conditional distribution of kappa in some detail, we may simulate a screening model for the examination process with fixed $\{\delta_{ij}\}$ and $\{s_{jk}\}$ as follows. Subjects are assumed to belong to "true" categories (specified in the simulation but assumed unknown to the examiners). Given a subject in true category k^*, we suppose examiner j scores the subject in category k with probability $\pi_{jk}*_k$, where $\pi_{jk}*_1 + \cdots + \pi_{jk}*_c = 1$ for all (j,k). The classification arrays $\pi_j = \{\pi_{jk}*_k : (k^*, k) = 1, \ldots, c\}$ contain the examiners' multiple sensitivity–specificity operating characteristics. Then, given a specification of true categories, say θ_i, for each subject i, and the m classification arrays π_j, we generate, for examiner j, n_j multinomial responses $\{Y_{ij}: \delta_{ij} = 1\}$ from the conditional version of the polytomous logistic regression model

$$\log \frac{P[Y_{ij} = k \mid \theta_i]}{P[Y_{ij} = 1 \mid \theta_i]} = \alpha_{jk} + \beta_{j2k} I[\theta_i = 2] + \cdots$$

$$+ \beta_{jck} I[\theta_i = c] \quad (k = 2, \ldots, c) \quad (5)$$

In Eq. 5, α_{jk} is the log odds on examiner j scoring a subject who is in true category 1 in category k versus category 1; and $\beta_{jk}*_k$ is the difference in log odds (on scoring in category k versus category 1) between a subject in true category $\theta_i = k^*$ versus true category 1. The log odds ratios $\beta_{jk}*_k$ alone are sufficient to determine the conditional distribution $Z_{ijk} = I[Y_{ij} = k]$ given $\{\delta_{ij}\}$ and $\{s_{jk}\}$. An efficient algorithm for random sampling of Y_{ij} from the conditional distribution follows from Levin,[6] and details omitted here are contained in Levin.[7] Once we have Z_{ijk} for $\delta_{ij} = 1$ and set $Z_{ijk} = 0$ for $\delta_{ij} = 0$, we obtain the simulated values of X_{ik} and d; since e_0 is constant, we obtain finally $\kappa = 1 - d/e_0$.

Many parameter configurations $\{\pi_j\}$ and $\{\theta_i\}$ may be of interest for experimentation. For simulations most relevant to a given data set, we use for $\beta_{jk}*_k$ some multiple of the log odds ratios obtained from the empirical probabilities $\{(s_{jk}*_k + \frac{1}{2})/\sum_k (s_{jk}*_k + \frac{1}{2})\}$, where $s_{jk}*_k$ is the sum of terms $\delta_{ij} Z_{ijk}$ over those subjects i for whom $\theta_i = k^*$. The "true" categories θ_i may be assigned by consensus classification from the observed scores, such that $X_{ik}* = \max_k X_{ik}$, with arbitrary breaking of modal ties. Generally with a few hundred simulations, we can estimate the conditional distribution of κ and its moments. We find the distributions to be left skewed for large kappa, so that it may be desirable to estimate confidence limits empirically from the tails of the simulated values. This tends to produce narrower confidence intervals than does the jackknife. An illustration follows.

Example: The scores of $n = 26$ children by $m = 7$ examiners on the $c = 3$ category item "Gets up off floor to standing" are displayed in the first seven columns of EXHIBIT 1. A zero indicates $\delta_{ij} = 0$; $1 = $ yes; $2 = $ no; $3 = $ not assessed/not in state. Column 8 gives the consensus classification (there were no modality ties). Column 9 reports values of $d_i = \sum_k X_{ik}(m_i - X_{ik})$, and column 10 gives $e_0(i) = m_i^2 \sum_k p_k(i) q_k(i) - \sum_j \delta_{ij} \sum_k p_{jk} q_{jk}$ such that $e_0 = \sum_i e_0(i)$. Columns 11–13 provide $p_k(i)$ for $k = 1, 2, 3$. The value of kappa for this item is $\kappa = 1 - d/e_0 =$

EXHIBIT 1. Calculation of Kappa for Item "Gets off Floor to Standing"[a]

Subject	Examiners 1 2 3 4 5 6 7	Consensus (8)	d_i (9)	$e_0(i)$ (10)	$p_k(i)$ (11)	(12)	(13)
1	2 2 0 2 1 2 2	2	10	16.502	0.5808	0.3308	0.0885
2	2 2 0 2 2 2 2	2	0	16.502	0.5808	0.3308	0.0885
3	2 2 0 2 1 2 2	2	10	16.502	0.5808	0.3308	0.0885
4	2 2 0 2 3 2 2	2	10	16.502	0.5808	0.3308	0.0885
5	2 2 0 2 3 2 2	2	10	16.502	0.5808	0.3308	0.0885
6	2 1 0 2 1 2 2	2	16	16.502	0.5808	0.3308	0.0885
7	2 2 0 2 3 2 2	2	10	16.502	0.5808	0.3308	0.0885
8	1 1 0 1 1 1 1	1	0	16.502	0.5808	0.3308	0.0885
9	1 1 0 1 1 1 1	1	0	16.502	0.5808	0.3308	0.0885
10	1 1 0 1 1 1 1	1	0	16.502	0.5808	0.3308	0.0885
11	1 1 0 1 0 1 1	1	0	10.479	0.5769	0.3769	0.0462
12	1 1 0 1 0 1 1	1	0	10.479	0.5769	0.3769	0.0462
13	3 1 0 3 0 3 3	3	8	10.479	0.5769	0.3769	0.0462
14	2 2 0 2 0 2 2	2	0	10.479	0.5769	0.3769	0.0462
15	1 1 1 3 0 1 1	1	10	15.043	0.6197	0.3419	0.0385
16	1 1 1 3 0 1 1	1	10	15.043	0.6197	0.3419	0.0385
17	1 1 1 1 0 1 1	1	0	15.043	0.6197	0.3419	0.0385
18	1 1 1 1 0 1 1	1	0	15.043	0.6197	0.3419	0.0385
19	1 1 1 1 0 1 1	1	0	15.043	0.6197	0.3419	0.0385
20	2 2 2 2 0 2 2	2	0	15.043	0.6197	0.3419	0.0385
21	1 1 1 1 0 1 1	1	0	15.043	0.6197	0.3419	0.0385
22	1 1 1 1 0 1 1	1	0	15.043	0.6197	0.3419	0.0385
23	1 1 1 1 0 1 1	1	0	15.043	0.6197	0.3419	0.0385
24	2 2 2 2 0 2 2	2	0	15.043	0.6197	0.3419	0.0385
25	1 1 1 1 0 1 1	1	0	15.043	0.6197	0.3419	0.0385
26	1 1 1 1 0 1 1	1	0	15.043	0.6197	0.3419	0.0385

$$d = \sum_i d_i = 94 \qquad 387.46 = \sum_i e_0(i) = e_0$$
$$\kappa = 1 - d/e_0 = 1 - 94/387.46 = 0.7574$$

[a] Coding of subject scores: 0 = not scheduled ($\delta_{ij} = 0$); 1 = yes; 2 = no; 3 = not assessed/not in state.

1 − 94/387.46 = 0.7574, excellent agreement in the phraseology of Landis and Koch[8]; (see also Fleiss,[3] p. 218). The sums $\{s_{jk}\}$ are given in the first three columns of EXHIBIT 2, and the corresponding $\{p_{jk}\}$ are given in the final three columns.

The jackknifed estimate of kappa is $\kappa_J = 0.7631$ with $se_J = 0.0578$. The lower one-sided 95% confidence limit K_L for kappa based on the Student critical value $t_{.05,25} = 1.708$ is $K_L = \kappa - t_{.05,25} se_J = 0.6644$, and the lower limit based on the normal critical value $z_{.05} = 1.645$ is $\kappa - z_{.05} se_J = 0.6680$.

EXHIBIT 3 gives the empirical classification arrays for each examiner. These give rise to the $\beta_{jk}^*{}_k$ parameters, also shown. We first multiplied each of the latter values by 1.5 in order to partly offset the shrinking toward zero that results when one-half is added to each cell frequency in the calculation of the empirical classification probabilities. Using these parameters and the consensus classifications from column 8 of EXHIBIT 1, we simulated 400 replications from the conditional distribution given fixed $\{\delta_{ij}\}$ and $\{s_{jk}\}$. The resulting histogram is shown in EXHIBIT 4. Note the negative skewness of the distribution. The mean value of kappa in the simulations was 0.7306, not far from the actual estimate of kappa from these

EXHIBIT 2. Marginal Distribution of Classification

Examiner	Classification $\{s_{jk}\}$				Probability $\{p_{jk}\}$		
	$k = 1$	2	3	n_j	1	2	3
1	15	10	1	26	0.5769	0.3846	0.0385
2	17	9	0	26	0.6538	0.3462	0
3	10	2	0	12	0.8333	0.1667	0
4	13	10	3	26	0.5000	0.3846	0.1154
5	6	1	3	10	0.6000	0.1000	0.3000
6	15	10	1	26	0.5769	0.3846	0.0385
7	15	10	1	26	0.5769	0.3846	0.0385

data, and the standard deviation of the simulated kappas was 0.0289, substantially smaller than the unconditional jackknife estimate se_J. The proportion of simulated values of κ greater than or equal to 0.7574 was 79/400 = 0.1975. To estimate the conditional lower 95% confidence limit from the empirical distributions, we require that value of K for which the proportion of simulated values in excess of 0.7574 is 5%. Toward this end, we repeated the simulation experiment with values of $\beta_{jk}{^*}_k$ inflated by only 1.25, and again with no inflation. Lagrange interpolation of

EXHIBIT 3. Empirical Classification Probabilities $\{(s_{jk}{^*}_k + \frac{1}{2})/\sum_k(s_{jk}{^*}_k + \frac{1}{2})\}$ and Log Odds Ratio Parameters $\{\beta_{jk}{^*}_k\}$

Examiner j			Classification Probabilities			Log Odds Ratio Parameters		
		$k =$	1	2	3	$k =$	2	3
1		1	0.9394	0.0303	0.0303			
	$k^* =$ True	2	0.0435	0.9130	0.0435	2	6.4785	3.4340
		3	0.2	0.2	0.6	3	3.4340	4.5326
2		1	0.9395	0.0303	0.0303			
		2	0.1304	0.8261	0.0435	2	5.2798	2.3354
		3	0.6	0.2	0.2	3	2.3354	2.3354
3		1	0.9130	0.0435	0.0435			
		2	0.1430	0.7143	0.1429	2	4.6540	3.0445
		3	0.3333	0.3333	0.3333	3	3.0445	3.0445
4		1	0.8182	0.0303	0.1515			
		2	0.0435	0.9130	0.0435	2	6.3404	1.6864
		3	0.2	0.2	0.6	3	3.2958	2.7850
5		1	0.7778	0.1111	0.1111			
		2	0.4118	0.1765	0.4118	2	1.0986	1.9459
		3	0.3333	0.3333	0.3333	3	1.9459	1.9459
6		1	0.9394	0.0303	0.0303			
		2	0.0435	0.9130	0.0435	2	6.4785	3.4340
		3	0.2	0.2	0.6	3	3.4340	4.5326
7		1	0.9394	0.0303	0.0303			
		2	0.0435	0.9130	0.0435	2	6.4785	3.4340
		3	0.2	0.2	0.6	3	3.4340	4.5326

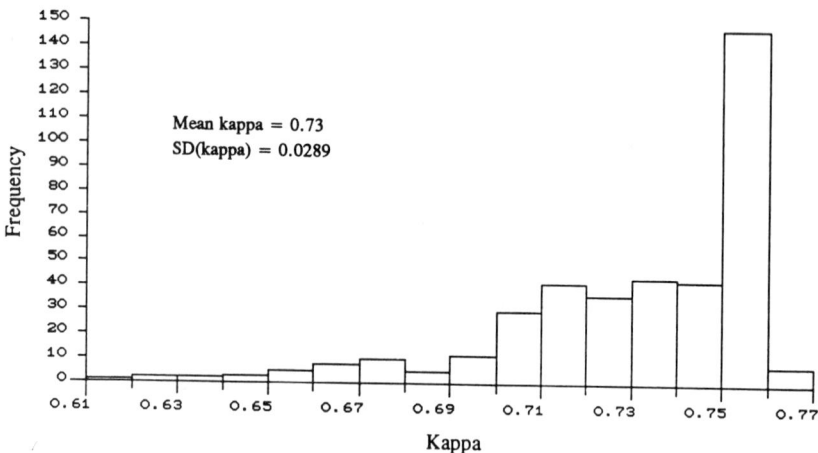

EXHIBIT 4. Histogram of simulated kappas.

the three simulation means by the proportions in excess of 0.7574 yielded at 5% the lower limit as $K_L = 0.6823$.

REFERENCES

1. COHEN, J. 1960. A coefficient of agreement for nominal scales. Educ. Psychol. Meas. **20:** 37–46.
2. DAVIES, M. & J. L. FLEISS. 1982. Measuring agreement for multinomial data. Biometrics **38:** 1047–1051.
3. FLEISS, J. L. 1981. Statistical Methods for Rates and Proportions. 2nd edit. Wiley. New York.
4. MILLER, R. G. 1964. A trustworthy jackknife. Ann. Math. Statist. **35:** 1594–1605.
5. QUENOUILLE, M. H. 1956. Notes on bias in estimation. Biometrika **43:** 352–360.
6. LEVIN, B. 1987. Conditional likelihood analysis in stratum-matched retrospective studies with polytomous disease states. Comm. Stat. **B16(3):** 699–718.
7. LEVIN, B. 1992. Sampling from the conditional polytomous logistic regression model. Technical Report B-80, Division of Biostatistics, Columbia University. New York.
8. LANDIS, J. R. & G. G. KOCH. 1977. The measurement of observer agreement for categorical data. Biometrics **33:** 159–174.

Assessing Neurobehavioral Changes in HIV+ Infants and Children

A Methodological Approach

EILEEN B. FENNELL

Department of Clinical and Health Psychology
University of Florida
Gainesville, Florida 32610

EPIDEMIOLOGY OF PEDIATRIC HIV INFECTION AND PEDIATRIC AIDS

In 1982, the first case of pediatric AIDS was reported by the Centers for Disease Control (CDC).[1] One years later, the first case of transfusion-associated AIDS was described.[2] Since that time, there has been a steady increase in the number of children reported to the CDC who are HIV seropositive or who present with evidence of immunosuppression and any of the many manifestations of pediatric AIDS.[3,4] Currently, children and adolescents represent about 2% of the total reported cases of AIDS, with children under 5 years representing the largest percentage at about 67%.[5] Although the incidence of transfusion or coagulation product acquired HIV infection has stabilized since the development of blood-screening tests, the incidence of perinatally acquired HIV infection is on the rise.[3] For example, it is estimated that approximately 6000 infected women of child-bearing age are delivering infants annually in the United States. If the vertical transmission rate is about 30%, this would lead to 1600 to 1800 children becoming infected per year.[6] By January, 1993, there will be more than 4000 cases of pediatric AIDS reported to the CDC, with approximately 85% of these cases acquired through vertical transmission from an infected mother. Epidemiological data on adolescents is still scarce, but it is estimated that there are currently 20,000 infected adolescents. Of these cases, 75% occur between the ages of 17 and 19 years, with a 4:1 male-to-female ratio as compared to adult sex ratios of 10:1 male to female and a suspected 1:1 ratio in infants.[6,7] The largest number of pediatric HIV cases occur in African–American, Hispanic, or other recently immigrated minorities.

Routes of Transmission

Among infants, it is likely that the predominant form of transmission will be vertically acquired HIV infection. The precise route of vertical transmission remains to be determined. Suggested routes include either intrauterine via transplacental mechanisms, intrapartum via exposure to maternal blood or vaginal secretions, or postpartum via breast milk or colostrum.[6] Among adolescents, i.v. drug abuse, homosexual or bisexual contact, and heterosexual contact with an infected person remain the likely modes of transmission. There remains that small percentage of cases where infection occurred via blood or coagulation factor products.[5]

Characteristics of Pediatric HIV Infection

In 1985 and again in 1987, the CDC published clinical criteria for the diagnosis of pediatric AIDS. This classification scheme recognized the observed differences in both the presentation and in the course of HIV infection between children and adults (TABLE 1). As TABLE 1 describes, the clinical manifestations of HIV infection in children is variable but can include skin, pulmonary, gastrointestinal, cardiovascular, lymphatic, hepatic, and central nervous system involvement. With dis-

TABLE 1. CDC Classification for HIV in Children

Class P-O Indeterminate Infection

    Infants below age 15 months born to infected mothers but without evidence of HIV infection or AIDS

Class P-1 Asymptomatic Infection

    Normal immune function (subclass A)
    Abnormal immune function (subclass B)
    Immune function not tested (subclass C)

Class P-2 Symptomatic Infection

    Nonspecific findings (two or more for two or more months); fever, failure to thrive, generalized lymphadenopathy, hepatomegaly, splenomegaly, enlarged parotid glands, persistent or recurrent diarrhea (Subclass A)

    Progressive neurologic disease: loss of developmental milestones or intellectual ability, impaired brain growth or progressive symmetrical motor deficits (Subclass B)

    Lymphoid interstitial pneumonitis (subclass C)
    Secondary infectious diseases (subclass D)

    D-1: Opportunistic infections in the CDC case definition (bacterial, fungal, parasitic, viral)
    D-2: Unexplained, recurrent serious bacterial infections (two or more in a two-year period)
    D-3: Other infectious diseases such as oral candidiasis, recurrent herpes stomatitis or multidermatomal or disseminated herpes zoster

    Secondary Cancers (subclass E)

    E-1: Cancers in the AIDS case definition
    E-2: Other malignancies possibly associated with HIV

    Other conditions possibly due to HIV infection such as hepatitis, cardiopathy, nephropathy, hematologic disorders, or dermatologic diseases

TABLE 2. Comorbidity Factors in Pediatric HIV Infection

> Intrauterine exposure to illicit drugs
> Poor maternal health and prenatal care
> Prematurity or low birth weight
> Low socioeconomic status
> Maternal neglect
> Language/ethnic minority
> Foster care placement
> Compliance with treatment

ease progression, neurological and neurodevelopmental symptoms may be the most prominent feature of the clinical picture.[8–11] The course of the illness from initial infection to symptomatic state in adult cases appears to be quite protracted, with some estimates of up to 10 years. In contrast, estimates from some early studies of pediatric cases were of an incubation period as short as 8 to 10 months.[6,7] Current experience suggests that children with HIV infection probably have a longer life expectancy up until the development of AIDS. Once a diagnosis of AIDS is made, progression may be quite rapid. Comparisons of the course of transfusion or coagulation factor acquired cases of pediatric AIDS with the course of vertically acquired infection suggest that the incubation period is longer for infections resulting from blood or blood products.[3,4]

Comorbidity Factors in Pediatric HIV Infection

In 1984, the federal government began to establish funding for AIDS research centers. Many of these centers designed longitudinal studies that were intended increase understanding of the natural history of the course of the disease.[13] Most of these centers were established in areas with high numbers of HIV-infected patients, so-called epicenters. Some included studies of cohorts of children with vertically acquired or transfusion-acquired HIV infection. A major thrust of these early centers was an examination of the neurological course of HIV infection. This thrust was in response to evidence that neurological and neurobehavioral changes were a primary manifestation of the disease process. It was in these centers that many large-scale early treatment efficacy studies were also undertaken. In 1988, the National Institutes of Health (NIH) established 13 clinical trials groups for pediatric AIDS.[13] As a result, the focus of much research was shifted from natural history studies to studies of the effectiveness of monotherapy or combinations of drugs that showed promise in halting the progression of HIV infection in children.[14,15] With the emergence of drug therapies, the focus of many clinical trials shifted to assessing treatment efficacy by both immunological parameters and neurobehavioral endpoints. These studies are still under way.

As experience grew with studies of the natural history of pediatric HIV infection and AIDS, a number of comorbidity factors began to be identified (TABLE 2). These factors had an impact in the types of assessments used, the types of control groups used, and even in the interpretation of the meaning of results. For example, did children born to i.v. drug-abusing mothers really have a worse developmental outcome because of the HIV infection or could some of the variance be accounted for by polydrug exposure *in utero,* nutritional factors, prenatal care, foster care placement, or examination procedures that were not typically standardized on lower socioeconomic, nonnative-English-speaking children. The impact of these comorbidities on efficacy of drug therapy is still under examination.

NEUROLOGICAL MANIFESTATIONS OF PEDIATRIC HIV INFECTION AND AIDS

It is estimated that between 78% and 93% of HIV-infected children will have neurological manifestations of the disease.[8,16,17] Clinical manifestations of neurological involvement include encephalopathy; acquired microcephaly; cognitive deficits; pyramidal, extrapyramidal, and cerebellar signs; seizures; developmental delays; myopathies; and peripheral neuropathies. These abnormalities can result from opportunistic viral and nonviral infections of the central or peripheral nervous system, neoplasms, and cerebrovascular lesions from hemorrhagic episodes or vasculitis.[18,19] The clinical course of the neurological manifestations of HIV infection and AIDS has been described as having at least three patterns: an acutely progressive course, a course characterized as typical of static encephalopathy, and a course described as a plateau (indolent) course. The characteristic features of each of these clinical pictures is described by Dr. Anita Belman in an earlier chapter in this volume.[20] As her paper and that of Dr. Ram Kairam[21] have noted, there are a number of findings in the neurological examination and in the neuroimaging studies of these children. Among the pathological findings reported in studies of children with AIDS are lower brain weights; diffuse gliosis of cortical and subcortical nuclei; focal necrosis of gray and white matter; perivascular inflammation; calcification of the basal ganglia, centrum ovale, and frontal lobes; atrophy; and ventricular dilation.

NEUROPSYCHOLOGICAL STUDIES OF PEDIATRIC HIV INFECTION

Neuropsychological studies of HIV-infected children and adolescents can be broadly divided into studies of vertically acquired HIV-infected infants and children and those that have studied children and adolescents who have acquired the HIV infection through transfusions or coagulation factor blood products. Studies of infants and children with vertically acquired infection have reported a number of problems in their development[22-24] (TABLE 3). In contrast, studies of transfused or hemophiliac children and adolescents have generally reported no significant differences between HIV-seropositive and HIV-seronegative subjects until the children become symptomatic.[25] Studies of children who have received treatment with antiretroviral drugs such as ziduvodine (AZT) and dideoxycytidine (DDI) alone or in combination, while preliminary, suggest that these drugs may prevent progression or even lead to improvements in cognitive functioning in small groups

TABLE 3. Common Problems Reported in Children with Perinatally Acquired HIV Infection

Cognitive delays
Language delays
Gross motor problems
Fine motor problems
Attentional disorders
Hyperactivity
Need for special education
Emotional withdrawal
Apathy

of children.[14,15] Even these findings, however, are not without some controversy.[26]

METHODOLOGICAL PROBLEMS IN CURRENT PEDIATRIC AIDS STUDIES

This section addresses only studies of vertically acquired pediatric HIV infection. Any attempt to develop a comprehensive picture of our understanding of pediatric HIV infection and its effects on the developing brain is hampered by a number of methodological issues that have complicated interpretation of published work. Somewhat similar concerns have been raised about adult studies in HIV-1 infection and AIDS.[27]

As summarized in TABLE 4, these problems develop from the use of different neuropsychological measures across study sites, the absence of appropriate control or contrast groups, the absence of culturally sensitive normative data or test translations, the need for better assessment of home/environmental factors that could affect development, the complications of embedding treatment aims in longitudinal studies, and the nature of the analytical approaches employed to interpret the clinical data that has been obtained. Unfortunately, to date no published large-scale studies in pediatric AIDS have attempted to correlate findings from repeated neuropsychological or cognitive assessments with the neurological findings on clinical examination or with the CT scan or MRI imaging studies of these children.

TABLE 4. Methodological Problems in Current Pediatric HIV-1 and AIDS Studies

Lack of common testing instruments
Lack of appropriate test translations or minority normative data
Testing often embedded in visits for medical treatments
Missing data due to illness or compliance problems
No or limited control/comparison groups
Personnel problems
Absence of measures of general adjustment/psychopathology
Traditional analytic approaches emphasizing levels of performance

Instead, data is generally presented by staging group. As a result, it is very difficult to draw clinicopathological relationships between changes in cognitive or neuropsychological performance and changes in clinical state. A second problem relates to the meaning of so-called "delays" in development, given the presence of many comorbidity factors in these children and the relative paucity of information about control groups that share similar risk factors. A third issue is the analytic approach generally employed in published studies. Most commonly, data is analyzed by a level of performance approach such as analysis of variance. Although such an approach allows one to describe the typical performance on a measure of a given group, it is relatively less sensitive to individual differences among members of that group compared to another. In addition, such statistical approaches are relatively unforgiving of missing data points—an unfortunately common event in many studies owing to illness (too ill to be tested) to compliance (did not show for the examination), or to procedure (examiner or patient unavailability because of conflicting protocol demands). These problems become more acute if, as in many current treatment protocols, the endpoint is change in neurobehavioral findings. One final concern is the problem of the natural evolution of the illness itself such that a child entering a longitudinal protocol will inevitably change patient group membership as the disease progresses. If the intent of a study is to assess changes on selected dependent measures, one consequence of this phenomenon is instability of comparison group membership, which can result in loss of power with multiple outcome measures.

DEVELOPMENT OF ACTG PROTOCOL 188: NEURODEVELOPMENTAL AND NEUROLOGICAL STUDY OF INFANTS AND CHILDREN WITH HIV INFECTION AND AIDS IN CLINICAL TRIALS

In response to these concerns, in 1990 a series of conferences were convened by the National Institute of Mental Health (NIMH). These conferences were designed to evaluate current methods in studies of pediatric HIV infection. Experts in the areas of pediatric behavioral nosology, pediatric neurology, child neuropsychology, and longitudinal design methods were given the task of critically examining ways in which future studies of pediatric HIV might optimize the approaches from these various disciplines. A goal of these meetings was to develop a research approach that was sensitive to the problems of clinical treatments in longitudinal studies of children who may develop neurobehavioral disorders as a consequence of their illness (NIMH Neurological and Neurobehavioral Task Force in Pediatric AIDS). With the subsequent support of the NIMH, National Institute of Childhood Health and Development (NICHD), and National Institute of Allergy and Infectious Diseases (NIAID), a methodological study was designed. Subsequent meetings with the ACTG Pediatric Groups eventually led to the development of the present Protocol 188, to its acceptance by the Clinical Trials Group, and to its initiation, linked for purposes of recruitment of subjects to a current protocol. This linked protocol is a three-arm clinical trial of AZT and DDI (ACTG No. 152). The goal of the present study is to assess neurodevelopment as a primary endpoint in ACTG clinical trials research. Unlike previous protocols, this study uses assessment methods that are conceptually related to domains of brain development and uses growth curve analytic methods in order to capture changes in development that might occur as the illness progresses. Domains to be assessed are those that represent functional abilities that emerge over the course of growth, development, and school experiences. These domains include cognition, language, gross and fine motor skills, constructional skills, attention, and achievement. The age span to be examined ranges from infancy to adolescence. Tests that have been shown to be sensitive to changes that accompany other chronic diseases of children were chosen within each domain across age groupings. Two assessment methods will be employed: frequent brief assays of behaviors that are state-responsive (monitoring battery) and less frequent assays of behaviors that are more closely related to the attainment of developmental growth (comprehensive battery). In addition, a brief neurological examination was developed that was designed to be closely linked to the neurobehavioral/neuropsychological assessments. Problems of multicultural assessment were addressed by developing Spanish translations and norms for all tests and procedures as well as requiring a bilingual examiner. Parallel testing of several different control/contrast groups are also a part of this study. These groups will allow the study to more precisely address comorbid factors such as socioeconomic status. Procedures for training and certifying all examiners at each of the six currently participating sites were developed. Site-specific needs were addressed in order to enhance the likelihood of enrollment and compliance with the protocol. Included among these was the need for full-time, dedicated personnel on the project and the development of on-site entry and computerized scoring of all examinations.

ANALYTIC METHOD OF PROTOCOL 188

A unique feature of this study is the planned approach to data analysis. Based on the recommendations of a number of experts, a three-phase data analysis plan was developed. Following data screening and reduction, a traditional general linear model approach will be employed in which analysis will focus on either the level of attainment (ANOVA, MANOVA, MANCOVA) or on time-linked analysis (trends over time). In this phase, demographic, immunological, and neurological factors will be addressed as they relate to effects in level of performance over the multiple assessments. This will allow for direct comparison with other ongoing studies. In the next phase, growth curve analysis of change will be employed.[28,29] In this approach, the individual rather than the group becomes the object of study as individual patterns of attainment on scores are developed. This approach allows us to study more precisely potential heterogeneity between subjects in patterns of change. As such, the emphasis is not on group differences but on individual differences in change. Finally, correlates of changes in individual growth parameters are then examined. This individual growth perspective, which views analysis of the process of change as the primary focus, allows us to describe the process of change at the individual and at the group level. Such an approach would allow the redefinition of endpoints in clinical treatment from such traditional clinical endpoints as change in CDC classification or loss of two standard deviations in

IQ to parameters of rapid change, positive or negative, in a developing skill. It will also permit the analysis of subtypes of responses to HIV infection at different stages in the course of the disease. This subtype analytical approach has been applied in other childhood disorders, such as learning disabilities, with considerable success. As a result, the different neurological abnormalities, age-dependent neuropsychological deficits, and developmental course of dyslexia as compared to attention deficit disorder (ADD) have now become apparent. It is our hope that a similar outcome will occur in studies of HIV-infected children. From such a knowledge base, better and potentially earlier treatments (biological, psychological, educational) can be effectively instituted.

SUMMARY

The rationale and development of a developmental approach to assessing neurobehavioral changes in infants and children exposed to or infected with the HIV-1 virus is presented. Methodological problems in earlier approaches to assessment are reviewed. Among these are measures employed, impact of different treatments on measures of outcome, multicultural differences between samples, and analytic approaches to developmental data. The assessment protocol developed by the Pediatric Neurobehavioral Study Group of NIMH/NICHD/NIAID is described.

THE PROTOCOL 188 TEAM

The following is a complete listing of those persons who are members of the Protocol 188 team with their roles listed in parentheses: Barbara Wilson, Ph.D., Northshore University Hospital (Project Investigator); Anita L. Belman, M.D., SUNY Stony Brook (Co-P.I.).: Jack Fletcher, Ph.D., University of Houston (Methodologist); David Francis, Ph.D., University of Houston (Methodologist); Susan Landry, Ph.D., University of Texas, Infant Studies (Consultant to NIMH); Eileen B. Fennell, Ph.D., University of Florida, Child Studies (Consultant to NIMH); Ena Vasquez-Nuttal, Ph.D., Boston University (Multicultural); Jack Moye, M.D. (NIAID/NICHD); Mary Glenn Fowler, M.D. (NIAID/NICHD); and Willo Pequegnat, Ph.D. (Project Officer).

REFERENCES

1. CENTERS FOR DISEASE CONTROL. 1982. Unexplained immunodeficiency and opportunistic infection in infants—New York, New Jersey, California. Morbid. Mortal. Wkly. Rep. **31:** 665–667.
2. AMMANN, A. J., M. J. COWAN, D. W. WARA, P. WEINTRAUB, S. DRITZ, H. GOLDMAN & H. A. PERKINS. Acquired immunodeficiency in an infant: Possible transmission by means of blood products. Lancet April **30:** 956–958.
3. OXTOBY, M. J. 1990. Perinatally acquired HIV infection. *In* Pediatric AIDS: The Challenge of HIV Infection in Infants, Children and Adolescents. P. A. Pizzo & C. A. Wilfert, Eds.: 3–21. Williams & Wilkins. Baltimore.
4. EYSTER, M. E. 1990. Transfusion and coagulation factor acquired disease. *In* Pediatric

AIDS: The Challenge of HIV Infection in Infants, Children and Adolescents. P. A. Pizzo & C. A. Wilfert, Eds.: 22–37. Williams & Wilkins. Baltimore.
5. HENGGELER, S. W., G. B. MELTON & J. R. RODRIGUEZ. 1992. Pediatric and Adolescent AIDS: Research Findings from the Social Sciences. Sage Publications. Newbury Park, CA.
6. BOYLAND, L. & Z. A. STEIN. 1991. The epidemiology of HIV infection in children and their mothers. Epidemiol. Rev. 13: 143–177.
7. GAYLE, H. D. & L. J. D'ANGELO. 1990. The epidemiology of AIDS and HIV infection in adolescents. In Pediatric AIDS: The Challenge of HIV Infection in Infants, Children and Adolescents. P. A. Pizzo & C. A. Wilfert, Eds.: 38–50. Williams & Wilkins. Baltimore.
8. BELMAN, A. L. 1992. Acquired immunodeficiency syndrome and the child's central nervous system. Pediatr. Clin. North Am. 39(4): 691–714.
9. EPSTEIN, L. G., J. GOUDSMIT, D. A. PAUL, S. H. MORRISON, E. M. CONNOR, J. M. OLESKE & B. HOLLAND. 1987. Expression of human immunodeficiency virus in cerebral spinal fluid of children with progressive encephalopathy. Ann. Neurol. 21: 397–401.
10. SCOTT, G. B., B. E. BUCK, J. G. LETERMAN, F. L. BLOOM & W. P. PARKS. 1984. Acquired immunodeficiency in infants. N. Engl. J. Med. 310: 76–81.
11. ULTMANN, M. H., A. L. BELMAN, H. A. RUFF, B. E. NOVICK, B. CONE-WESSON, H. J. COHEN & A. RUBINSTEIN. 1989. Developmental abnormalities in infants and children with acquired immune deficiency syndrome (AIDS) and AIDS-related complex. Dev. Med. Child Neurol. 27: 563–571.
12. AYLWARD, E. H., A. M. BUTZ, N. HUTTON, M. L. JOYNER & J. W. VOGELHUT. 1992. Cognitive and motor development in infants at risk for human immunodeficiency virus. Am. J. Dis. Child. 146: 218–222.
13. NOVELLO, A. & P. H. WISE. 1990. Public policy issues. In Pediatric AIDS: The Challenge of HIV Infection in Infants, Children and Adolescents. P. A. Pizzo & C. A. Wilfert, Eds.: 745–755. Williams & Wilkins. Baltimore.
14. PIZZO, P. A., J. EDDY, J. FALLOON, F. M. BALIS, R. F. MURPHEY, H. MOSS, P. WOLTERS, P. BROUWERS, P. JAROSINSKI, M. RUBIN, S. BRODER, R. YARCHOAN, A. BRUNETTE, M. MAHA, S. NUSINOFF-LEHRMAN & D. POPLACK. 1988. Effect of continuous intravenous infusion of zidovudine (AZT) in children with symptomatic HIV infection. N. Engl. J. Med. 319: 889–896.
15. WOLTERS, P., P. BROUWERS, H. MOSS, D. EL AMIN, F. BALIS, K. BUTLER & P. A. PIZZO. 1991. The effect of dideoxyinosine (DDI) on the cognitive functioning of infants and children with infection after six and 12 months of treatment. VII International Conference on AIDS, Padua, Italy. Abstract no. 194.
16. SCHWARCZ, S. K. & G. W. RUTHERFORD. 1989. Acquired immunodeficiency syndrome in infants, children and adolescents. J. Drug Iss. 19: 75–92.
17. EPSTEIN, L. G., L. R. SHARER, V. V. JOSHI, M. M. FOJAS, M. R. KOENIGSBERGER & J. M. OLESKE. 1984. Progressive encephalopathy in children with acquired immunodeficiency syndrome. Ann. Neurol. 17: 488–496.
18. BROUWERS, P., A. L. BELMAN & L. G. EPSTEIN. Central nervous system involvement: Manifestations and evaluation. Pediatric AIDS: The Challenge of HIV Infection in Infants, Children and Adolescents. P. A. Pizzo & C. A. Wilfert, Eds.: 318–335. Williams & Wilkins. Baltimore.
19. SCOTT, G. B. & C. HUTTO. 1990. Prognosis in pediatric HIV infection. In Pediatric AIDS: The Challenge of HIV Infection in Infants, Children and Adolescents. P. A. Pizzo & C. A. Wilfert, Eds.: 187–198. Williams & Wilkins. Baltimore.
20. BELMAN, A. L. 1993. Neurologic syndromes. Ann. N. Y. Acad. Sci. This volume.
21. KAIRAM, R. 1993. Reliability of neurologic assessment in a collaborative study of HIV infection in children. Ann. N. Y. Acad. Sci. This volume.
22. HITTELMAN, J. 1990. Neurodevelopmental aspects of HIV infection. In Brain in Pediatric AIDS. P. B. Kozlowski, D. A. Souder, P. M. Vietze & H. M. Wisniewski, Eds.: 64–71. S. Karger. Basel.
23. DIAMOND, G. W., P. GURDIN, A. A. WIZNIA, A. L. BELMAN & H. J. COHEN. 1990.

Effects of congenital HIV infection on neurodevelopmental status of babies in foster care. Dev. Med. Child Neurol. **32:** 999–1004.
24. HITTELMAN, J., A. WILLOUGHBY, N. NELSON, J. GONG, H. MENDEZ, S. HOLMAN, J. GOEDERT & S. LANDESMAN. 1991. Neurodevelopmental outcome of perinatally acquired HIV infection in the first 24 months of life. VII International Conference on AIDS, Padua, Italy. Abstract no. 65.
25. WHITT, J. K., S. R. HOOPER & M. B. TENNISON. 1991. Longitudinal patterns of neuropsychologic functioning in HIV-infected children with hemophilia. VII International Conference on AIDS, Padua, Italy. Abstract no. 66.
26. NOZYCE, M., M. WEISBERGER, S. ARPADI, G. LAMBER & A. WIZNIA. 1991. Oral AZT therapy on neurodevelopmental functioning. VII International Conference on AIDS, Padua, Italy. Abstract no. 206.
27. VAN GORP, N., D. G. LAMB & F. A. SCHMITT. 1993. Methodological issues in neuropsychology research with HIV-spectrum disease. Arch. Clin. Neuropsychol. **8:** 17–34.
28. FLETCHER, J. M., D. J. FRANCIS, W. PEQUEGNAT, S. W. RADENBUSH, M. H. BORNSTEIN, F. SCHMIDT, P. BROUWERS & E. STOVER. 1991. Neurobehavioral outcomes in diseases of childhood. Am. Psychol. **46:** 1267–1277.
29. FRANCIS, D. J., J. M. FLETCHER, K. K. STUEBING, K. C. DAVIDSON & N. M. THOMPSON. 1991. Analysis of change: Modeling individual growth. J. Consult. Clin. Psychol. **59:** 27–37.

Intravenous Gammaglobulin for Pediatric HIV-1 Infection

Effects on Infectious Complications, Circulating Immune Complexes, and CD4 Cell Decline

ARYE RUBINSTEIN,[a] THERESA CALVELLI, AND
R. RUBINSTEIN

*Department of Pediatrics, Microbiology, and Immunology
Albert Einstein College of Medicine
Bronx, New York 10461*

The use of intravenous gammaglobulin (IVIG) in the treatment of HIV-1 infected children was initially introduced by us in 1979. Between 1978 and 1981, before the acquired immunodeficiency syndrome (AIDS) was a known entity, we identified a cluster of immunodeficient children with recurrent bacterial infections, including sepsis and meningitis. Paradoxically, these patients exhibited a hypergammaglobulinemia despite their clinical picture, suggesting a humoral immune defect.[1,2] We have, therefore, treated these children monthly with 100 to 200 mg/kg body weight IVIG as employed for agammaglobulinemic patients.[3-5] By 1981 it became evident that these children probably were suffering from AIDS, that their immunodeficiency was much broader than was initially appreciated and was accompanied by autoimmune phenomena and T-cell aberrations. In order to address these additional issues, a modified IVIG regimen of a biweekly infusion of 300 mg/kg was introduced.[6] In our preliminary reports in 1985 and 1986, we demonstrated that this new regimen reduced the incidence of infections, decreased hospital admission days, and resulted in beneficial immunomodulatory effects that were not as obvious with the monthly regimen.[6]

Following our reports, several additional uncontrolled studies in HIV-1 infected children seemed to confirm the reduction of infectious complications by IVIG.[7-10] The first attempt by Swiss investigators[10] to blind IVIG treatment against intravenous albumin failed when health care personnel were able to identify placebo-treated children, who did not fare as well as IVIG-treated patients. In 1988, the

---

[a] Address for correspondence: Arye Rubinstein, M.D., Albert Einstein College of Medicine, Department of Pediatrics, Microbiology & Immunology, 1300 Morris Park Avenue, Bronx, New York 10461.

National Institutes of Child Health and Human Development (NICHD) in the United States embarked on a multicenter, placebo-controlled, randomized IVIG trial.[11] Although this study confirmed the benefit of IVIG for HIV-1 infected children with $CD4^+$ T-cell counts over $200/mm^3$, many issues remained unresolved. In the present paper we will address these issues in the context of our own 14-year experience with this therapy.

STUDY POPULATION

Between 1982 and 1992, 93 patients have received Gamimune (Cutter Laboratories, New Haven, CT) IVIG at 2-week intervals at a dose of 300 mg/kg. The data from 71 of these patients who have completed a 2- to 10-year treatment course was analyzed. Entry criteria included the following:

1. A history of one or more serious bacterial infections such as meningitis, sepsis, pneumonia with positive bacterial culture, or which responded promptly to antibiotic treatment.
2. Three or more recurrent "minor" bacterial infections such as otitis, pharyngitis, bronchitis, urinary tract infection, or recurrent febrile episodes without specific organ manifestations (FUO).
3. No history of prior bacterial infection but abnormal *in vitro* lymphocyte mitogenic responses to pokeweed mitogen and to staphylococcal Cowan A antigen and poor antibody responses to current vaccinations or to phage OX174 immunization.[2-6]
4. A cohort of 27 HIV-infected, age-matched children for whom no consent was given for participation in the IVIG trials was used as control.

MONITORING OF RESPONSE TO IVIG

The study was not placebo controlled. Nevertheless, clinical data were analyzed by persons who were unacquainted with the patients, and all laboratory tests were blinded. The evaluations were based on the following:

1. Clinical data comparing the number of bacterial and viral infections per year before and after institution of IVIG and to the control group;
2. Circulating immune complex measured by the Raji cell assay as previously reported[3,6]; and
3. $CD4^+$ cell, percentages and absolute values measured by flow cytometric analysis.[6]

RESULTS

Effect on Infectious Complications

Overall, a 42% reduction of serious and minor bacterial infections was noted. Eleven patients who were enrolled in the IVIG trial because of their B-cell defect,

TABLE 1. CD4+ Cells and IVIG in HIV-1 Infected Children >2 Years of Age

Percent Change of CD4+ Cell Counts/mm^3	Control[a]		IVIG[a]	
	First Year	Fourth Year	First Year	Fourth Year
>10% Decrease/year	59%	100%	28%	90%
<10% Decrease/year	31%	0	29%	10%
>10% Increase/year	10%	0	43%	0

[a] Figures express the percent of patients showing a change in CD4+ cells in the first and fourth years of either treatment with IVIG or no treatment with IVIG (controls).

but who had no history of prior serious or recurrent bacterial infections, were not included in the clinical outcome analysis because of the absence of an appropriate placebo-controlled group. Their response to IVIG was monitored exclusively by the modulation of previously abnormal immunological parameters. Patients with previous serious or recurrent minor bacterial infections were subdivided into three groups: (i) those with an *in vitro* and/or *in vivo* documented B-cell defect and CD4+ T cells over 200/mm^3, (ii) those with an *in vitro* and/or *in vivo* documented B-cell defect and CD4+ T cells <200/mm^3 but no history of an opportunistic infection (OI), and (iii) same as group ii, but with a history of an OI. Reduction in infectious complication rates were noted in all three groups. However, a longer lasting benefit of four years or longer was noted only in groups i and ii.

Effect on CD4+ T Cells

As seen in TABLE 1, in the first year of treatment, increases in CD4+ T-cell counts were four times more frequent in IVIG-treated patients. A decrease in CD4+ T cells greater than 10% was almost twice as frequent in untreated patients in the first year of treatment. By four years of follow-up, no difference was noted between the control and the IVIG group except for the observation that 10% of IVIG-treated patients (versus none of untreated patients) have maintained a stable CD4+ T-cell count.

Circulating Immune Complexes

Using both the Raji cell assay and the C_{1q} assay,[3,6,12,13] patients without OI had much higher CICs (TABLES 2 and 3). In a pilot study in 1982–83, we could

TABLE 2. Circulating Immune Complexes (Raji Cell Assay) in 37 HIV-Infected Children

Patient Group	CD4 Cells/mm^3	Elevated CIC[a]	CIC $x \pm$ 1SD (μg/ml)
With OI	<200	11%	186 ± 80
Without OI	619 ± 404	82%	673 ± 288

[a] CIC: circulating immune complexes; OI: opportunistic infection; $p < 0.05$.

TABLE 3. Circulating Immune Complexes (c_{1q} Assay) in 50 HIV-Infected Children

Patient Group	Elevated CIC[a]	CIC $x \pm$ 1SD (μg/ml)
With OI	0%	3 ± 3.1
Without OI	90%	58 ± 28

[a] CIC: circulating immune complexes; OI: opportunistic infection; $p < 0.01$.

TABLE 4. Circulating Immune Complexes (c_{1q} Assay μg Eg/ml)

	IVIG Untreated	IVIG Treated
CIC at study entry	65 ± 32	81 ± 31
Decrease of CIC in μg Eg/ml per 12 months	4.1 ± 12[a]	17 ± 35[a]

[a] $p < 0.01$.

not demonstrate a reduction in CIC in six patients receiving three infusions of 300 mg IVIG/kg at 4-week intervals. In contrast, six patients receiving 300 mg/kg IVIG at biweekly intervals all showed a significant decrease in CIC levels after the third dose. In the study expanded to 50 patients receiving 300 mg/kg IVIG biweekly, there was a significant decrease in CIC as measured by the Raji cell and C_{1q} assay (TABLE 4).

DISCUSSION

We have previously reported the presence of a functional humoral immunodeficiency early in the course of congenital HIV-1 infection in infants and children.[1-5,14] This B-cell defect may be due to hyperactivation of B cells, among other possible causes,[15-17] or to direct inhibition of B and T cells by HIV-1 proteins.[18] The excessive B-cell activation in HIV-1 infected children is also manifested in an increase of total B cells with a reduction in virgin B cells available for mitogen- or antigen-driven stimulation.[1,2,14,16,17] Furthermore, immunization of HIV-1 infected children with B- and T-cell-dependent antigens elicits diminished antibody responses[2,19] and formation of low affinity/avidity antibodies incorporated into CIC in antigen excess.[12]

The rationale for the use of IVIG in HIV-1 infection is therefore manifold. First and foremost, IVIG contains a pool of specific antibodies that react with a variety of microbial agents and can thus prevent infections. We have previously reported a reduction in the incidence of serious infections, of febrile episodes, and in hospital admission days in HIV-1 infected children receiving biweekly IVIG.[4,6] These observations have been confirmed in the present expanded study and by other studies in relatively small numbers of patients.[7-10,20] A subsequent large, controlled NICHD study, administering 400 mg/kg IVIG every 4 weeks, has shown that the time free from serious laboratory-proven bacterial or clinically diagnosed serious infections was significantly prolonged by IVIG only in children with entry

CD4$^+$ T-cell counts above 200/mm^3.[11] Further analysis of this cohort has shown a beneficial effect of IVIG across multiple infectious outcome measures including minor viral and bacterial infections.[21] In our present study we have documented reduction in serious and minor infections also in patients with CD4$^+$ T-cell counts below 200/mm^3 as long as they had no history of an OI. The difference in outcome between our study and the NICHD study may be related to the divergent IVIG treatment regimen, with the shorter IVIG intervals of two weeks employed by us. In fact, Mofenson *et al.* have recently reported from the NICHD study[22] "that the greatest reduction in serious bacterial infections, minor bacterial infections and viral infection rates occurred early in the interval following infusion, with attenuation of benefit late in the interval."

The potential for reduced benefit from longer IVIG intervals (4 weeks) was also indicated in a pilot study conducted by us in 1982–83 showing that CIC decreased exclusively in patients with the two-week IVIG interval, but not in those with the 4-week IVIG interval. In our expanded study, CIC were analyzed in a cohort of 50 children treated biweekly with IVIG. A significant decrease of CIC was noted over prolonged periods of time (TABLE 4). Similar findings have been reported by Schaad *et al.* using 400 mg/kg IVIG biweekly.[10] The clearance of CIC may have important biological consequences. In the presence of CIC in antigen excess,[12] CIC as well as free antigens may exert unwanted immunoregulatory events with a potential for activation of viral (HIV-1) replication. Conversely, antibodies in IVIG preparations may restore immune functions by shifting the antigen-to-antibody ratio in CIC towards equivalence, promoting their clearance by the reticuloendothelial system. In fact, the present study demonstrates that the reduction in CIC is accompanied by a decreased rate of CD4$^+$ T-cell depletion in patients receiving IVIG.

Other mechanisms may, however, also account for the observed beneficial effects of IVIG including anti-inflammatory effects by binding of C3b to the Fc fragment of IgG,[23] Fc receptor blockade,[24,25] induction of suppressor T cells,[26–29] and restoration of the idiotypic network.[30,31] Finally, IVIG may exert a "specific" effect on HIV-1 through the recently shown presence of soluble CD4 in commercial IVIG preparations.[32] We reported as early as 1985, that generic IVIG as well as hyperimmune IVIG (with documented reactivity to gp120 and gp41), reduced serum concentrations of p17, p24, gp41, and gp120.[33,34] This effect of generic IVIG on gp120 may now theoretically be attributed among others also to the binding of free gp120 on HIV-1 with its ligand, soluble CD4 present in IVIG preparation.

Taken together, our studies indicate that IVIG at a two-week interval may have an advantage over the four-week interval as demonstrated by (1) improved reduction of serious and minor bacterial and viral infections and extension of this benefit to a subpopulation of children without OI but with CD4$^+$ T cell counts below 200/mm^3, and (2) improved clearance of CIC with subsequent delay of immunological attrition.

Several issues remain unresolved. The optimal dose and interval of IVIG has to be further fine-tuned and prospective "best" responders versus "nonresponders" should be better characterized. Finally, it is evident from this long-term study of 71 patients that the beneficial effects of IVIG may wane with time. Therefore, endpoints of treatment should be better defined using a broader range of parameters, such as activation markers, as well as criteria for viral loads and other immunomodulatory effects.

REFERENCES

1. RUBINSTEIN, A., M. SICKLICK, A. GUPTA, L. BERNSTEIN, et al. 1983. Acquired immunodeficiency with reversed T4/T8 ratios in infants born to promiscuous and drug-addicted women. JAMA 249: 2352-2356.
2. BERNSTEIN, L., H. OCHS, R. J. WEDGWOOD & A. RUBINSTEIN. 1985. Defective humoral immunity in pediatric AIDS. J. Pediatr. 107: 352-357.
3. RUBINSTEIN, A., M. SICKLICK, L. BERNSTEIN & B. SILVERMAN. 1984. Treatment of AIDS with intravenous gammaglobulin. Pediatr. Res. 18: 264A.
4. RUBINSTEIN, A. 1983. AIDS in infants (editorial). Am. J. Dis. Child. 137: 825-827.
5. SILVERMAN, B. & A. RUBINSTEIN. 1985. Serum LDH levels in adults and children with AIDS and ARC. Possible indicator of B cell lymphoproliferation and disease activity. Effect of intravenous gammaglobulin on enzyme levels. Am. J. Med. 78: 728-735.
6. CALVELLI, T. A. & A. RUBINSTEIN. 1986. Intravenous gammaglobulin in infant AIDS. Pediatr. Infect. Dis. 5: S207-210.
7. SIEGEL, F. P. & J. A. OLESKE. 1986. In Clinical use of intravenous immunoglobulin. A. Morell & U. E. Nydegger, Eds.: 373-385. Academic Press, New York.
8. PAHWA, S., K. BIRON, W. LIM, et al. 1988. Continuous varicella-zoster infection associated with acyclovir resistance in a child with AIDS. JAMA 260: 19.
9. PAHWA, S. 1989. Intravenous immune globulin in patients with AIDS. J. Allergy Clin. Immunol. 84: 625-631.
10. SCHAAD, U. B., A. GIANELLA-BORRADORI, B. PERRET, P. IMBACH & A. MORELL. 1988. Intravenous immune globulin in symptomatic pediatric HIV infection. Eur. J. Pediatr. 147: 300-303.
11. NICHD IVIG COLLABORATIVE GROUP. 1991. Efficacy of intravenous immunoglobulin for the prophylaxis of serious bacterial infections in symptomatic HIV-infected children. N. Engl. J. Med. 325: 73-80.
12. ELLAURIE, M., T. A. CALVELLI & A. RUBINSTEIN. 1990. Human immunodeficiency virus (HIV) circulating immune complexes in infected children. AIDS Res. Hum. Retrovir. 6: 1437-1441.
13. ELLAURIE, M., T. CALVELLI & A. RUBINSTEIN. 1990. Immune complexes in pediatric human immunodeficiency virus infection. Am. J. Dis. Child. 144: 1207-1209.
14. RUBINSTEIN, A. 1986. Pediatric AIDS. Curr. Probl. Pediatr. 16: 361-409.
15. PAHWA, S. 1989. Intravenous immune globulin in patients with AIDS. J. Allergy Clin. Immunol. 845: 625-631.
16. SCHNITTMAN, S. M., H. C. LANE, S. E. HIGGINS, et al. 1986. Direct polyclonal activation of human B lymphocytes by the AIDS virus. Science 233: 1084-1086.
17. YARCHOAN, R., R. R. REDFIELD & S. BRODER. 1986. Mechanisms of B cell activation with AIDS and related disorders. J. Clin. Invest. 78: 439-447.
18. CHIRMULE, N. B., V. KALYANARAMA, N. OYAIZU & S. PAHWA. 1988. Inhibitory influences of envelope glycoproteins of HIV-1 on antigen specific responses. J. AIDS 1: 425-430.
19. BORKOWSKY, W., C. STEELE, S. GRUBMAN, et al. 1986. Antibody responses to bacterial toxoids in children infected with HIV. J. Pediatr. 110: 563-569.
20. HAGUE, R. A., P. L. YAP, J. Y. MOK, O. B. EDEN, N. A. COUTTS, J. G. WATSON, F. D. HARGREAVES & J. M. WHITELAW. 1989. Intravenous immunoglobulin in HIV infection: Evidence for efficacy of treatment. Am. J. Dis. Child. 68: 1146-1150.
21. MOFENSON, L. M., J. MOYE, JR., J. BETHEL, et al. 1992. Prophylactic intravenous immunoglobulin in HIV-infected children with CD4$^+$ counts of 0.20×10^9/L or more. JAMA 268(4): 483-488.
22. MOFENSON, L. M., J. MOYE, H. W. LISCHNER, et al. 1992. Occurrence of infections and time from infusion in HIV-infected children in a clinical trial of intravenous

immunoglobulin (IG). 32nd ICAAC, Anaheim, California. American Society for Microbiology.
23. BASTA, M., P. H. LANGLOIS, M. MARGUES, M. M. FRANK & L. H. FRIES. 1989. High-dose intravenous immunoglobulin modifies complement-mediated in vivo clearance. Blood **4(1):** 326–333.
24. FEHR, J., V. HOFFMAN & U. KAPPELER. 1982. Transient reversal of thrombocytopenia in ITP by high-dose IVIG. N. Engl. J. Med. **306:** 1254–1258.
25. BUSSEL, J. B. 1989. Modulation of Fc receptor clearance and antiplatelet antibodies as a consequence of intravenous immune globulin infusion in patients with immune thrombocytopenic purpura. J. Allergy Clin. Immunol. **84:** 566–579.
26. HASHIMOTO, F., Y. SAKIYAMA & S. MATSUMOTO. 1986. The suppressive effect of gammaglobulin preparations on in vitro PWM-induced immunoglobulin productions. Clin. Exp. Immunol. **65:** 409.
27. KAWADA, K. & P. I. TERASAKI. 1987. Evidence for immunosuppression by high-dose gammaglobulin. Exp. Hematol. **15:** 133–136.
28. BALLOW, M., W. WHITE & C. DESBONNET. 1989. Modulation of in vitro synthesis of immunoglobulin and the induction of suppressor activity by therapy with intravenous gammaglobulin. J. Allergy Clin. Immunol. **84:** 595–602.
29. GUPTA, A., G. NOVICK & A. RUBINSTEIN. 1986. Restoration of suppressor T cell functions in children with AIDS following intravenous gammaglobulin treatment. Am. J. Dis. Child. **140:** 146.
30. NYDEGGER, U. E., Y. SULTAN & M. D. KAZATCHKINE. 1989. The concept of anti-idiotypic regulation of selected autoimmune diseases by intravenous gammaglobulin. Clin. Immunol. Immunopathol. **53:** 572–582.
31. SULTAN, Y., M. D. KAZATCHKINE, P. MAISONEUVE & U. E. NYDEGGER. 1989. Anti-idiotype suppression of autoantibodies to factor VIII by high-dose intravenous gammaglobulin. Lancet **2:** 765–768.
32. BLASCZYK, R., U. WESTHOFF & H. GROSSE-WILDE. 1993. Soluble CD4, CD8 and HLA molecules in commercial immunoglobulin preparations. Lancet **341:** 789–790.
33. RUBINSTEIN, A., B. KRIEGER, M. SICKLICK, L. BERNSTEIN, G. NOVICK & A. WIZNIA. 1985. Treatment of AIDS with hyperimmune serume to LAV. Proc. 1st Int. Conf. AIDS. p41.
34. ELLAURIE, M., T. CALVELLI & A. RUBINSTEIN. 1987. Reduction of HIV-1 antigens in the serum of HIV-infected children following treatment with IVIG. Blood **70:** Abstract No. 333.

Opportunistic Infections in Pediatric HIV Disease[a]

RUSSELL B. VAN DYKE[b]

*Section of Pediatric Infectious Diseases
and
Tulane/LSU Pediatric
AIDS Clinical Trials Unit
Department of Pediatrics
Tulane School of Medicine
New Orleans, Louisiana 70112*

Before the identification of HIV, the clinical syndrome of AIDS was recognized by the unusual occurrence of opportunistic infections in persons not believed to be at risk for these infections. AIDS was first recognized by a clustering of *Pneumocystis carinii* pneumonia in young gay males in southern California. Soon thereafter, other opportunistic infections were observed, including disseminated mycobacterial infections, toxoplasmosis, and cytomegalovirus retinitis. When pediatric AIDS was recognized, many of these same opportunistic infections were found in children. Indeed, the occurrence of opportunistic infections remains the cornerstone of the case definition of AIDS. The recognition that HIV-infected persons are at increased risk for certain specific opportunistic pathogens allows for prophylaxis against these agents. Prevention of opportunistic infections remains a mainstay in the management of HIV infection. At the present time, the use of single agents in the prophylaxis of multiple organisms is being investigated. I will review several opportunistic infections that are particular problems for HIV-infected children, with emphasis on the prevention.

In both children and adults, *Pneumocystis carinii* pneumonia is the most common AIDS-defining diagnosis, occurring in one-third to one-half of all cases[1] (see TABLE 1). Other common opportunistic infections in children include cytomegalovirus infections (CMV), chronic and recurrent mucosal and esophageal candadiasis, herpes zoster, nontuberculous mycobacteria (principally *Mycobacterium avium* complex), *Cryptosporidium enteritis,* and mucocutaneous herpes simplex virus infections. HIV-infected children also have a higher number of common

---

[a] Supported in part by Grant No. AI32913-01 from the National Institute of Allergy and Infectious Diseases.

[b] Address for correspondence: Russell B. Van Dyke, M. D., Department of Pediatrics, Tulane School of Medicine, 1430 Tulane Ave., New Orleans, LA 70112.

TABLE 1. Pediatric AIDS in the USA—1991: AIDS-Defining Diseases[a]

Number of cases	683
Pneumocystis carinii pneumonia	33%
LIP	21%
Candidiasis, esophageal or pulmonary	19%
Multiple/recurrent bacterial infections	18%
HIV encephalopathy	14%
Failure to thrive	12%
CMV	5%
Cryptosporidiosis	3%
Nontuberculous mycobacteria	3%
Herpes simplex virus	2%
Tuberculosis, disseminated	1%
CNS toxoplasmosis	1%
Lymphoma	1%

[a] Data taken from the CDC HIV/AIDS Surveillance Report.[1]

childhood infections such as otitis media, sinusitis, viral respiratory infections, bacterial pneumonia, bacteremia, and meningitis. A recent survey of the NIH-funded AIDS Clinical Trials Group pediatric units provides estimates of the incidence of opportunistic infections and other common infections in HIV-infected children[2] (TABLE 2). The incidence of some AIDS-defining opportunistic infections in children in the United States is changing as the epidemic evolves.[3] Mycobacterial infections are increasing in frequency, presumably as a result of the longer survival of HIV-infected children. In contrast, the frequency of recurrent bacterial infections is dropping, perhaps owing to prophylaxis with antibiotics and intravenous immunoglobulin. There has been little change in the incidence of *Pneumocystis*, CMV, and candidiasis.

TABLE 2. Incidence of Infections in HIV-Infected Children[a]

	Cases/100 Child Years	
	Age 0–12	Age 12–18
Pneumocystis pneumonia	6.4	2.5
Herpes zoster	5.0	3.8
Nontuberculous mycobacteria	2.6	3.8
CMV	2.4	1.2
Cryptosporidiosis	1.1	1.2
Tuberculosis	1.0	2.5
Otitis media	57	29
Upper respiratory	47	25
Sinusitis	15	20
Bacterial pneumonia	11	10
Bacteremia	8.2	3.8
Varicella	4.7	0
UTI	3.7	6.3
Meningitis	1.1	0

[a] Data taken from the pediatric units of the AIDS Clinical Trials Group, Summer, 1992.[2]

TABLE 3. Indications For PCP Prophylaxis in Children[a]

I. Following an episode of PCP, *or*
II. CD4 < 20% at any age, *or*
III. Age-adjusted CD4 thresholds: • Age < 1 year: CD4 cell count < $1500/mm^3$ • Age 1–2 years: CD4 cell count < $750/mm^3$ • Age 2–6 years: CD4 cell count < $500/mm^3$ • Age > 6 years: CD4 cell count < $200/mm^3$ Consider prophylaxis in any child less than 12 months of age with a confirmed HIV infection.

[a] Adapted from the *Morbidity and Mortality Weekly Report*.[4]

PNEUMOCYSTIS CARINII PNEUMONIA

Pneumocystis carinii pneumonia (PCP) remains the most common opportunistic infection in HIV-infected children. PCP presents at a much younger age than do other opportunistic infections, peaking at 5 months of age. PCP in children has a much more rapidly progressive course than in adults, with a mortality rate as high as 40 to 50%. The major risk factor for the development of PCP in both adults and children is a depressed CD4 lymphocyte count. Children are known to have substantially higher normal values for both CD4 cell number and percentage than do adults, and guidelines for initiation of PCP prophylaxis in children based on age-adjusted CD4 values have been published[4] (TABLE 3). Because PCP occurs at an early age, infants at risk of HIV infection must be identified, lymphocyte subsets measured in the first few months of life, and PCP prophylaxis initiated when indicated. Identification of infants at risk will require widespread HIV testing of pregnant women and newborn infants, and this should be encouraged as a part of routine prenatal and newborn care. Infants born to HIV-infected mothers may be started empirically on PCP prophylaxis at two months of age if lymphocyte subsets have not been obtained. Prophylaxis may then be discontinued if subsequent testing determines that it is not required.

The drug of choice for both prophylaxis and treatment of PCP is trimethoprim/sulfamethoxazole (TMP/SMX) (TABLE 4). A substantial number of children are intolerant to TMP/SMX, and intravenous pentamidine is the alternative drug of choice for treatment of PCP. Both oral dapsone and intravenous pentamidine are alternatives for PCP prophylaxis in children, and published guidelines should be consulted.[4] M-atovaquone (BW 566C80) is a promising new drug that is currently

TABLE 4. PCP Prophylaxis in Children

Agent of choice: TMP/SMX (75 mg/m^2 of TMP per dose) given twice daily for 3 consecutive days per week.
Alternatives: • Dapsone, 1–2 mg/kg p.o. once daily.   • Aerosol pentamidine, 300 mg monthly (age > 5 years).   • Parenteral (i.v.) pentamidine, 4 mg/(kg·dose) every 2–4 weeks

being evaluated for both prophylaxis and treatment of PCP.[5] Potential advantages of atovaquone include a long half-life, low toxicity, and the ability to kill *Pneumocystis* in an animal model while pentamidine and TMP/SMX only suppress the organism. Early initiation of corticosteroid therapy has been shown to reduce morbidity in adults with PCP.[6,7] Although anecdotal reports suggest a similar efficacy in children, a definitive pediatric trial has not been performed. Nevertheless, many authorities believe that the early initiation of corticosteroids is beneficial to children with PCP. The recommended regime is methylprednisolone for 5 days at 2 mg/(kg·day) divided every 6 hours, followed by 3 days at 1 mg/(kg·day) divided every 12 hours, then 2 days at 0.5 mg/(kg·day) as a single dose.

NONTUBERCULOUS MYCOBACTERIAL INFECTIONS

Disseminated infections with the *Mycobacterium avium* group of environmental mycobacteria (MAC) have long been recognized as a problem in adults with AIDS. The incidence of MAC infection in children is increasing, presumably as a result of the longer survival of HIV-infected children. In a recent report from the Children's Hospital of New Jersey, 10% of 139 children with AIDS had a documented infection with a nontuberculous mycobacterium, of which most were caused by MAC[8] (TABLE 5). The mean age of these infected children was 54 months. As with adults, children infected with MAC have extremely low CD4 counts; in this report, the mean CD4 count was 29 cells/mm^3. Ninety-three percent of the infected children had a CD4 count of less than 100 cells/mm^3 or less than 20%, suggesting that these might be useful criteria for the initiation of prophylaxis.

MAC infection is associated with failure to thrive, anorexia, abdominal pain,

TABLE 5. Nontuberculous Mycobacteria in Children with AIDS[a]

Prevalence	10%
Median age	54 months
Male	30%
Median CD4 count	29 cells/mm^3
Median % CD4 cells	4.8%
CD4 < 100 or < 20%	93%
M. avium complex	93%
M. kansasii	7%
Positive blood culture	86%
Symptoms	
Failure to thrive	100%
Anorexia	90%
Abdominal pain/tenderness	90%
Chronic fever	80%
Anemia—transfusion dependent	70%
Diarrhea	60%
Night sweats	25%
Mortality @ 10 months	75%

[a] Data taken from Hoyt *et al.*[8]

TABLE 6. Rifabutin for MAC Prophylaxis in Adults with Fewer Than 200 CD4 Cells[a]

	Rifabutin	Placebo	
MAC bacteremia	10.2%	17.6%	($p < 0.01$)
Mortality	7.0%	7.8%	
Adverse events	48%	48%	

[a] Adapted from Cameron et al.[9] and Gordin et al.[10]

and chronic fever (TABLE 5). Because these children have extremely low CD4 counts, their length of survival is very short. In this report, 75% of children died within 10 months of identification of their MAC infection. Two adult studies have demonstrated the ability of rifabutin to delay or prevent the onset of MAC bacteremia in adults with CD4 cell counts of fewer than 200 cells/mm^3.[9,10] Mortality rate did not decrease in either of these studies (TABLE 6). There are as yet no studies of MAC prophylaxis in children. On the basis of these adult data, however, it is reasonable to initiate prophylaxis with rifabutin when the CD4 count falls below 100 cells/mm^3 or 20%. Treatment of established MAC infection is extremely difficult and results in doubtful long-term benefit. Prolonged therapy with multiple drugs is required.[11]

TUBERCULOSIS

Cases of tuberculosis are increasing at an alarming rate among HIV-infected adults, and it is anticipated that a similar increase will occur in children. Both HIV-infected children and uninfected children living in the household of an adult with tuberculosis are at high risk of infection. Of particular concern is the increasing incidence of multiple-drug-resistant tuberculosis. In a recent report, 12 children in a clinic population of 300 HIV-infected children were infected with tuberculosis.[12] Two of the children acquired multiple-drug-resistant tuberculosis from a household contact. The mean age of infected children was 51 months, and they had a mean CD4 count of 811 cells/mm^3, substantially higher than that found in children with MAC. Most of the children had pulmonary disease; disseminated disease was seen in only one child. All of the children had a PPD reaction of greater than 5 mm, and 75% had greater than 10 mm. Obviously, PPD testing remains an important part of the routine care of all children. In children living in high-risk environments such as households with HIV-infected adults, use of 5 mm as the criteria for a positive PPD is appropriate. Children with a reactive tuberculin skin test should receive a course of suppressive treatment. Because of the increasing risk of tuberculosis in childhood, there is a renewed interest in the use of the BCG vaccine in high-risk children, and clinical trials are now being developed.

CYTOMEGALOVIRUS

Cytomegalovirus infection is common in HIV-infected children, with active CMV present in as many as 20 to 45% of children with symptomatic HIV disease.[13]

CMV may accelerate the progression of HIV disease. The most common clinical manifestations of CMV disease are interstitial pneumonitis, chorioretinitis, hepatitis, neutropenia, thrombocytopenia, and gastrointestinal disease. Less is known about the frequency of CMV encephalitis, but CMV may contribute substantially to the central nervous system disease found in HIV-infected children. Although cytomegalovirus retinitis is less common in children than adults, it is an equally devastating disease that can rapidly lead to loss of vision. Consequently, routine fundascopic examination by an experienced ophthalmologist is an important part of the care of CMV-seropositive children with AIDS. Diagnosis of active CMV disease is difficult because asymptomatic viurea is common in children, but detection of virus in blood and tissues by virus isolation or PCR suggests active CMV disease. Ganciclovir is the drug of choice for treatment of established CMV disease in children. Long-term suppression therapy following treatment of acute CMV retinitis is required to prevent relapse.[14] Foscarnet has been shown to be effective in adults, but little information is available on its use in children.

CANDIDIASIS

Chronic and recurrent *Candida* infections of skin and mucous membranes is frequently the presenting infection in HIV-infected children. These infections generally respond to topical or oral therapy but may promptly recur once therapy is discontinued. Esophageal candidiasis, characterized by dysphasia and pain on swallowing, should be considered in a child who is eating poorly. Interestingly, disseminated candidiasis is relatively uncommon in HIV-infected children in the absence of an indwelling central venous catheter. Oral candidiasis may be confused with oral hairy leukoplakia, but this disease is unusual in children. Endoscopy is necessary to confirm the diagnosis of esophageal candidiasis and to rule out other agents including herpes simplex virus, CMV, and mycobacteria. Oral candidiasis usually responds to topical therapy with nystatin or clotrimazole; refractory cases may require long-term oral ketoconazole. Esophageal candidiasis requires systemic therapy with either an imidazole (fluconazole or ketoconazole) or amphotericin B. Hepatotoxicity is a common complication of imidazole therapy in HIV-infected children.

LYMPHOCYTIC INTERSTITIAL PNEUMONITIS

Lymphocytic interstitial pneumonitis (LIP) is a common chronic pulmonary disease of HIV-infected children. It results from the proliferation of lymphoid tissue in the interstitium of the lung parenchema and produces tachypnea, hypoxia, and clubbing of the digits. The chest radiograph demonstrates diffuse reticulonodular infiltrates, often associated with hilar lymphadenopathy. LIP occurs during the lymphoproliferative stage of HIV disease, which includes generalized lymphadenopathy, hepatosplenomegaly, and parotid enlargement. It is associated with a relatively good prognosis; children with LIP have a mean survival of 6 years.[15] The etiology of LIP is not well understood. The genome of Epstein-Barr virus and HIV have both been demonstrated in the lungs of children with LIP, and the disease may result from either or both of these agents.[16,17] Children with symptomatic LIP frequently improved with the initiation of antiretroviral therapy. Those who fail to respond may benefit from a course of corticosteroids (prednisone 2 mg/kg daily for 2–4 weeks, then taper over several weeks to 0.5 mg/(kg·day).

REFERENCES

1. CENTERS FOR DISEASE CONTROL. 1992. HIV/AIDS Surveillance Report January: 16.
2. WEI, L. J. 1992. Personal communication.
3. MASCOLA, L., T. FREDERICK, A. ELLER, et al. 1992. Trends in AIDS-defining conditions in pediatric HIV infection. Program and Abstracts of the 32nd Interscience Conference on Antibicrobial Agents and Chemotherapy (Anaheim, CA: no. 902. Oct. 11–14.
4. CENTERS FOR DISEASE CONTROL. 1991. Guidelines for prophylaxis against *Pneumocystis carinii* pneumonia for children infected with human immunodeficiency virus. Morbid. Mortal. Wkly. Rep. **40**(No. RR-2): 1–13.
5. FALLOON, J., J. KOVACS, W. HUGHES, et al. 1991. A preliminary evaluation of 566C80 for the treatment of *Pneumocystis* pneumonia in patients with the acquired immunodeficiency syndrome. N. Engl. J. Med. **325**: 1534–1538.
6. BOZZETTE, S. A., F. R. SATTLER, J. CHIU, et al. 1990. A controlled trial of early adjunctive treatment with corticosteroids for *Pneumocystis carinii* pneumonia in the acquired immunodeficiency syndrome. N. Engl. J. Med. **323**: 1451–1457.
7. NATIONAL INSTITUTES OF HEALTH—UNIVERSITY OF CALIFORNIA EXPERT PANEL FOR CORTICOSTEROIDS AS ADJUNCTIVE THERAPY FOR *PNEUMOCYSTIS* PNEUMONIA. 1990. Consensus statement on the use of corticosteroids as adjunctive therapy for pneumocystis pneumonia in the acquired immunodeficiency syndrome. N. Engl. J. Med. **323**: 1500–1504.
8. HOYT, L., J. OLESKE, B. HOLLAND & E. CONNOR. 1992. Nontuberculous mycobacteria in children with acquired immunodeficiency syndrome. Pediatr. Infect. Dis. J. **11**: 354–60.
9. CAMERON, W., P. SPARTI, N. PIETROSKI, et al. 1992. Rifabutin prevents *M. avium* complex bacteremia in patients with AIDS and CD4 ≤ 200. Program and Abstracts of the 32nd Interscience Conference on Antibicrobial Agents and Chemotherapy (Anaheim, CA): no. 888. Oct. 11–14. American Society for Microbiology. Washington, D.C.
10. GORDIN, F., S. NIGHTINGALE, B. WYNNE, et al. 1992. Rifabutin monotherapy prevents or delays *Mycobacterium avium* complex bacteremia in patients with AIDS. Program and Abstracts of the 32nd Interscience Conference on Antibicrobial Agents and Chemotherapy (Anaheim, CA): no. 889. Oct. 11–14. American Society for Microbiology. Washington, D.C.
11. HOY, J., A. MIJCH, M. SANDLAND, et al. 1990. Quadruple-drug therapy for *Mycobacterium avium*-intracellulare bacteremia in AIDS patients. J. Infect. Dis. **161**: 801–805.
12. MCSHERRY, G., G. BERMAN, H. AGUILA, et al. 1992. Tuberculosis in HIV-infected children in Newark 1981–1992. Program and Abstracts of the 32nd Interscience Conference on Antibicrobial Agents and Chemotherapy (Anaheim, CA): no. 905. Oct. 11–14. American Society for Microbiology. Washington, D.C.
13. FRENKEL, L. D., S. GAUR, M. TSOLIA, et al. 1990. Cytomegalovirus infection in children with AIDS. Rev. Infect. Dis. **12**(Suppl. 7): S820–S826.
14. JACOBSON, M. A., J. J. O'DONNELL, H. R. BRODIE, et al. 1988. Randomized prospective trial of ganciclovir maintenance therapy for cytomegalovirus retinitis. J. Med. Virol. **25**: 436–440.
15. SCOTT, G. B., C. HUTTO, R. MAKUCH, et al. 1988. Survival of children with perinatally acquired human immunodeficiency virus type 1 infection. N. Engl. J. Med. **321**: 1791–1796.
16. ANDIMAN, W. A., R. EASTMAN, K. MARTIN, et al. 1985. Opportunistic lymphoprolifera-

tion associated with Epstein-Barr viral DNA in infants and children with AIDS. Lancet **2:** 1390–1392.
17. CHAYT, K. J., M. E. HARPER, L. M. MARSELLE, et al. 1986. Detection of HTLV-III RNA in lungs of patients with AIDS and pulmonary involvement. JAMA **256:** 2356–2359.

Antiviral Therapy for HIV Infection in Infants and Children[a]

ANNE A. GERSHON[b]

Department of Pediatrics
Columbia University College of Physicians and Surgeons
New York, New York 10032

A number of antiviral drugs are now available to treat HIV-infected children, and more are under investigation and in the process of development. Much research needs to be done before a cure for HIV is achieved, however, and a number of questions remain, in part because HIV infection in children is somewhat different than it is in adults. This manuscript will review several outstanding questions with regard to treatment of HIV infection in infants and children.

WHAT IS THE BEST MEANS OF EVALUATING EFFICACY OF ANTIVIRAL DRUGS?

In evaluating an antiviral drug, clinical endpoints such as return to function and/or prolongation of life are considered optimal. Such endpoints, for example, have been used successfully to evaluate antiviral drugs against herpes simplex and respiratory virus infections which normally have rather short clinical courses. In adults with HIV infection, however, the necessity for rapid recognition of an effective drug to treat an infection that may be quiescent for many years has to a large extent precluded the use of clinical markers. Therefore, surrogate markers, such as $CD4^+$ and p24 antigen levels, have been developed and used. The problem with surrogate markers, however, is that they may not necessarily reflect the efficacy of a given drug. For example, rising $CD4^+$ levels and falling p24 antigen levels may or may not occur during long-term drug therapy for HIV infection, despite an apparent positive clinical effect of the drug.

With respect to use of clinical markers to judge drug efficacy, dealing with the pediatric HIV-infected population has an advantage over studying HIV-infected adults. In children, growth and development, which normally are constantly

---

[a] Supported by National Institutes of Health Grant AI 27562.
[b] Address for correspondence: Department of Pediatrics, Anne A. Gershon, M.D., Columbia University College of Physicians and Surgeons, 650 West 168th Street, New York, NY 10032.

changing and expanding at rapid, well-standardized, and measurable rates have proven to be extremely useful clinical markers of efficacy of drugs against HIV. For example, in an early study of intravenously administered zidovudine (ZDV) by Pizzo et al.,[1] it was found that treated children had considerable weight gain and a significant improvement in neurologic symptoms as measured by developmental testing. Other successful drug trials in HIV-infected children have yielded similar data.[2,3] In contrast, in children with advanced HIV infection, it was concluded that a suboptimal dose of ZDV was used, because no changes in height, weight, and neurologic status were observed after 1 year of therapy.[4] At present, a major study of the efficacy of ZDV in children, being conducted by the AIDS Clinical Trials Group (ACTG) of the National Institutes of Health, Protocol 128, explores two different doses (320 mg/m^2 and 720 mg/m^2 daily) of orally administered ZDV. One aim of anti-HIV therapy in children is to protect the developing central nervous system (CNS) from the deleterious effects of HIV. In Protocol 128, the efficacy of ZDV is being judged by determining whether there are differences in neurological development in the children who received one of these two doses of ZDV. It has been reasoned that, if tolerable, high doses of ZDV may be more useful in children than low doses, in that the central nervous system (CNS) may be better protected from the effects of HIV. Because it is possible to measure neuropsychiatric developmental parameters and compare their progression between children over a relatively short period of time, clinical endpoints can be used successfully for this study of efficacy of ZDV.

Another reason that children may be ideal subjects for whom clinical endpoints may be used as an indication of drug efficacy is the compressed time scale of disease progression in children compared with adults. This is particularly true for those children, believed to constitute about 25% of vertically infected infants, who present with serious symptoms of HIV infection early in infancy. A bimodal peak of development of AIDS has been observed in children, one group presenting at 1 to 2 years of age and another, often associated with lymphoid interstitial hyperplasia (LIP), developing AIDS at about 6 years of age.[5] Particularly for those children who develop AIDS in infancy, it should be possible to examine prolongation of life as a clinical endpoint for evaluation of drug efficacy. In ACTG Protocol 152, a comparison of monotherapy with ZDV or didanosine (ddI) and combination therapy with both, primary endpoints are survival and disease progression (indicated by development of opportunistic infections, growth, and neuropsychological maturation). Such endpoints are not so easily applied to adults in judging drug efficacy against HIV, although weight gain and Karnofsky scores are used.

Despite the shortcomings of surrogate markers, however, they are being used increasingly to evaluate HIV-infected children in addition to markers of clinical progression of disease. A good deal more is known about surrogate markers in adults, however, than in children, and it is crucial that additional research be directed toward exploring the validity of such markers in infants and children. It has become clear that infants and children have higher levels of CD4$^+$ cells than adults, and that normal adult levels are not reached by children until they are

TABLE 1. CD4⁺ Counts in Healthy Children of Various Ages

	Age				
	1–6 months	7–12 months	13–24 months	25–74 months	Adults
Denny & Palumbo[6]					
CD4⁺ cells					
Median	3211	3128	2601	1668	1027
5–95 percentile	1153–5285	967–5289	739–4463	505–2831	237–1817
Percentage					
Median (%)	51.6	47.9	45.8	42.1	50.9
5–95 percentile (%)	36.3–67.1	32.8–63.0	31.2–60.4	32.2–52.0	34.7–67.1
Erkeller-Yuksel et al.[26]					
CD4⁺ cells					
Median	1900		1600		800
5–95 percentile	1500–2400		1000–1800		700–1100
Percentage					
Median (%)	35		37		42
5–95 percentile (%)	28–42		30–40		38–46

about 6 years old[6,7] (TABLE 1). This variability of CD4⁺ cells according to age in childhood must be considered whenever surrogate markers are used in pediatric studies of drug efficacy against HIV and in planning therapy for children not on treatment protocols. They were, for example, strongly considered when developing a protocol for prevention of *Pneumocystis carinii* pneumonia (PCP) for HIV-infected children.[8]

HOW IMPORTANT IS RESISTANCE OF HIV TO ANTIVIRALS?

The first studies that identified resistance of HIV to ZDV came from clinical trials in adult patients.[9] These studies revealed that development of resistance to ZDV correlates directly with the length of time that the patient has been taking the drug. Resistance to ZDV appears to develop in about 50% of patients who have taken it for 1 year, and 100% of patients have high-level resistance after 2 years. In the initial studies, although resistant HIV was present, the patients had not experienced an increase in HIV-related symptoms.[9] Because it is recognized that clinical deterioration of HIV-infected patients also occurs inevitably with time, whether there is a causal relationship between these two phenomena has not been answered for certain. Clearly the analysis is extremely complicated. It is recognized that other variables may confound the meaning of development of drug resistance to ZDV, such as low CD4⁺ counts (which predispose a patient to rapidly multiplying virus), high degrees of viral burden, and the phenotype of the infecting virus itself, all of which favor selection of drug-resistant HIV. More recently, however, when adult patients who had been treated with ZDV for at least one year and who had similar initial CD4⁺ levels were divided into groups, those with ZDV-resistant HIV and those with ZDV-susceptible HIV, there was clinical deterioration mainly in those with drug-resistant virus.[10]

In a study to evaluate the importance of resistance of HIV to ZDV in pediatric patients, virus isolates from HIV-infected children, whose average age at beginning ZDV was 4 years, were tested for sensitivity to ZDV after 9 to 39 months of therapy. Over the next 6 months, there was a highly significant difference in clinical outcome in those whose virus isolates were sensitive to ZDV compared with those whose isolates were resistant. Resistant viruses were more likely to be isolated from those who deteriorated or died in comparison to those who remained stable.[11] The authors suggested that since children who deteriorated clinically were likely to have resistant HIV after prolonged monotherapy, it would be reasonable to administer another antiretroviral drug. They acknowledge, however, that their study did not allow them to conclude whether increased replication of HIV leads to enhanced recovery of resistant virus or whether resistance leads to progression of disease. They nevertheless cite the fact that in another study, because an increased HIV burden was found in children *after* they developed resistant HIV, they favor the hypothesis that resistance may indeed lead to disease progression. Obviously, more information will be necessary to clarify the role of drug resistance on the course of HIV, but it seems highly likely that there is a cause and effect relationship in both adults and children.

WHAT DRUGS ARE NOW APPROVED FOR CHILDREN?

Drugs that treat HIV infection mainly work by attempting to interfere with the replication of HIV. Points in the growth cycle of the virus most amenable to interference with multiplication of virus include the following: blockage of virus entry (soluble $CD4^+$ preparations), prevention of transcription of RNA to DNA (RT inhibitors), interference with translation (agents acting on regulatory genes or their proteins), inhibition of assembly (protease inhibitors), and release of virus (interferon). TABLES 2 and 3 list clinical trials in children in the published literature (TABLE 1) and ACTG treatment protocols, most of which remain ongoing and are unpublished (TABLE 2).

The first drug to be approved for treatment of HIV infection for adults and children was ZDV, a synthetic thymidine analogue that acts as a competitive inhibitor of viral RT and as a chain terminator of viral DNA synthesis. In adults, early therapy with ZDV (500 mg daily) has been shown to delay progression of disease and to prolong life.[12] Although in another study delayed progression to AIDS but not prolongation of life were observed with early ZDV, a dose of 1500 mg of ZDV daily had been given, which may have resulted in increased toxicity, obscuring a survival effect.[13] Toxicity of ZDV is mainly evidenced by bone marrow depression, which is more commonly seen in patients who have AIDS and which can be controlled to some extent by erythropoetin and colony-stimulating factors, particularly in adults. Other toxicities include abnormalities of liver function tests, nausea, vomiting, headache, anorexia, and malaise. The FDA has approved ZDV for use in HIV-infected patients (including children) with or without symptoms who have $CD4^+$ levels of <500 cells/mm^3.

TABLE 2. Published Studies of Antiviral Therapy in Children

Author, year	Title
Pizzo et al. 1988	Effect of continuous intravenous infusion of zidovudine (AZT) in children with symptomatic HIV infection[1]
Balis et al. 1989	Pharmacokinetics of zidovudine administered intravenously and orally in children with human immunodeficiency virus infection[16]
Balis et al. 1989	The pharmacokinetics of zidovudine administered by cutaneous infusion in children[17]
McKinney et al. 1990	Safety and tolerance of intermittent intravenous and oral zidovudine therapy in human immunodeficiency virus-infected pediatric patients (ACTG Protocol 003)[18]
Pizzo et al. 1990	Dideoxycytidine alone and in an alternating schedule with zidovudine (AZT) in children with symptomatic human immunodeficiency virus infection[21]
Blanche et al. 1991	Low-dose zidovudine in children with human immunodeficiency virus infection acquired in the perinatal period[4]
McKinney et al. 1991	A multicenter trial of oral zidovudine in children with advanced human immunodeficiency virus disease (ACTG Protocol 043)[2]
Butler et al. 1991	Dideoxyinosine in children with symptomatic human immunodeficiency virus infection[3]
Balis et al. 1992	Clinical pharmacology of 2′,3′-dideoxyinosine in human immunodeficiency virus-infected children[20]
Husson et al. 1992	Phase 1 study of continuous-infusion soluble CD4 as a single agent and in combination with oral dideoxyinosine therapy in children with symptomatic human immunodeficiency virus infection[22]

Early trials in adults focused on dose finding; it was determined that a dose of 500 to 600 mg/day yielded the highest degree of safety and efficacy.[14,15] In subsequent studies in adults, there has been more and more of a tendency toward therapy at earlier and earlier stages of HIV infection. This is an additional reason why it is important to understand how resistance to HIV develops; it is possible, although it seems unlikely because of the interplay of the immune system with HIV, that earlier therapy might lead to earlier development of resistance. On the other hand, if it does not, early therapy for HIV infection may be more efficacious than waiting until AIDS has developed. Of the two possibilities, this seems more likely. In addition, while another argument against early therapy is possible drug toxicity, the experience in adult patients has been that therapy early in HIV disease is better tolerated than it is later in the infection.

How data from studies in adults translate into use of ZDV for children is problematic. As has been mentioned, it is still not clear what the best dose of ZDV is for children, although the issue is being studied. Moreover, as has also been mentioned, CD4$^+$ levels are highest in infancy and gradually fall with time. Therefore, one cannot reliably use a level of 500 CD4$^+$ cells/mm^3 to begin therapy in an asymptomatic child, except in those who are more than 6 years old. This is one reason why low CD4$^+$ lymphocyte counts were not a major criterion for entry into ACTG Protocol 128; HIV-infected children with CD4$^+$ lymphocyte counts above 500/mm^3 could enter the study as long as they had symptoms such as chronic

TABLE 3. Pediatric ACTG Studies of Antiviral Therapy against HIV

ACTG Number	Title of Protocol
Protocol 003	Phase I evaluation of ZDV in children with AIDS or ARC
Protocol 043	Multicenter trial to evaluate oral ZDV in treatment of children with symptomatic HIV infection
Protocol 049	Multicenter, Phase I trial to evaluate the safety and pharmacokinetics of intravenous and oral ZDV in infants with perinatal HIV exposure
Protocol 076	Phase III randomized, placebo-controlled trial to evaluate the efficacy, safety, and tolerance of ZDV for the prevention of maternal–fetal HIV transmission
Protocol 082	Phase I trial to evaluate ZDV in HIV-1 infected pregnant women and their offspring and a Phase I pharmacokinetic and safety trial of ZDV in laboring women and their offspring
Protocol 091	Phase I safety and pharmacokinetics study of ddI administered twice daily to infants and children with AIDS or symptomatic HIV infection
Protocol 103	Randomized trial to evaluate the impact of maintaining steady-state concentrations in ZDV versus and intermittent schedule of ZDV delivery versus intermittent ddI in children with symptomatic HIV infection
Protocol 128	Randomized, blinded trial to evaluate the safety and tolerance of high versus low dose of ZDV administered to children with HIV (320 vs. 720 mg/m^2 daily)
Protocol 138	Trial of two doses of ddC in treatment of children with symptomatic HIV infection who are intolerant of ZDV or show progressive disease while on ZDV (0.02 ddC vs. 0.03 ddC mg/kg daily)
Protocol 144	Randomized, comparative trial of two doses of ddI in children with symptomatic HIV infection who are either unresponsive to ZDV or who are intolerant to ZDV (100 vs. 300 mg/m^2 daily)
Protocol 152	Randomized, comparative trial of ZDV vs. ddI vs. ZDV plus ddI in symptomatic HIV-infected children
Protocol 153	Safety and tolerance of ZDV and interferon α in HIV-infected children
Protocol 176	Phase I study to evaluate the safety and toxicity of the combination of ZDV and ddI in children with HIV infection
Protocol 180	Niverapine (BiRG 587) Phase I plus ZDV
Protocol 182	Phase III study to evaluate the safety, tolerance, and efficacy of early treatment with ZDV in asymptomatic infants with HIV infection
Protocol 190	Phase II study to evaluate pharmacokinetics, safety, tolerance, and activity of ddC administered in combination with ZDV in pediatric patients with HIV infection

pneumonitis (including LIP), HIV-associated hepatitis, cardiomyopathy, and nephropathy. In contrast, ACTG Protocol 182, a placebo-controlled study of administration of ZDV (or placebo) to infants and young children who are proven to be HIV-infected but who have no symptoms, is addressing the issue of whether early therapy will be helpful to children. In this study, infants must be less than 9 months of age at study entry, and they must have total CD4$^+$ counts of more than 2000/mm^3 with more than 20% total lymphocytes.

A number of studies of ZDV in HIV-infected infants and children have been published. Most have been Phase I (or early Phase II) studies with the goal of obtaining pharmacokinetic data, to explore the issues of safety, toxicity, and dose finding, after intravenous and/or oral dosing.[1,4,16–18] A multicenter study of oral

ZDV, 720 mg/(m^2·day) given to 88 children with advanced HIV infection for a median of 56 weeks, has recently been reported.[2] On this dosage of ZDV, 61% of the children experienced at least one episode of hematologic toxicity that was usually treatable by dose modification or transfusion. This dosage is comparable to a dose of 250 mg 6 times per day in adults (1500 mg/day). Because in addition almost three-fourths of these children had AIDS, this degree of toxicity is not surprising. On the other hand, most of these children clearly benefited from ZDV, as evidenced by an increase in growth and cognitive function, decreases in p24 antigen in cerebrospinal fluid (CSF), and fewer positive cultures for HIV in CSF. Based on historical controls, it appeared that there may have been prolongation of life in these children. Although the levels of CD4$^+$ lymphocytes increased during the first 12 weeks of therapy, this improvement was not lasting.

At present, the approach to treatment of an HIV-infected child who is not participating in a clinical trial protocol is to a large extent up to the judgment of the individual physician; however, it seems prudent that drug-naive, HIV-infected children with low CD4$^+$ counts for their ages and/or HIV-related symptoms, such as failure to thrive, encephalopathy, opportunistic infection(s), cardiomyopathy, nephropathy, or malignancy, should be treated with ZDV. At this time most experts would not treat the child with isolated adenopathy, hepatosplenomegaly, parotitis, or mild LIP with a normal CD4$^+$ count. The most reasonable orally administered dose at this time would be 720 mg/(m^2·day), based on the study of McKinney *et al.*[2] Treated children need close follow-up every few months, with monitoring of clinical symptoms, CBC and serum chemistries for monitoring of possible toxicity, CD4$^+$ counts, and the dosage of ZDV adjusted if necessary. In addition, these children should be receiving prophylaxis against PCP. There is a growing sentiment that asymptomatic HIV-infected children with low CD4$^+$ levels for their ages should also be treated, but as yet no consensus document has been published on this issue.

Like ZDV, ddI is a purine nucleoside analogue that inhibits the RT of HIV. It is less toxic than ZDV, and it has a longer plasma half-life, so it can be administered every 12 hours. Because it is unstable in acid, however, it must be given along with antacid medication. In studies in HIV-infected adults (ACTG 116/117) ddI therapy was found to be associated with decreases in p24 antigen levels, increases in CD4$^+$ lymphocyte levels, and clinical improvement such as weight gain. Toxicity included pancreatitis and painful peripheral neuropathy; bone marrow depression was not a significant problem. A recently published study of this protocol in adult patients who had previously received ZDV for a median of 13.9 months and then were either switched to ddI or continued on ZDV for an average of 55 weeks, revealed that those switched to ddI had a lower chance of developing AIDS or dying than those who remained on ZDV.[19] They also had increased CD4$^+$ levels and decreased p24 antigen levels. These patients either were symptomatic and had <300 CD4$^+$ cells/mm^3 or were asymptomatic and had <200 CD4$^+$ cells/mm^3. Two different daily doses of ddI were studied, and the lower dose (500 mg) proved superior.

Published studies of ddI in children include one dealing with clinical pharmacology[20] and one Phase I/II study.[3] In the latter study, 43 children were given five dosages of ddI ranging between 60 and 540 mg/m^2 daily for 24 weeks. Approximately two out of three of these children had not previously received antiretroviral therapy. Pancreatitis occurred in two children who were receiving the highest dosages of ddI, but neuropathy has not been a problem. In general, increases in $CD4^+$ cell counts, decreases in p24 antigenemia and increases in IQ scores were observed. There was considerable variability in bioavailability of ddI in these children, however, and one of the authors' conclusions was that it might be necessary to monitor levels of drug in ddI-treated children. At present, orally administered ddI, 200 mg/m^2 daily has been approved for HIV-infected children who do not tolerate or do poorly on ZDV.

Additional clinical trials of orally administered ddI are currently being conducted in children. In ACTG 144, which is a "salvage" protocol for children who are either intolerant or unresponsive to ZDV, ddI (100 compared with 300 mg/m^2 daily) is being administered. In ACTG 152, a comparison is being made between ZDV (720 mg/m^2 daily) alone, ddI (240 mg/m^2 daily) alone, and a combination of both drugs (360 mg/m^2 of ZDV and 240 mg/m^2 of ddI daily). Results of these studies will not be available for several years.

Zalcitabine (ddC), another nucleoside analogue RT inhibitor, is also being studied in children, in ACTG Protocol 138, in which two doses (0.015 mg/kg vs. 0.03 mg/kg daily) are being compared for tolerance and efficacy against HIV. In adults, ddC is not as effective as ZDV; the FDA did not approve it for monotherapy in the spring of 1992. It was approved, however, for use in adults with advanced HIV infection. ($CD4^+$ less than 300/mm^3), when given along with ZDV. ACTG Protocol 138 is also a "salvage" protocol, for children who have not benefited or cannot tolerate ZDV. Unfortunately, ddC does not penetrate into the CNS as well as either ZDV or ddI, which might seriously hamper its use for children. Its main toxicity in adults has been peripheral neuropathy; hematologic toxicity is minimal. A published clinical trial of orally administered ddC in children suggested an antiviral effect, in that during an 8-week course of ddI therapy, over 50% of treated children had a decrease in p24 blood antigen level and/or an increase in $CD4^+$ lymphocyte count.[21] Observed adverse effects included rashes and mouth sores but no dose-limiting hematologic effects or peripheral neuropathy. Children in this study were also given ZDV on an alternating drug basis. Monotherapy with ddC is not approved by the FDA for use in children and is available only on a study basis.

Another category of RT inhibitors that are being studied are non-nucleoside drugs such as Nevirapine (BiRG 587). Drugs of this category have been found to be highly potent *in vitro* against HIV but extremely rapid development of drug resistance by HIV has also been noted. Therefore, these drugs are currently hypothesized to be potentially useful only when given in conjunction with other anti-HIV agents. ACTG Protocol 180 is a Phase I study in children, examining safety and tolerance of this drug alone and in combination with ZDV. If the two drugs are found to be well tolerated when given together, future efficacy studies may be carried out in children, as combination therapy. At present, because soluble $CD4^+$ preparations have not shown good evidence of antiviral activity *in vivo*, studies involving this therapy are not currently being continued.[22]

WHAT ABOUT THE FUTURE?

Combinations of drugs given concurrently may decrease the problem of viral resistance, be less toxic, be synergistic against HIV, and lead to better efficacy. Drug therapy for cancer, in which monotherapy is rarely used, is the model on which this approach is based. Ideally, for combination therapy, each drug should have antiviral activity but have a unique mechanism of action and no shared cross resistance. In addition, primary toxicities should not overlap, so the drugs can be used at full therapeutic doses, and there should be preclinical evidence of additive or synergistic action.

Results of combination therapy studies are now emerging from adult ACTG protocols. These suggest that concurrent therapy with two drugs yields better results than alternating the drugs, which had been predicted from results of cancer chemotherapy protocols.[23] In general, the studies so far in patients with advanced HIV infection indicate that it is safe to take this approach; data on efficacy remain inconclusive, mainly because a low dose of ZDV (150 mg/day) was given to comparison groups. In adult ACTG Protocol 106, for example, there were six comparison groups receiving various doses of ZDV and ddC, compared to ZDV alone. Those receiving combination therapy maintained higher $CD4^+$ counts, and the therapy was well tolerated without significant toxicity. In groups receiving higher dosages [e.g., ZDV 600 mg/day plus ddC 0.03 mg/(kg·day)], there were improvements in weight, $CD4^+$ counts, and p24 antigenemia.[24] Combination therapy ACTG Protocol 143 in adults was similar to Protocol 106, but compared the effects of ZDV alone, ddI alone, and a combination of both drugs given concurrently, in dosages similar to those employed in Protocol 106, with similar results.[25] In April 1992, the FDA Antiviral Drug Products Advisory Committee approved the use of ZDV and ddC combination therapy for adults with advanced HIV infection.

Combination therapy cannot be recommended at this time for HIV-infected children (other than those participating in clinical trials) since there are no data on which to base recommendations. However, a number of clinical trials in HIV-infected children are in progress. In addition to ACTG Protocol 152, other protocols in which combination therapy is being evaluated in children include ACTG 153 (ZDV plus interferon α), ACTG Protocol 180 (ZDV plus Nevirapine), and ACTG Protocol 190 (ZDV plus ddC). Most of these are Phase I studies, evaluating tolerance and safety. The long-range prediction for treatment of HIV-infected patients is that eventually medications will be administered on the basis of the susceptibility of HIV to the specific drug.

Newer drugs, protease and TAT inhibitors, are projected to be studied in clinical trials in children. If they can be given with nucleoside analogues such as ZDV, using the model of cancer chemotherapy, there may be greater efficacy against HIV.

In HIV-infected cells, virus-induced proteases are needed to cleave the HIV gag polyprotein into functional structural proteins; these are necessary for virus assembly and budding. Protease inhibitors, therefore, have the potential to interfere with multiplication of HIV in chronically infected cells, and released viral particles have markedly decreased infectivity. Until now, protease inhibitors have been poorly soluble with resultant poor bioavailability, but recently improved compounds have been developed, and clinical trials with these compounds have begun.

Another projected form of antiviral therapy is by inhibition of the HIV regulatory protein TAT (*trans*-activator of transcription). TAT protein is required for virus transcription and replication. Like protease inhibitors, TAT inhibitors are be effective in chronically HIV-infected cells, but TAT inhibitors have a further advantage in that they can protect cells that are already infected with HIV from progressing beyond latency. Another advantage of TAT inhibitors is that, in contrast to other anti-HIV drugs, resistant viruses against TAT inhibitors have not developed in laboratory testing, probably because all virus multiplication is shut off so that resistant mutants cannot develop. These aspects of TAT inhibitors make them potentially highly advantageous in treating HIV infection and also ideal for use in combination therapy with RT inhibitors. A Phase I study of the compound RO-24-7429, a TAT inhibitor, has begun in adults with advanced HIV infection. This drug is a benzodiazepine; no children have yet received it.

One final clinical trial of ZDV involving infants deserves mention, ACTG Protocol 076, which is attempting to determine whether administration of ZDV to pregnant women can interrupt transmission of HIV from a mother to her offspring. This is a double-blind, placebo-controlled study in women whose $CD4^+$ counts are above $200/mm^3$, for whom use of AZT is considered optional during pregnancy. These women are being treated during the second and/or third trimesters of pregnancy, through delivery, and their infants are then given the same treatment as the mother orally for the first 6 weeks of life. The infants are followed up closely for whether they are infected with HIV or not. Any that are infected can then be placed on ACTG Protocol 182. Protocol 076 is a major effort in pediatric AIDS because if ZDV is successful in preventing vertical transmission of HIV, it will be a significant clinical and scientific advance.

REFERENCES

1. Pizzo, P. A., J. Eddy, J. Falloon, F. Balis, R. Murphy, H. Moss, *et al.* 1988. Effect of continuous intravenous infusion of zidovudine (AZT) in children with symptomatic HIV infection. N. Engl. J. Med. **319:** 889–899.
2. McKinney, R., M. Maha, J. Connor, J. Feinberg, G. Scott, M. Wulfson, K. Macintosh, W. Borkowsky, J. Modlin, P. Weintrub, K. O'Donnell, R. Gelber, G. Rogers, S.N. Lehrman, C. Wilfert & Protocol 043 Study Group. 1991. A multicenter trial of oral zidovudine in children with advanced human immunodeficiency virus disease. N. Engl. J. Med. **324:** 1018–1025.
3. Butler, K. M., R. N. Husson, F. M. Balis, P. Brouwers, J. Eddy, D. Elamin, J. Gress, M. Hawkins, *et al.*, 1991. Dideoxyinosine in children with symptomatic human immunodeficiency virus infection. N. Engl. J. Med. **324:** 137–144.
4. Blanche, S., D. A-M., M. S. Navarette, M. Tardieu, M. Debre, C. Rouzioux, J. Seldrup, S. Kouzan & C. Griscelli. 1991. Low dose zidovudine in children with human immunodeficiency virus infection acquired in the perinatal period. Pediatrics **88:** 364–370.
5. Connor, E. & C. McSherry. 1991. Antiviral treatment of human immunodeficiency virus infection in children. Sem. Ped. Infect. Dis. **2:** 285–300.
6. Denny, T. N. & P. Palumbo. 1992. Laboratory tools for diagnosis and monitoring HIV-infected women and children. *In* Management of HIV Infection in Infants and

Children. R. Yogev & E. Connor, Eds.: 129–161. Mosby Year Book. St. Louis, MO.
7. YANASE, Y., T. TANGO, K. OKUMURA, *et al.* 1986 Lymphocyte subsets identified by monoclonal antibodies in healthy children. Pediatr. Res. **20:** 1147–1151.
8. CENTERS FOR DISEASE CONTROL. 1991. Guidelines for prophylaxis against *Pneumocystis carinii* pneumonia for children infected with human immunodeficiency virus. Morbid. Mortal. Wkly. Rep. **40**(March 15): 1–9.
9. LARDER, B. A., G. DARBY & D. RICHMAN. HIV with reduced sensitivity to zidovudine (AZT) isolated during prolonged therapy. 1989. Science **243:** 1731–1734.
10. SINGER, J. *et al.* 1991. Clinical significance of in-vitro HIV resistance to zidovudine in early HIV-infected individuals after four years of therapy. Paper presented at the Seventh International Conference on AIDS. June, 1991. Florence, Italy.
11. TUDOR-WILLIAMS, G., M. ST. CLAIR, R. E. MCKINNEY, M. MAHA, E. WALTER, S. SANTACROCE, M. MINTZ, *et al.* 1992. HIV-1 sensitivity to zidovudine and clinical outcome in children. Lancet **339:** 15–19.
12. GRAHAM, N., S. ZEGER, L. PARK, S. VERMUND, R. DETELS, C. RINALDO & J. PHAIR. 1992. The effects on survival of early treatment of human immunodeficiency virus infection. N. Engl. J. Med. **326:** 1037–1042.
13. HAMILTON, J. D., P. HARTIGAN, M. SIMBERKOFF, P. DAY, G. DIAMOND, G. DICKINSON, G. DRUSANO, *et al.* 1992. A controlled trial of early versus late treatment with zidovudine in symptomatic human immunodeficiency virus infection. Results of the Veterans Affairs Cooperative Study. N. Engl. J. Med. **326:** 437–443.
14. FISCHL, M., D. RICHMAN, N. HANSEN, A. C. COLLIER, J. CAREY, M. PARA, D. HARDY, *et al.* 1990. The safety and efficacy of zidovudine (AZT) in the treatment of subjects with mildly symptomatic human immunodeficiency virus type 1 (HIV) infection. Ann. Int. Med. **112:** 727–737.
15. VOLBERDING, P. A., S. LAGAKOS, M. A. KOCH, *et al.* 1990. Zidovudine in asymptomatic human immunodeficiency virus infection. A controlled trial in persons with fewer than 500 CD4-positive cells per cubic millimeter. N. Engl. J. Med. **322:** 941–949.
16. BALIS, F. M., P. A. PIZZO, J. EDDY, C. WILFERT, R. MCKINNEY, G. SCOTT, R. F. MURPHY, P. JAROSINSKI, J. FALLOON & D. POPLACK. 1989. Pharmacokinetics of zidovudine administered intravenously and orally in children with human immunodeficiency virus infection. J. Pediatr. **114:** 880–884.
17. BALIS, F. M., P. A. PIZZO, R. F. MURPHY, *et al.* 1989. The pharmacokinetics of zidovudine administered by cutaneous infusion in children. Ann. Int. Med. **110:** 279–285.
18. MCKINNEY, R., P. PIZZO, G. SCOTT, *et al.* 1990. Safety and tolerance of intermittent intravenous and oral zidovudine therapy in human immunodeficiency virus-infected pediatric patients. J. Pediatr. **116:** 640–647.
19. KAHN, J. O., S. W. LAGAKOS, D. D. RICHMAN, A. CROSS, C. PETTINELLI, L. SONG-HENG, M. BROWN, *et al.* 1992. A controlled trial comparing continued zidovudine with didanosine in human immunodeficiency virus infection. N. Engl. J. Med. **327:** 581–587.
20. BALIS, F. M., P. A. PIZZO, K. M. BUTLER, M. E. HAWKINS, P. BROUWERS, R. N. HUSSON, F. JACOBSEN, S. M. BLANEY, J. GRESS, P. JAROSINSKI & D. G. POPLACK. 1992. Clinical pharmacology of 2',3'-dideoxyinosine in human immunodeficiency virus-infected children. J. Infect. Dis. **165:** 99–104.
21. PIZZO, P., K. BUTLER, F. BALIS, E. BROUWERS, M. HAWKINS, J. EDDY, M. EINLOTH, J. FALLOON, R. HUSSON, *et al.* 1990. Dideoxycytidine alone and in an alternating schedule with zidovudine in children with symptomatic human immunodeficiency virus. J. Pediatr. **117:** 799–808.
22. HUSSON, R. N., Y. CHUNG, J. MORDENTI, K. BUTLER, S. CHEN, A.-M. DULIEGE, P. BROUWERS, *et al.* 1992. Phase 1 study of continuous-infusion soluble CD4 as a single agent and in combination with oral dideoxyinosine therapy in children with symptomatic human immunodeficiency virus infection. J. Pediatr. **121:** 627–633.
23. YARCHOAN, R., J. M. PLUDA, C. F. PERNO, H. MITSUYA, R. V. THOMAS, K. M. WYVILL & S. BRODER. 1990. Initial experience with dideoxynucleosides as single agents and in combination. Ann. N. Y. Acad. Sci. **616:** 328–343.

24. MENG, T.-C., M. FISCHL, A. M. BOOTA, S. SPECTOR, D. BENNETT, Y. BASSIAKOS, S. LAI, B. WRIGHT & D. RICHMAN. 1992. Combination therapy with zidovudine and dideoxycytidine in patients with advanced human immunodeficiency virus infection. Ann. Int. Med. **116:** 13–20.
25. COLLIER, A. C. 1991. Effect of combination therapy with zidovudine and didanosine (ddI) on surrogate markers. Paper presented at the Seventh International Conference on AIDS. June, 1991. Florence, Italy.
26. ERKELLER-YUKSEL, F. M., V. DENEYS, B. YUKSEL, I. HANNET, F. HULSTAERT, C. HAMILTON, H. MACKINNON, L. T. STOKES, V. MUNHYESHULI, F. VANLANGENDONCK, M. DEBRUYERE, B. A. BACH, P. M. LYDYARD. 1992. Age-related changes in human blood lymphocyte subpopulations. J. Pediatr. **120:** 216–222.

The Clinical Evaluation of Cytokines and Immunomodulators in HIV Infection

ARTHUR J. AMMANN

*The Ariel Project for Prevention of
HIV Transmission from Mother to Infant
Pediatric AIDS Foundation
Novato, California 94949*

INTRODUCTION

The availability of large amounts of highly purified recombinant proteins has revolutionized therapeutic approaches to disease. Previously, biologic factors were identified on the basis of relatively crude *in vitro* or *in vivo* assays and identified by a specific biologic effect. For example, macrophage activating factor (MAF) was discovered primarily by its effect on macrophages *in vitro*. It was not clear if the effects were due to a single factor or to the presence of small amounts of contaminants. Subsequently, it was shown that MAF was identical to interferon-γ (IFN-γ).[1] This was possibly because recombinant IFN-γ had been isolated and purified; specific monoclonal antibodies were developed along with bioassays; and, therefore, immunologic and biologic identity could be confirmed.

Advances also brought new challenges. It became clear that once sufficient amounts of a factor became available for animal studies, the biologic effects of a factor might be much broader than anticipated, more toxic, or have primary effects that differed significantly from its originally assigned name. Tumor necrosis factor (TNF; originally called cachetin), for example, does not have significant antitumor effects *in vivo* in humans, but does have significant toxic effects.[2] It is now known that it is a major mediator of endotoxin shock. Rather than regarding it as a potential therapeutic agent for cancer treatment, it is now felt that major benefits might be derived from blocking the acute effects of TNF in endotoxin shock and the chronic effects in the wasting syndrome of AIDS.

The discussion that follows describes the evaluation of those cytokines that have undergone the most extensive evaluation in HIV-infected patients. Most of these have been evaluated exclusively in adults. Only interferon-α (IFN-α) has proven to be successful in controlled trials in AIDS.

Several generalizations can be made following an analysis of the success or failure of cytokines in clinical trials.

1. Cytokines that have limited and specific biologic effects are more likely to be clinically useful. Interferon-α has activity that is restricted to antiviral activity and has been efficacious against several chronic viral infections. On the other hand, interferon-γ, which has broad biologic effects that trigger the production of multiple cytokines, has only limited application at this time.

2. The name or designation of a cytokine, often based on *in vitro* observations, does not necessarily predict *in vivo* biologic activity. The effect of TNF on malignancy in humans has not been significant because severe toxicity occurs related to the role of TNF in mediating endotoxin shock.

3. More information is needed in understanding the pharmacokinetics of cytokines. The usefulness of interleukin-2 (IL-2) is limited by its short half-life and the need to treat *ex vivo* in order to stimulate lymphokine-activated killer (LAK) cells. In contrast, the biologic effects of IFN-γ are observed with injections of small amounts given as infrequently as three times per week.

INTERFERON-α

At least 14 subtypes of IFN-α exist, with two recombinant forms currently approved for clinical use.[3,4] IFN-α is species specific, which makes trials in animals difficult. The major biologic activity of IFN-α is antiviral, although it will also stimulate natural killer (NK) cells and expression of class I and II antigens on cell membranes. The effect of IFN-α on HIV-1 is to interfere with the release of mature virions.[5]

Before the availability recombinant IFN-α, clinical trials were performed with leukocyte-derived interferon. After some initial confusing results, a number of more recent studies using recombinant interferons have provided more convincing evidence that IFN-α is effective in both the treatment of Kaposi's sarcoma (KS) and HIV-1.[6,7]

Doses of IFN-α range between 15 and 20 million units/m^2 daily. At the highest levels, most patients experience side effects that include malaise, headache, muscle pain, nausea, diarrhea, leukopenia, hepatic toxicity, and mental status alterations. The side effects, and the requirement for parental administration, have limited the usefulness of IFN-α.

The efficacy of IFN-α is apparent in patients with higher CD4 counts, suggesting that IFN-α does not have a direct action. The response rate in patients treated for KS has varied from 30 to 50% of patients, with improved responses observed in patients with mild disease and no opportunistic infection.[6,7]

IFN-α has *in vitro* synergism with zidovudine (ZDV) and recombinant CD4.[8] Synergism has been more difficult to demonstrate in clinical trials, since ZDV alone will result in improvement of surrogate markers of HIV-1 infection. Results of clinical trials have not yet been conclusive, with some trials demonstrating an early reduction in plasma p24 antigen and viral burden, and others describing only transient effects.

Three forms of IFN-α have been used clinically: lymphoblastoid, recombinant IFN-α-2a and recombinant IFN-α-2b. The latter two differ in structure by two amino acids. Many patients who receive recombinant IFN-α develop neutralizing antibodies that can interfere with biologic effects.

IFN-α has several antiviral effects, including activity against rhinovirus (topical papillomavirus, and hepatitis A and B. It is approved for use in hairy cell leukemia, papilloma virus warts, and chronic hepatitis.[9-11]

A single AIDS Clinical Trial Group (ACTG) protocol for evaluation of IFN-α in children is in progress. This compares IFN-α to ZDV plus IFN-α. Other studies in progress in adults include IFN-α in combination with interleukin-2 (IL-2) or granulocyte-macrophage colony stimulating factor (GM-CSF).

INTERFERON-γ

Unlike IFN-α and IFN-β, IFN-γ has a broad range of biologic activities, only one of which is an antiviral effect.[12] IFN-γ has antiproliferative effects against several tumors *in vitro* and acts synergistically with TNF. The antitumor effect is currently under investigation. A variety of microbial agents are inhibited *in vitro* and *in vivo* by IFN-γ and include chlamydia, toxoplasma, leishmania, plasmodium, cytomegalovirus (CMV), and HIV-1.[13] IFN-γ also enhances the expression of class I and II histocompatibility antigens and induces oxidative metabolism in monocytes and macrophages.[14]

Clinical trials using IFN-γ have evaluated its effectiveness as an antitumor agent and as an antimicrobial agent. Conclusions concerning its efficacy as an antitumor agent cannot be made as yet. In studies evaluating KS, questions have been raised as to whether IFN-γ may have caused an acceleration of KS.

IFN-γ is approved for use in patents with chronic granulomatous disease (CGD).[15] Patients with CGD have a genetic defect in oxidative metabolism of monocytes and macrophages. IFN-γ, given three times per week, reduced the number of serious infections and hospitalizations in a controlled trial. The successful use of IFN-γ in CGD patients, at low doses and infrequent administration, stands in contrast to the lack of efficacy in other trials using high doses (1 to 10 million units per m^2 per day) given on a daily basis. This points out the need for more pharmacokinetic information on the use of cytokines.

A single trial of IFN-γ in HIV-1 infected children is planned. On a theoretical basis, the use of IFN-γ as a prophylactic agent has considerable merit based on its broad *in vitro* and *in vivo* antimicrobial activity and the potential lack of emergence of resistant organisms.

INTERLEUKIN-2

IL-2 is one of 10 well-described cytokines that have been designated interleukins. The term "interleukin" was adopted to classify various diverse cytokines (substances derived from cells) that are derived from white blood cells and that act between cells. As the biology of interleukins was studied in more detail, however, it became apparent that many interleukins are produced by cells such as endothelial cells and may act on other cells of nonleukocyte origin.

IL-2 was one of the first recombinant proteins to be evaluated clinically. Because of its potent *in vitro* effects on the immune system, it was anticipated that it would result in marked stimulation of the immune system *in vivo*. IL-2, *in vitro*, stimulated T cells, increased the release in various cytokines, and was a potent T-cell growth factor. Adding IL-2 to cell cultures resulted in the infectability of T cells and growth of HIV-1. *In vivo*, IL-2 enhanced the primary immune response of animals, restored T cell responsiveness of athymic mice, generated NK cell activity, and had some activity toward malignancies that was most likely mediated by LAK cells.[16]

The *in vitro* and *in vivo* evidence of a T-cell stimulatory effect of IL-2 made this cytokine a primary candidate for T-cell reconstitution in primary and secondary immunodeficiency. Although some success was observed in the acceleration of reconstitution of immunity after bone marrow transplantation, the improved immunity observed in patients with AIDS was only transient. This may have been related to the dose of IL-2 used, the method of administration, or the short half-life of IL-2. It is more likely, however, that as T-cells were stimulated *in vivo* by IL-2, they became targets for new HIV-1 infection.

More recent clinical protocols in HIV-1 infection employ IL-2 PEG, which has a longer half-life, used concomitantly with antiretroviral treatment such as ZDV.[17] Preliminary results show more persistent increases in CD4 counts, associated with decreases in circulating virus.

IL-2 is administered over a wide range of doses (1000 to 10 million units/m^2 daily). Large doses result in significant toxicity, especially the "capillary leak" syndrome. This has resulted in studies using *ex vivo* exposure of leukocytes to IL-2 in order to generate tumoricidal LAK cells. Although this method has met with some success, it is difficult and expensive to perform. Currently, IL-2 is approved for the treatment of renal cell carcinoma in adults. There are no clinical trials in children with HIV-1 infection.

TUMOR NECROSIS FACTOR

A tumor necrosis factor was first described in 1931 after Gratia and Linz observed that endotoxins were capable of inducing hemorrhagic necrosis in transplanted animal tumors. It was not, however, until recombinant tumor necrosis factor (TNF) became available that the specific biologic functions of this molecule could be identified. A closely related molecule, lymphotoxin, was found to bind to the TNF receptor and mediate identical biologic effects. It was renamed TNF-β. Another factor, cachectin, was also extensively studied as a substance that resulted in wasting disease in animals. It was found to be identical to TNF-α.

TNF is a potent cytokine produced primarily by macrophages and monocytes after a variety of stimuli. It is produced acutely during endotoxin shock and, along with IL-1, is a major mediator of the physiologic events in endotoxin shock.[18,19] Monoclonal antibodies to TNF neutralize the major toxic effects of TNF. Recently, it has also been found that pentoxyfyline neutralizes the *in vitro* and *in vivo* effects of TNF.

In addition to pronounced antitumor effects in animals, TNF has protective effects in a variety of experimental infections, including herpes and HIV. Nevertheless, an initial study demonstrating an anti-HIV-1 *in vitro* effect has not been confirmed, and recent studies indicate that TNF actually increases HIV-1 replication.[20]

Studies in HIV-1 infection indicate that TNF is present in increased amounts in plasma and the cerebrospinal fluid of patients with AIDS. Based on the biologic activities of TNF, it has been postulated that TNF plays a role in the progression of HIV-1 infection, the chronic wasting syndrome, and central nervous system abnormalities. Paradoxically, clinical trials of TNF have taken opposite approaches, either administration of TNF or attempts to block TNF, thus illustrating the incomplete knowledge that exists for many cytokines.

TNF has been administered to HIV-1 infected patients to treat HIV-1 infection and/or KS. It has been used in Phase I studies, either alone or in combination with IFN-γ. Overall, the antitumor and anti-HIV-1 effects were disappointing; and, in some instances, it was suspected that KS lesions may have progressed. Direct inoculation of TNF into KS lesions, however, has resulted in improvement, but because of TNF toxicity and the availability of other agents, this form of treatment has not been pursued.

Pentoxyfyline has the ability to inhibit the physiologic effects of TNF *in vitro* and *in vivo*. It is currently under evaluation in adult trials. No pediatric trials currently exist. If the wasting syndrome and central nervous system disorders of adults and children have similar immunopathologic mechanisms, it would be important to investigate the potential benefit of this agent in neutralizing the effect of TNF.

GROWTH HORMONE AND INSULIN-LIKE GROWTH FACTOR

A relationship between growth hormone (GH) and the immune system has been postulated since the 1960s. It has been difficult to prove, however, that GH is an essential cytokine in the regulation of immunity. Studies have shown that lymphocytes have receptors for GH, cells of the immune system proliferate in response to GH *in vitro*, growth hormone-deficient mice have reduced amounts of thymic and lymphoid tissue, and insulin-like growth factor (IGF-1) increases the size of the thymus and spleen in hypophysectomized rats to a greater extent than other organs.[21,22] More recently, it has been shown that GH accelerates immunologic reconstitution after bone marrow transplantation in severe combined immunodeficient mice.[23]

In addition to *in vitro* and *in vivo* effects of GH and IGF-1 on the immune system, both molecules have anabolic effects. When administered to patients in negative nitrogen balance, they result in nitrogen retention, weight gain, and increased muscle mass. These effects, coupled with a potential for improving immune functions, make both molecules attractive candidates for the treatment of HIV-1 infected patients with wasting and immunodeficiency.

Unfortunately, neither GH or IGF-1 has been evaluated in children with HIV-1 infection in spite of several Phase I studies in adults suggesting a beneficial effect. This is particularly distressing because growth hormone was first evaluated and approved for children and has also enjoyed orphan drug status since the mid 1980s. It is to be hoped that trials of GH and IGF-1 will be initiated in HIV-1 infected infants and children in the near future.

CONCLUSIONS

The optimism concerning the potential of cytokines for the treatment of HIV-1 infections and its complications has not been fully realized. With a few exceptions, many well-defined cytokines remain under investigation even after years of clinical evaluation. Some of the reasons for delay include toxicity that was greater than originally anticipated (TNF), biologic effects that were more diffuse than originally anticipated (IL-2), and *in vitro* anti-HIV-1 efficacy that has not been confirmed *in vivo* (IFN-γ).

Nevertheless, some of the cytokines offer considerable promise. IFN-γ has been shown to be effective as a general antimicrobial prophylactic agent in chronic granulomatous disease. It is possible that it could also be used in HIV-1 infection. IFN-α has been approved for the treatment of KS. It also has a beneficial effect on ITP and, *in vitro* and *in vivo*, causes a decrease in HIV-1 replication. It has potential as a synergistic agent when combined with other antiretroviral agents.

As new cytokines are studied in detail, it is apparent that more information is needed concerning the pharmacokinetics and the most effective means of administering these molecules. Traditional approaches to therapy, such as dose escalation until toxicity is achieved, may not be appropriate for cytokine therapy. IFN-γ was found to be effective when given only three times per week at doses that had minimal toxicity.

A major obstacle to the rapid evaluation of new agents in HIV-1 infected infants and children is the continued exclusion of this population from early trials. Several steps must be taken to remedy this situation. Legislation is needed to encourage, or require, Phase I pharmacokinetic and safety studies in infants and children (and women) with life-threatening diseases. Such legislation should provide incentives to the pharmaceutical industry, since some disincentives might cause pharmaceutical companies to abandon drug development for rare diseases in children and women.

Another area that may be an obstacle is that of liability. Although a pharmaceutical company claimed that liability was the primary reason for withdrawing from passive antibody trials in HIV-1 infected pregnant women and children, there has been no substantiation that any liability judgments have been awarded in the experimental phase of drug evaluation for life-threatening illnesses. Therefore, if liability protection is required, it should be limited to approved drugs. It has been suggested that additional liability protection could be modeled after the childhood vaccine liability act.

Finally, it is apparent that there are insufficient numbers of HIV-1 infected children to evaluate all potential therapeutics for efficacy. This is especially true for combination treatments in which the estimated numbers for efficacy in a clinical trial exceed 800. It is therefore essential that strict priorities be established for drug and cytokine evaluation in children. Phase I and II pharmacokinetic and safety trials should receive priority. Phase III and IV efficacy trials should be performed only if the study has the power to answer the question of efficacy or if the question can be uniquely or more rapidly answered in the pediatric population, for example, prevention of HIV-1 transmission from mother to infant, prevention of HIV-1 in infants born to HIV-infected mothers when treatment is instituted at birth, reversal of dementia and wasting syndrome. The hope for the future is that early diagnosis and routine screening of newborns will permit earlier access of HIV-1 infected infants to life-saving therapy and increase the number of HIV-1 infected infants who will have access to clinical trials.

REFERENCES

1. TALMADGE, K. W., H. GALLATI, F. SINIGAGLIA, A. WALZ & G. GAROTTA. 1985. Identity between human interferon-γ and macrophage-activating factor produced by human T lymphocytes. Eur. J. Immunol. **16:** 1471–1477.
2. BEUTLER, B. & A. CERAMI. 1989. The biology of cachectin/TNF—a primary mediator of the host response. Annu. Rev. Immunol. **7:** 625–655.
3. FINTER, N. B., S. CHAPMAN & P. DOWD. 1991. The use of interferon-α in virus infections. Drugs **42:** 749–765.
4. MITSUYASU, R. T. 1992. AIDS-associated Kaposi's sarcoma and the mechanisms of interferon-α activity: A riddle within a puzzle. J. Intern. Med. **231:** 321–325.
5. LAI, P. K., Y. TAMURA & W. G. BRADLEY. 1991. Cytokine regulation of the human immunodeficiency virus (HIV). Int. J. Immunopharmacol. **13:** 55–61.
6. EDLIN, B. R., R. A. WEINSTEIN & S. M. WHALING. 1992. Zidovudine–interferon-α combination therapy in patients with advanced human immunodeficiency virus type 1 infection: Biphasic response of p24 antigen and quantitative polymerase chain reaction. J. Infect. Dis. **165:** 793–798.
7. GILL, P. S. 1991. Phase I/II trials of α-interferon alone or in combination with zidovudine as maintenance therapy following induction chemotherapy in the treatment of acquired immunodeficiency syndrome-related Kaposi's sarcoma. Semin. Oncol. **18:** 53–57.
8. PAN, X. Z., Z. D. QIU & P. A. BARON. 1992. Three-drug synergistic inhibition of HIV-1 replication *in vitro* by 3'-fluoro-3'-deoxythymidine, recombinant soluble CD4, and recombinant interferon-α. AIDS Res. Hum. Retrovir. **8:** 589–595.
9. HANDLY, J. M., T. HORNER & R. D. MAW. 1991. Subcutaneous interferon-α-2a combined with cryotherapy vs. cryotherapy alone in the treatment of primary anogenital warts: A randomized observer blind placebo controlled study. Genitourin. Med. **67:** 297–302.
10. GWALTNEY, J. M., JR. 1992. Combined antiviral and antimediator treatment of rhinovirus colds. J. Infect. Dis. **166:** 776–782.
11. GINTER, N. B., S. CHAPMAN & P. DOWD. 1991. The use of interferon-α in virus infections. Drugs **42:** 749–765.
12. DEMAEYER, E. & J. DEMAEYER-GUIGNARD, Eds. 1988. Interferon and Other Regulatory Cytokines. John Wiley & Sons. New York.
13. MURRAY, H. W. 1988. Interferon-γ, the activated macrophage, and host defense against microbial challenge. N. Engl. J. Med. **108:** 595–608.
14. GRAY, P. W. & D. V. GOEDDEL. 1987. Molecular biology of interferon-γ. Lymphokines **13:** 151–162.
15. DINAUER, M. C. & S. H. ORKIN. 1992. Chronic granulomatous disease. Annu. Rev. Med. **43:** 117–124.
16. MALKOVSKY, M., P.M. SONDEL & W. STROBER. 1988. The interleukins in acquired disease [Review]. Clin. Exp. Immunol. **74:** 151–161.
17. CLARK, A. G., M. HOLONDIY & D. H. SCHWARTZ. 1992. Decrease in HIV provirus in

peripehral blood mononucler cells during zidovudine and human rIL-2 administration. J. Acq. Immun. Defic. Syndr. **5:** 52–59.
18. PALLADINO, M. A. & A. J. AMMANN. 1988. Tumor necrosis factors alpha and beta. A family of biochemically related cytokines. *In* Leucolysins and Cancer. J. H. Ransom & J. R. Ortaldo, Eds.: 235–244. Human Press. Clifton, NJ.
19. CERAMI, A. & B. BEUTLER. 1988. The role of cachetin/TNF in endotoxic shock and cachexia. Immunol. Today **9:** 28–31.
20. WONG, G. H. W. & J. F. KROWKA. 1988. *In vitro* anti-human immunodeficiency virus activities of tumor necrosis factor-α and interferon-γ. J. Immunol. **140:** 120–124.
21. BINZ, K., P. JOLLER & P. FROESCH. 1990. Repopulation of the atrophied thymus in diabetic rats by insulin-like growth factor I. Proc. Natl. Acad. Sci. USA **87:** 3690–3694.
22. VERLAND, S. & S. GAMMELTOFT. 1989. Functional receptors for insulin-like growth factors I and II in rat thymocytes and mouse thymona cells. Mol. Cell. Endocrinol. **67:** 207–216.
23. MURPHY, W. J., S. K. DURUM & D. L. LONGO. 1992. Growth hormone accelerates peripheral T cell reconstitution in mice with severe combined immune deficiency (SCID) (Abstract). Weston Society Clinical Research. Carmel, CA.

Passive Immunity in the Prevention of Maternal–Fetal Transmission of Human Immunodeficiency Virus Infection

JOHN S. LAMBERT[a]

Departments of Medicine and Pediatrics
University of Rochester School of Medicine and Dentistry
Rochester, New York 14642

E. RICHARD STIEHM

Department of Pediatrics
UCLA School of Medicine
Los Angeles, California 90024

INTRODUCTION

Human immunodeficiency virus (HIV) infection of women is increasing, and maternal transmission of HIV to children is a growing problem. As of December 1991, the Centers for Disease Control reported 20,739 cases of AIDS among women in the United States, which represents 10.4% of cumulative cases in adults. During this same time period, 3426 cases were reported in children.[1] By the end of 1992, it is predicted that worldwide about 4 million infants will have been born to HIV-infected women.[2] Factors influencing HIV transmission in pregnancy are under intensive investigation with the focus on multiple factors, including the mechanisms and timing of transmission, the role of the maternal and fetal immune systems, and the role of the placenta, as well as HIV viral tropism and virulence. It appears that women who have low CD4 cell counts, who are p24 antigen positive, and who lack the ability to neutralize their infants' viruses are more likely to transmit HIV.[3-9]

A number of interventions have been proposed to interrupt the maternal–fetal transmission of HIV. These include antiretroviral drug therapy during pregnancy, active immunotherapy with candidate AIDS vaccines, monoclonal antibodies, and a hyperimmune anti-HIV globulin (HIVIG), which is the focus of this paper.

---

[a] Address for correspondence: John S. Lambert, M.D., Assistant Professor of Medicine & Pediatrics, University of Rochester School of Medicine & Dentistry, Box 689, 601 Elmwood Ave., Rochester, NY 14642.

RATIONALE FOR HIVIG THERAPY

Immune globulins have been used for treatment or prophylaxis against multiple human pathogens, including cytomegalovirus (CMV), varicella zoster virus (VZV), hepatitis B virus (HBV), measles, rabies virus, and vaccinia virus, among others.[10-15] At least two nonhuman retroviral infections have been treated with specific immune globulin.[16,17] In one study, six-month-old kittens inoculated with feline leukemia virus (FeLV) all became persistently viremic. However, when kittens were treated six days post virus inoculation with goat anti-FeLV or with antiserum to purified Friend leukemia virus (FLV) gp71, 75% of them were protected. In another study, FLV was injected into mice: All control animals became viremic and died at 8 to 12 weeks. Mice given goat anti-FLV gp71 seven days post inoculation did not become viremic and remained disease-free throughout their lifespan.

Three human clinical trials have been performed with an immune globulin taken from donors who were HIV infected and asymptomatic.[18-20] When these products were administered to patients with AIDS, plasma p24 antigen cleared, and some patients showed clinical improvement. In the only controlled clinical trial to date, performed by Vittecoq et al.,[20] 18 patients received either HIV immune or HIV negative plasma. The donors of the HIV immune plasma remained asymptomatic after one year. Over a 34-week study period, with a total of seven infusions administered every two weeks, two out of nine opportunistic infections developed in the study group compared to eight out of nine in the control group ($p = 0.016$ by t test). p24 Antigen dramatically declined in the group receiving HIV-immune plasma, but not in the control group. After cessation of the immune plasma infusions, patients who received the HIV-immune plasma experienced deterioration in their clinical status, but stabilized with reintroduction of the HIV-immune plasma.

THE ABBOTT HIVIG PRODUCT

HIVIG is a preparation of highly purified human immune globulin that contains high titers of antibody to HIV structural proteins with activity in virus neutralization and antibody-dependent cytotoxicity (ADCC) assays.[21] HIVIG is prepared from plasma of HIV-seropositive donors who are clinically asymptomatic and have CD4-positive lymphocytes ≥ 400 cells/mm^3. The plasma has high-titer anti-p24 antibody, has high neutralizing antibody activity against MN V3 loop peptides, and is not infectious for HIV, as determined by p24 antigen measurement, HIV viral coculture, and chimpanzee challenge. Purification of the HIVIG product includes multiple steps to inactivate HIV, including treatment with solvent/detergent, fractionation by the cold-ethanol procedure of Cohn-Oncley, and further purification by ion-exchange chromatography. Lots of HIVIG contain anti-p24 antibody titers $\geq 100,000$, anti-gp41 titers >4000, and anti-gp120 titers >1000. Neutralization titers of 1:160 to 1:1280 to HIV IIIb and MN strain have been demonstrated. HIVIG is active in ADCC assays and contains antibodies to V3 loop peptides in four strains tested (IIIB, MN, WMJ, SC). At a concentration of 500 µg/ml, HIVIG prevents *in vitro* infection of T cells. *In vitro* enhancement of HIV infection of lymphocytes by anti-HIV antibodies has been demonstrated. HIVIG concentrations of less than 10^{-3} µg/ml mediated enhancement of HIV infection in monocyte–macrophage cell lines. To date, however, no correlation has been demonstrated clinically with this *in vitro* phenomenon. This antibody-dependent enhancement (ADE) effect is not found with higher concentrations of antibody. Other studies using human peripheral blood mononuclear cells (PBMC) and peritoneal macrophages did not demonstrate an ADE effect of HIVIG at either high or low concentrations. Antibody levels obtained after a 200 mg/kg i.v. dose of HIVIG are 10,000 times higher than those reported to be associated with *in vitro* ADE.

A human safety study with HIVIG involved a group of 13 patients, most of whom had advanced HIV infection.[22] The patients received four doses of HIVIG every four weeks, the first two infusions at a dose of 50 mg/kg, the last two infusions 200 mg/kg. HIVIG was well tolerated. p24 Antigen became undetectable in six patients who were p24 antigen positive at entry into the study. HIV culture positivity was delayed in three patients treated with HIVIG, from 8.9 days at study entry to 17.9 days after treatment with HIVIG. No ADE was observed.

Animal studies have supported the theory that HIVIG is a tenable means of therapy. Initial chimpanzee studies did not show protection when the animals were challenged with 400 $TCID_{50}$ of HIV.[23] However, 1000 mg/kg of HIVIG given to a chimpanzee protected against a 120-$TCID_{50}$ HIV challenge. In another study by Eichberg *et al.*, chimpanzees were protected against HIV viral challenge of 120 $TCID_{50}$, when first given 10 ml/kg of HIVIG. After infusion with HIVIG, an antibody titer of 1:400 was observed.[24]

In a cynomolgus monkey model, hyperimmune sera to HIV-2 and simian immunodeficiency virus of the sooty mangabe (SIV_{Sm}) obtained from vaccine-immunized monkeys administered 6 hours before intravenous challenge of cell-free HIV demonstrated the success of passive immunotherapy. In the HIV-2 animal model, a high immunoglobin dose of 9 ml/kg protected two of three animals from viral infection.[25,26] In another study, by Emini *et al.*,[27] a product containing a mouse–human chimeric IgG1 antibody specific for the PND of the V3 loop of gp120 of HIV-1 IIIb was administered to a chimpanzee. Twenty-four hours later the chimpanzee was given 75 chimpanzee infectious doses of an HIV-1 IIIb isolate. The antibody titer at time of challenge was 1:320. The control animal became infected, but the immunized animal remains uninfected.

Human and animal studies using passive immunotherapies to date have demonstrated a high possibility of success with HIVIG. Therapeutic trials with HIVIG have been considered in adults with advanced HIV infection who would not likely respond to active immunotherapy protocols that use AIDS vaccines, for which an intact immune system is necessary. Additionally, trials of post-exposure prophylaxis in occupationally exposed health care workers and in the interruption of the maternal–fetal transfer of HIV infection have been proposed.

PREVENTION OF MATERNAL–FETAL HIV-1 TRANSMISSION

Currently, an AIDS clinical trial group study (ACTG 185) sponsored by the National Institutes of Health (NIH) has been designed to interrupt the maternal–fetal transmission of HIV infection. HIVIG will be studied at a 200 mg/kg dose, based on the IgG levels achieved in human trials and *in vitro* studies performed with this product.[21] Syncytia formation has been inhibited at IgG concentrations of 375 to 1200 µg/ml, ADCC activity has been demonstrated at 2.5 to 250 µg/ml, and HIV replication in monocyte/macrophage lines was inhibited at 50 to 500 µg/ml. A dose of 200 mg/kg produces levels in excess of 2600 µg/ml. With a half-life of 15 days, HIVIG administered monthly will produce trough levels of IgG of >650 µg/ml, a hundred times higher than antibody levels producing the *in vitro* ADE phenomenon.

ACTG 185 is a phase-III randomized, double-blind controlled study of the use of HIVIG for the prevention of maternal–fetal transmission in pregnant women and newborns receiving zidovudine (ZDV). HIV-infected pregnant women who are receiving oral ZDV for medical indications will be administered HIVIG or IVIG (the control) monthly, beginning at 20 to 30 weeks' gestation. The newborn infant will receive a single dose of HIVIG or IVIG within 12 hours after birth. In addition the infant will receive oral ZDV for six weeks. We hypothesize that the HIVIG intervention will reduce vertical HIV transmission compared with the IVIG administered in an identical manner. The estimated sample size is a total of 400 mother–infant pairs, 200 in each arm of the study. A 50% treatment effect (reduction of transmission from 30% to 15%) can be detected with a power of 80% (HIVIG vs. IVIG). The women will be eligible for randomization to HIVIG or IVIG between 20 and 30 weeks of pregnancy and will be stratified by (1) CD4 count at the time of entry (CD4 <200/mm^3 or ≥200/mm^3, (2) whether ZDV therapy began before or after conception (as an initial surrogate for duration of ZDV therapy), and (3) clinical center.

Data relevant to the women's pregnancy and HIV disease status will be collected to evaluate the safety and tolerance of HIVIG when administered with ZDV and to evaluate the influence of HIVIG compared with IVIG on the progression of maternal disease. Follow-up of the women will occur up to 26 weeks postpartum to evaluate long-term safety and to assess whether HIVIG affects disease progression. Women will be provided access to other ACTG clinical trials and to standard medical care in their respective clinical centers.

"NESTED" STUDIES IN ACTG 185

It is hoped that additional information will be obtained from this clinical trial that will provide insight into (1) the factors subserving protection from HIV infection and (2) how to optimally diagnose HIV infection in infants born to HIV-infected pregnant women. One of the unique features of the maternal–fetal transmission model that makes it attractive in researching HIV pathogenesis is that pregnancy is a well-defined and limited period during which clinical, virological, and immunological factors can be investigated and correlated with outcomes in the infant. Answers to what factors subserve maternal–fetal transmission of HIV may also answer the question of what constitutes protective immunity in HIV infection. A secondary objective of ACTG 185 is to evaluate the maternal virologic and immunologic factors involved in HIV transmission from mother to infant and the influence of HIVIG on the following parameters: (1) HIV plasma viremia and quantitative cell culture results, p24 antigen levels, and CD4 cell counts compared between transmitting and nontransmitting mothers and (2) the role of HIV antibody in vertical transmission measured by quantitative anti-p24 HIV antibody, V3 loop antibody (MN and IIIb strain), and neutralizing antibody in transmitting and nontransmitting women and their infants. Another secondary objective is to compare the early sensitivity and specificity of various methods of diagnosing HIV infection in infants, including PCR detection of HIV DNA, HIV-IgA assays, and placental HIV RNA PCR, with that of standard HIV culture methods.

ETHICAL AND LEGAL CONSIDERATIONS

The development of an immunotherapeutic intervention in pregnancy poses many unique problems. Maternal therapy raises complex ethical and legal questions regarding the rights of the fetus.[28-30] Theoretical adverse effects of maternal immunization have been reviewed by Ukwu et al.,[31] and many of these concerns apply to passive immunotherapies: (1) immune complex–mediated injury to the placenta and compromise of the maternal–fetal blood flow; (2) induction of tolerance to HIV antigens in the newborn; (3) anti-idiotype antibody to gp160, leading to autoimmunity, interference with normal CD4 receptor function, or altered development of lymphocyte populations expressing CD4 in the infant; (4) antibody-mediated enhancement of HIV replication in the placenta or cord blood lymphocytes, leading to increased rates of fetal HIV infection; (5) ineffective HIV-specific immune responses that do not inhibit virus replication, leading to increasing amounts of HIV antigen and immune-mediated tissue injury; and (6) other unpredictable events, such as the HIV-specific, antibody-mediated suppression of lymphoproliferative responses caused by antibody against regions of gp41 homologous to certain HLA-DR phenotypes. The current legal climate is another obstacle for trials in the United States. Up to 3% of infants born in this country have major abnormalities, and the combined rate of spontaneous abortion and stillbirth approaches 20%. Rates may be even higher in HIV-infected women, and it may be difficult to establish a causal relationship between the proposed intervention (HIVIG) and the background of "normal" complications of pregnancy in HIV-infected women.

ACTG 185 has been on hold since July 1992 because of a liability dispute. The manufacturer of HIVIG (Abbott Laboratory, N. Chicago, IL) has requested complete indemnification from liability—which would require an act of Congress—before allowing use of its HIV immune globulin. Their major concern appears to be the theoretical risk of the ADE phenomenon, the case in which administration of HIVIG could enhance the transmission of HIV to an infant. The phenomenon of antibody-dependent enhancement of viral infection was first described in animal viruses by Hawkes in 1964[32] and since has been reported in numerous flavivirus systems.[33-36] Experiments have been performed with HIV *in vitro* that demonstrate this phenomenon, where subneutralizing HIV antibody levels can cause modest increases in HIV production, as detected in culture supernatants.[37] However, there has been no clinical correlation in the HIV system *in vivo*.

The issue of indemnification raised with the Abbott HIVIG product has raised serious concerns regarding our ability to modify pediatric HIV infection by intervening with potential therapeutic agents in pregnancy. Currently there are about 6000 births each year to women infected with HIV; about one-third of these children become infected.[38] Hyperimmune globulin products have proven safe and efficacious in the treatment and prophylaxis of many other viral infections. *In vitro* data, animal efficacy trials, and Phase I human trials have revealed this product to be safe, with a high potential for success. Medicolegal roadblocks have broad implications for access of therapies to a population infected with HIV, namely pregnant women, for whom we desperately need therapeutic interventions as well as intense scientific investigation into factors involved in maternal-fetal HIV transmission. The urgency of the problem necessitates current barriers be eliminated with great haste, so that interventional trials can be initiated. National and international implementation of passive immunotherapy trials, perhaps in conjunction with candidate AIDS vaccines (similar to the hepatitis B model "passive-active" approach for the interruption of maternal-fetal transmission of HBV), is one of the best opportunities we have with currently available therapies of giving hope for the elimination of pediatric HIV infection in countries where HIV has established itself in women of child-bearing age.

REFERENCES

1. CENTERS FOR DISEASE CONTROL. 1991. HIV/AIDS surveillance report December 11, 1991. Atlanta, GA.
2. CHIN, J. 1990. Current and future dimensions of the HIV/AIDS pandemic in women and children. Lancet **336:** 221–224.
3. EUROPEAN COLLABORATIVE STUDY. 1991. Children born to women with HIV infection: Natural history and risk of transmission. Lancet **339:** 1249–1253.
4. D'ARMINIO, M. A., M. RAVIZZA, M. L. MUGGIASCA, *et al.* 1991. HIV-infected pregnant women: Possible predictors of vertical transmission. VII International Conference on AIDS (Florence, Italy): Abstract no. WC 49.
5. BOUE, F., J. C. PONS, L. KEROS, *et al.* 1990. Risk for HIV-1 perinatal transmission varies with the mother's stage of HIV infection. VI International Conference on AIDS (San Francisco, CA): Abstract no. ThC 44.
6. EUROPEAN COLLABORATIVE STUDY. 1992. Risk factors for mother-to-child transmission of HIV-1. Lancet **339:** 1007–1012.
7. TIBALDI, C., E. PALOMBA, N. ZIARATI, *et al.* 1991. Maternal factors influencing vertical HIV transmission. VII International Conference on AIDS (Florence, Italy): Abstract no. WC 3277.
8. SCARLATTI, G., J. ALBERT, P. ROSSI, *et al.* 1992. Homologous and heterologous neutralization activity in sera of HIV-1 infected mothers: Correlation to transmission. Proceedings of VIII International AIDS Conference (Amsterdam, the Netherlands): Abstract no. WeC1061.
9. KLIKS, S.C., M. B. FADEM, D. W. WARA & J. A. LEVY. 1992. Evidence for the maternal transfer to neutralization-escape or enhancement variants into newborn infants. Proceedings of VIII International Conference on AIDS (Amsterdam, the Netherlands): Abstract no. PoA 2463.
10. STIEHM, E. R., E. ASHIDA, K. S. KIM, *et al.* 1987. Intravenous immunoglobulins as therapeutic agents. Ann. Intern. Med. **107:** 367–382.

11. STIEHM, E. R. 1986. Specific human immunoglobulins as therapeutic agents. *In* Clinical Use of Intravenous Immunoglobulins. A. Morell & U. E. Nydegger, Eds.: 237–252. Academic Press, Harcourt-Brace Jovanovich Inc. San Diego, CA.
12. ORENSTEIN, W. A., D. L. HEYMANN, R. J. ELLIS, *et al.* 1981. Prophylaxis of varicella in high-risk children: Dose–response effect of zoster immune globulin. J. Pediatr. **98**: 368–373.
13. SNYDMAN, D. R., B. G. WERNER, B. HEINZE-LACEY, *et al.* 1987. Use of cytomegalovirus immune globulin to prevent cytomegalovirus disease in renal-transplant recipients. N. Eng. J. Med. **317**: 1049–1054.
14. SEEFF, L. B. & J.H. HOOFNAGLE. 1979. Immunoprophylaxis of viral hepatitis. Gastroenterology **77**: 161–182.
15. BEASLEY, R. P., C. C. LIN, K. Y. WANG, *et al.* 1981. Hepatitis B immune globulin (HBIG) efficacy in the interruption of perinatal transmission of hepatitis B virus carrier state. Lancet **2**: 388–393.
16. DE NORONHA, F., W. SCHAFER, M. ESSEX & D. P. BOLOGNESI. 1978. Influence of antisera to ocoravirus glycoprotein (gp71) on infections of cats with feline leukemia virus Virology **85**: 617–621.
17. IGLEHART, J. D., M. J. WEINHOLD, E. C. WARD, *et al.* 1983. Prospects for immunological management of lethal tumors. Cancer Invest. **1**: 409–421.
18. JACKSON, G. G., J. T. PERKINS, M. RUBENS, *et al.* 1988. Passive immunoneutralization of human immunodeficiency virus in patients with advanced AIDS. Lancet **2**: 647–652.
19. KARPAS, A., F. HILL, M. YOULE, *et al.* 1988. Effects of passive immunization in patients with acquired immunodeficiency syndrome-related complex and acquired immunodeficiency syndrome. Proc. Natl. Acad. Sci. USA **85**: 9234–9237.
20. VITTECOQ, D., B. MATTLINGER, F. BARRE-SINOUSSI, *et al.* 1992. Passive immunotherapy in AIDS: A randomized trial of serial human imunodeficiency virus-positive transfusions of plasma rich in p24 antibodies versus transfusions of seronegtive plasma. J. Infect. Dis. **165**: 364–368.
21. CUMMINS, L.M., K. J. WEINHOLD, T. J. MATTHEWS, *et al.* 1991. Preparation and characterization of an intravenous solution of IgG from human immunodeficiency virus-seropositive donors. Blood **77(5)**: 1111–1117.
22. RHAME, F. S., R. N. GOODROAD, L.M. CUMMINS, *et al.* Safety and pharmacokinetics of human immunodeficiency virus immune globulin in persons with acquired immunodeficiency syndrome. (Submitted for publication in 1991.)
23. PRINCE, A. M., B. HOROWITZ, L. BAKER, *et al.* 1988. Failure of human immunodeficiency virus (HIV) immunoglobulin to protect chimpanzees against experimental challenge with HIV. Proc. Natl. Acad. Sci. USA. **85**: 6944–6948.
24. EICHBERG, J. W. 1990. Experience with thirteen HIV efficacy trials in chimpanzees. VI International Conference on AIDS (San Francisco, CA): Abstract no. Th. A338.
25. PUTKONEN, P., R. THORSTENSSON, L. GHAYAMIZADEH, *et al.* 1991. Prevention of HIV-2 and SIV($_{Sm}$) infection by passive immunization of cynomolgus monkeys. Nature: 436–438.
26. PUTKONEN, Z. P., R. THORSTENSSON, J. ALBERT, *et al.* 1991. Prevention of HIV-2 and SIVsm infection by passive immunization in cynomolgus monkeys. VII International Conferenced on AIDS (Florence, Italy): Abstract M.A. 21.
27. EMINI, E. A., W. A. SCHIEF, K. MURTHY, *et al.* 1991. Passive immunization with a monoclonal antibody directed to the HIV-1 gp120 principal neutralizing determinant confers protection against HIV-1 challenge in chimpanzees. VII International Conference on AIDS (Florence, Italy): Abstract no. Th.A.64.
28. GRAHAM, B. S. & D. T. KARZON. 1990. Development of an AIDS vaccine: Biological and ethical challenges. Infect. Dis. Clin. North Am. **4**: 223–243.
29. THE KEYSTONE CENTER. 1991. Final report of the Keystone AIDS vaccine liability project. Vaccine **9**: 703–709.
30. COHEN, J. 1992. Is liability slowing AIDS vaccines? Science **256**: 168–170.
31. UKWU, H. N., B. S. GRAHAM, J. S. LAMBERT & P. F. WRIGHT. 1992. Perinatal transmis-

sion of human immunodeficiency virus-1 infection and maternal immunization strategies for prevention. Obstet. Gynecol. **80:** 458–468.
32. HAWKES, R. A. 1964. Enhancement of the infectivity of arborviruses by specific antisera produced in domestic fowls. Aust. J. Exp. Med. Sci. **42:** 465–482.
33. HALSTEAD, S. B. & E. J. O'ROURKE. 1977. Antibody-enhanced dengue virus infection in primate leukocytes. Nature (London) **265:** 739–741.
34. HALSTEAD, S. B. & E. J. O'ROURKE. 1977. Dengue viruses and mononuclear phagocytes. I. Infection enhancement by non-neutralizing antibody. J. Exp. Med. **146:** 210–217.
35. SCHLESSINGER, J. J. & M. W. BRANDRISS. 1981. Growth of 17D yellow fever virus in a macrophage-like cell line, U937: Role of Fc and viral receptors in antibody-mediated infection. J. Immunol. **127:** 659–665.
36. PEIRIS, J. S. M. & J. S. PORTERFIELD. 1979. Antibody-mediated enhancement of flavivirus replication in macrophage-like cells. Nature (London) **282:** 509–511.
37. TAKEDA, A. & F. A. ENNIS. 1990. FcR-mediated enhancement of HIV-1 infection by antibody. AIDS Res. Hum. Retrovir. **6:** 999–1004.
38. GWINN, M., M. PAPPAIOANOU, J. R. GEORGE, *et al.* 1991. Prevalence of HIV infection in childbearing women in the United States. JAMA **265:** 1704–1708.

Prospects for Prevention of Vertical Transmission of Human Immunodeficiency Virus by Immunization

S. J. CRYZ, JR.,[a] H. GOLDSTEIN,[b] E. FÜRER,[a] J. U. QUE,[a]
T. HASLER,[a] B. ALTHAUS,[a] AND A. RUBINSTEIN[b]

[a] *Swiss Serum and Vaccine Institute*
CH-3001 Berne, Switzerland

[b] *Departments of Pediatrics and Microbiology and Immunology*
Albert Einstein College of Medicine
Bronx, New York 10461

INTRODUCTION

The incidence of pediatric AIDS has increased dramatically as the infection rate among women of child-bearing age has risen.[1,2] Vertical transmission of human immunodeficiency virus type-1 (HIV-1) is believed to be the primary route of infection, although perinatal infection cannot be ruled out.[3-6] Acquisition of HIV-1 has been shown to occur predominantly during the second trimester of pregnancy.[7] The rate of maternofetal transmission can vary from 13% to 65% depending on the study population.[8-10] In contrast to adulthood infection where overt disease is usually manifested only after a prolonged asymptomatic phase, infants infected *in utero* may show signs of illness as soon as the first year of life.[7] By 3 years of age, nearly all will present with AIDS. The comparatively rapid development of symptoms in this patient population presents a unique opportunity to study the feasibility of preventing HIV-1 transmission or blocking disease progression by immunological intervention.

FACTORS THAT MAY AFFECT VERTICAL TRANSMISSION OF HIV-1

The fact that *in utero* exposure to HIV-1 does not necessarily lead to infection strongly suggests the existence of a transmission-blocking maternal immune response. Identification of the factors that define a nontransmitting state would greatly facilitate vaccine development.

Initial studies addressing this issue found a modest degree of correlation between elevated antibody levels to the third hypervariable region (V3) of gp120 from the IIIB strain of HIV and a decreased rate of maternofetal transmission.[11,12] Therefore, between 31% and 46% of noninfected neonates had circulating anti-V3 antibodies, whereas those who became infected lacked such antibodies. Although inconclusive, these reports did indicate the existence of a humoral response that effectively prevented fetal infection. In addition, the critical domain of HIV-1 involved in this process was tentatively identified.

These findings were expanded on by Devash et al.[13] who used an antigen-limiting ELISA to detect high-affinity maternal antibody to a peptide (KRIHIGP-GRAFYT; residues 307–319) corresponding to the tip of the V3 loop from the MN strain of HIV-1. The MN strain was selected because it appears to be the predominant HIV-1 isolate in the United States.[14] The rationale for selecting this peptide is based on the fact that antibodies directed to this domain constitute the majority of neutralizing activity in anti-gp120 antiserum.[13] A total of 15 maternal–neonatal serum samples were analyzed retrospectively. All four noninfected neonates possessed high-affinity antibodies, whereas none of the 11 infected infants did so. No correlation was found between lack of transmission and parameters such as $CD4^+$ T-cell count, in vitro lymphoproliferative response to a mitogen, or circulating p24 antigen. Furthermore, the clinical status of the mother did not appear to influence virus transmission.

Two subsequent studies, however, found no correlation between high-affinity anti-V3 antibodies and decreased vertical transmission. Parekh et al.,[15] using the identical peptide as Devash et al.,[13] noted than neither total anti-peptide antibody nor the presence of high-affinity antibody influenced fetal infection rates. Robertson et al.,[16] using a 33-amino-acid peptide (residues 302–335), also found no beneficial effect conferred by antibodies recognizing this peptide. It is important to note that in the second study the results obtained could have been markedly influenced by conformational changes induced when the peptide was bound to the ELISA matrix. Such alterations may have rendered the KRIHIGPGRAFYT domain unavailable for antibody binding.

APPROACHES FOR THE PREVENTION OF VERTICAL TRANSMISSION OF HIV-1

Immunological means to prevent maternofetal transmission of HIV-1 could be based on either active, passive, or combined immunization. The following key factors must be taken into consideration when designing immunological intervention studies: (i) infection of the fetus occurs predominantly during the second trimester, (ii) the potential for fetal harm associated with active vaccination of pregnant women, (iii) a possible immunomodulating effect mediated by the immune response mounted to HIV-1 infection as regards active vaccination, and (iv) the limitations of passive therapy as concerns the onset and duration of immunity. Both approaches are dependent on the availability of an assay system capable of accurately measuring those factors that mediate protection.

Passive immunization offers the advantages of avoiding possible fetal harm and individual variations in response to active vaccination. In addition, assuming that vertical transmission can be blocked solely by relevant antibodies, the dosing regimen can be adjusted to ensure that protective levels of antibody are maintained. The major impediments to a passive approach are availability of product, logistics of a repeated dosing schedule, and cost.

Such a passive product could, in theory, be derived from plasma of HIV-infected persons, immunized donors, or monoclonal antibodies (mAb). The first approach has obvious safety concerns. Vaccination of healthy plasma donors with an HIV vaccine, while conceivable, may be constrained by social issues, especially if immunization renders those donors seropositive. The use of mAbs, especially if of human origin or humanized by recombinant DNA technology, would circumvent such problems. A chimeric mouse–human antibody directed against the V3 loop has been described.[17] This mAb was able to protect chimpanzees when given either before or shortly after an HIV-1 challenge. Regardless of whether human polyclonal antibodies or mAbs are eventually selected, such an approach is likely to be costly, thereby limiting its application primarily to developed countries.

Active vaccination has several distinct potential advantages over passive immunization, including (i) the ability to engender both a humoral and cell-mediated immune response, (ii) lower cost, and (iii) being simpler to implement, especially in underdeveloped areas of the world. The fetal harm issue could be avoided by the immunization of high-risk persons intraconceptually, which also offers numerous practical advantages. Additionally, vaccination may benefit the mother by impeding disease progression.

RELEVANT EPITOPES OF HIV-1: POTENTIAL VACCINE CANDIDATES

The structure of HIV-1 has been elucidated in great detail. The viral genome codes for four structural proteins/glycoproteins. The outer viral coat is composed primarily of gp160, which in turn consists of gp120 and gp41. gp120 extrudes from the viral surface while most of the gp41, being a transmembrane protein, is buried within the membrane. Two internal proteins, p17 and p24, are also present. Most attention relating to immunity has focused on gp120 and gp160 because of their surface exposure and role in mediating the initial phases of infection.

Antigenically, gp120 is characterized by five hypervariable regions (V1–V5), so designated because of frequent mutations within these areas. The most immunodominant of these regions concerning the elicitation of neutralizing antibodies is V3, which is also referred to as the principal neutralizing domain (PND). The PND, which generally spans amino acids 296–303 to 331–338 (depending on the HIV isolate), is configured as a loop owing to the formation of a disulfide bond.[18] This loop structure is believed to be universally conserved among HIV-1 isolates. The minimal epitope capable of inducing a neutralizing antibody response is composed of approximately 10 amino acids that reside at the tip of the loop.[18] At the center of these 10 amino acids is the highly conserved GPGR motif, which confers a β-turn configuration. Mutations within the primary sequence of this region can lead to so-called "escape mutants," which are no longer neutralized by antibodies directed against the original sequence.[19,20]

Anti-PND antibody has been shown to play a crucial role in protection against HIV-1 infection. In three independent chimpanzee challenge studies using gp120-based vaccines, protection was found to correlate with anti-PND antibody titers.[21-23] A human monoclonal antibody that bound to amino acid residues 313–322 (PGPGRAFYTT) was able to neutralize the homologous MN strain and several related variants.[18] Significantly, a single amino acid substitution at position 320 (Y to H) completely abrogated the neutralizing capacity of this antibody. Emini et al.[17] found that a chimeric mouse–human IgG1 mAb directed to the PND-protected chimpanzees when administered before or 10 min after challenge. Anti-PND antibodies can neutralize HIV-1 infectivity even after gp120-mediated binding to CD4 has occurred, presumably by inhibiting proteolytic cleavage of gp120 essential for virus internalization. Polyclonal antiserum derived from HIV-1 infected persons failed to protect chimpanzees when passively transferred even though it possessed substantial neutralizing activity.[23] Upon subsequent analysis, this preparation was found to block attachment of gp120 to CD4, but did not possess an appreciable amount of anti-PND antibodies.

Although some evidence indicates that anti-gp41 and anti-p17 antibodies may also confer protection, gp120/gp160-based vaccines appear to hold the most promise.

CANDIDATE HIV-1 VACCINES

Several types of HIV-1 vaccines are currently undergoing Phase I/II studies in humans (TABLE 1). The greatest experience to date has been with a nonglycosylated, recombinant gp160. Most (30/33) HIV-negative volunteers mounted a hu-

TABLE 1. HIV-1 Candidate Vaccines

Type	Description
Virus "core"	Beta-propiolactone-treated and irradiated, gp160-depleted viral core, complexed with Freund's complete adjuvant
gp160	Nonglycosylated protein produced in *Spodoptera frugiperda* cells
gp160	Entire protein produced in VERO cells
gp160	Recombinant vaccinia virus expressing gp160
gp120	Nonglycosylated protein produced in yeast cells
gp120	Recombinant BCG expressing gp120
gp120	Glycosylated glycoprotein produced in CHO cells combined with muramyl tripeptide adjuvant
gp41	Glycosylated glycoprotein produced in mammalian cells
gp41	Nonglycosylated protein produced in yeast cells
gp41	Recombinant BCG expressing gp41
Peptides	Numerous peptides from gp160 (primarily from PND, gp41, and p17). Many coupled to carrier protein (PPD, toxin A, KLH) or complexed with potent adjuvants (muramyl di- and tripeptides, monophoryl lipid A, oil in water mixtures).

moral immune response following multiple immunizations. No evidence of a T-cell response was observed. A Phase I study with this vaccine has also been performed in 30 patients with early-stage HIV-1 infection.[24] Both a humoral and a T-cell immune response was elicited in 63% of those immunized. No response was seen in seven (23%) of the patients. A more vigorous immune response was obtained in subjects whose $CD4^+$ cell count was ≥600 at the time of their first immunization and who received six versus three doses of vaccine. Vaccination did not exert any detectable adverse effect on the immune system. In four of five good responders, a cross-reactive neutralizing antibody response was seen. The $CD4^+$ cell count among those patients who responded remained stable over the 10-month observation period, although it declined an average of 7.2% in the non-responder group. This has been interpreted as a beneficial effect mediated by vaccination. A Phase II trial with this vaccine in 600 patients with $CD4^+$ cell counts >500 is under way.

Nonglycosylated gp120 formulated with an oil in water adjuvant (muramyl tripeptide linked to d-palmitoyl phosphatidylethanolamine [MTP-PE] mixed in Squalene and Tween-80) has been administered to healthy adults.[25] Only low levels of nonneutralizing antibodies were elicited even after six immunizations with 250 μg of gp120. In a subsequent study with a similar formulation, neutralizing antibodies were elicited.[26] The best response, however, was observed with adjuvant concentrations which caused severe, flulike reactions in ~20% of vaccines. Glycosylated gp120 has also been formulated with the above adjuvant and administered to healthy adults.[27] Although the neutralizing antibody response was superior, a high rate of adverse reactions was also noted.

The gene coding for gp160 has been cloned and expressed in vaccinia virus. The recombinant vaccine was used to immunize 18 healthy adults, 16 of whom were previously vaccinated against vaccinia.[28] Prior exposure to vaccinia significantly reduced the immune response. Therefore, only a transient T-cell proliferative response was seen in these persons. In contrast, both vaccinia-naive subjects mounted a long-lasting lymphoproliferative response. An anti-gp160 antibody response was detected in only one primed and two naive subjects, but only by Western blot.

The above studies show that native gp120 and gp160 are poorly immunogenic in both HIV-1 seronegative and seropositive subjects. Multiple doses of vaccine, in some cases combined with potent adjuvants, are needed to induce an immune response. Significantly, the induction of anti-gp160 antibodies in HIV-1 seropositive patients was not associated with any detrimental effects on the immune system.

Our approach toward development of an HIV-1 vaccine is based on the use of PND peptides to yield a multivalent, economic vaccine. As noted above, anti-PND antibodies can neutralize HIV-1 *in vitro* and protect against experimental infections. Serological studies using HIV-1 strains isolated in the United States have shown an unexpectedly high level of cross-reactivity. For example, approximately 65% of randomly selected sera from HIV-seropositive patients recognized the IHIGPGRAFY PND sequence.[29] Furthermore, the PND "core" motifs of IGPGRAF, IGPGRA, and GPGRAF were represented in more than 90% of HIV-1 isolates.[29] Of perhaps greatest importance was the finding that polyclonal antisera that recognized the GPGRAF sequence neutralized four of four clinical isolates expressing this motif. This is not surprising because the MN family of HIV predominates in the United States. Nevertheless, divergent strains, insofar as the PND sequence is concerned, can be found in the United States and Europe. African and Far Eastern isolates, however, share little PND sequence homology with the MN HIV-1 family. Finally, although cross-reacting antibodies may mediate a degree of protection, strain-specific antibodies are generally far more active.

The PND peptides we have chosen represent amino acid residues 307–319 (tip of the V3 loop) from the MN ARV-2/SF2, NY5, SC, CDC42/CDC4, and Thailand 1 strains. To render these peptides immunogenic, we have chosen two carrier molecules, the purified protein derivative (PPD) of *Mycobacterium tuberculosis* and toxin A from *Pseudomonas aeruginosa*, which possess unique and complementary attributes. PPD was selected for the following reasons: (i) it contains a number of T-cell epitopes that could function to recruit lymphocytes primed by prior immunization with bacille Calmette-Guérin (BCG) vaccine, thereby enhancing the response to the PND peptide; (ii) PPD is nonimmunogenic, thereby avoiding the potential for carrier-based epitopic suppression; (iii) PPD is widely used as a human skin test reagent; (iv) immunization with BCG, outside of North America and certain European countries, is routinely performed during childhood, giving rise to a primed population; and (v) consideration is now being given to vaccinating HIV-seropositive persons with BCG due to the prevalence of tuberculosis in AIDS patients and the recent emergence of multiresistant strains. Nevertheless, only PPD-positive persons would be expected to respond to PPD-based vaccines. To circumvent this potential problem, we have also selected another carrier, toxin A, where anti-carrier priming is not a prerequisite for mounting an immune response to the PND peptide hapten. Toxin A was selected on the basis of the following: (i) it has been successfully used as a carrier protein for a variety of experimental human conjugate vaccines[30–32]; (ii) naturally acquired antitoxin A antibodies among the general population are low, avoiding the issue of carrier-based epitopic suppression[33]; (iii) toxin A-based conjugates have been well tolerated in a number of clinical trials; and (iv) toxin A is classified as a superantigen.

PND peptides have been covalently coupled to PPD by reaction with glutaraldehyde and to toxin A by use of adipic acid dihydrazide serving as a spacer molecule with carbodiimide as the coupling agent. Both conjugates were found to be immunogenic in BCG-primed guinea pigs. The kinetics of the immune responses, however, were different. Near-maximal titers of anti-PND antibodies were achieved after primary immunization with the toxin A construct, whereas several booster doses of PPD-based vaccines were required. Immunization with both vaccines engendered high-affinity and neutralizing antibodies. Immunization with MN PND vaccines elicited antibodies that cross-reacted extensively with the SC PND, but only modestly with the PNDs of other strains, even though some possessed the GPGRAF motif.

A monovalent MN-PND-PPD conjugate vaccine has been evaluated in PPD-positive and PPD-negative, HIV-seronegative adults. The vaccine, which contained 0.65-μg PND and 50-IU PPD, was administered intradermally at two sites. The majority (10/12) of PPD-positive subjects responded with a humoral response, whereas there was no evidence of a response among the 10 PND-negative subjects.

Immunization evoked a high-affinity antibody response in most responders. Serum from responders was able to neutralize the MN strain *in vitro*. Cross-neutralization studies are now in progress.

The MN-PND-toxin A vaccine is now being evaluated for safety and immunogenicity in healthy seronegative adults, and a Phase I study of the MN-PND-PPD vaccine in seropositive patients with a $CD4^+$ cell count ≥ 400 is under way.

A pentavalent PND vaccine has been produced by combining equal amounts of monovalent vaccines. The immune response to this polyvalent vaccine as compared to its individual components is being tested in animals.

REFERENCES

1. NEW YORK STATE DEPARTMENT OF HEALTH. 1988. AIDS among New York State children. Epidemiol. Notes **10**: 1–2.
2. NOVICK, L. F., D. BERNS, R. STRICKOFF & R. STEVENS. 1988. HIV seroprevalence in newborn infants in New York State (Abstr.). Program and Abstracts: IV International Conference on AIDS (Stockholm, Sweden). Bio-Data. Washington, D.C.
3. FALLOON, J., J. EDDY, L. WIENER & P. PIZZO. 1989. Human immunodeficiency virus in children. J. Pediatr. **114**: 1–30.
4. WIZNIA, A. & A. RUBINSTEIN. 1988. Acquired immunodeficiency syndrome in infants and children. Ann. Nestle **46**: 154–175.
5. RUBINSTEIN, A. 1986. Pediatric AIDS. Curr. Prob. Pediatr. **16**: 361–409.
6. ZIEGLER, J. B., D. A. COOPER, R. D. JOHNSON & J. GOLD. 1985. Postnatal transmission of AIDS-associated retrovirus from mother to infant. Lancet **1**: 896–898.
7. SOEIRO, R., A. RUBINSTEIN, W. K. RASHBAUM & W. D. LYMAN. 1992. Maternofetal transmission of AIDS: Frequency of human immunodeficiency virus type 1 nucleis acid sequences in human fetal DNA. J. Infect. Dis. **166**: 699–703.
8. BLANCHE, S., C. ROUZIOUX, M. L. G. MOSCATO, *et al.* 1989. A prospective study of infants born to women seropositive for human immunodeficiency virus type 1. N. Engl. J. Med. **320**: 1643–1648.
9. EUROPEAN COLLABORATIVE STUDY. 1991. Children born to women with HIV-1 infection: Natural history and risk of transmission. Lancet **337**: 253–260.
10. RYDER, R. W., W. NSA, S. E. HASSIG, *et al.* 1989. Perinatal transmission of the human immunodeficiency virus type 1 to infants of seropositive women in Zaire. N. Engl. J. Med. **320**: 1637–1642.
11. BROLIDEN, P., V. MOSCHESE, K. LJUNGGREN, *et al.* 1989. Diagnostic implication of specific immunoglobulin G patterns of children born to HIV-infected mothers. AIDS **3**: 577–582.
12. ROSSI, P., V. MOSCHESE, P. A. BROLIDEN, *et al.* 1989. Presence of maternal antibodies to human immunodeficiency virus type 1 envelope glycoprotein gp120 epitopes correlate with the uninfected status of children born to seropositive mothers. Proc. Natl. Acad. Sci. USA **8**: 8055–8058.
13. DEVASH, Y., T. A. CLAVELLI, D. G. WOOD, K. J. REAGAN & A. RUBINSTEIN. 1990. Vertical transmission of human immunodeficiency virus is correlated with absence of high-affinity/avidity maternal antibodies to the gp120 principal neutralizing domain. Proc. Natl. Acad. Sci. USA **87**: 3445–3449.
14. DEVASH, Y., T. J. MATTHEWS, J. E. DRUMMOND, *et al.* 1990. C-terminal fragments of gp120 and synthetic peptides from five HTLV-III strains: Prevalence of antibodies to the HTLV-III-MN isolate in infected individuals. AIDS Res. Hum. Retrovir. **6**: 307–316.
15. PAREKH, B. S., N. SHAFFER, C. P. PAU, *et al.* 1991. Lack of correlation between maternal antibodies to V3 loop peptides of gp120 and perinatal HIV-1 transmission. AIDS **5**: 1179–1184.
16. ROBERTSON, C. A., J. Y. Q. MOK, K. S. FROEBEL, P. SIMMONDS, S. M. BURNS, H. S.

MARSDEN & S. GRAHAM. 1992. Maternal antibodies to gp120 V3 sequence do not correlate with protection against vertical transmission of human immunodeficiency virus. J. Infect. Dis. **166:** 704–709.
17. EMINI, E. A., W. A. SCHLIEF, J. H. NUNBERG, *et al.* 1992. Prevention of HIV-1 infection in chimpanzees by gp120 V3 domain-specific monoclonal antibody. Nature **355:** 728–730.
18. JAVAHERIAN, K., A. LANGLOIS, C. MCDANAL, *et al.* 1989. Principle neutralizing domain of the human immunodeficiency virus type 1 envelope protein. Proc. Natl. Acad. Sci. USA **86:** 6768–6772.
19. REITZ, M. S., JR., C. WILSON, C. NAUGLE, R. C. GALLO & M. ROBERT-GUROFF. 1988. Generation of a neutralization-resistant variant of HIV-1 is due to selection for a point mutation in the envelope gene. Cell **54:** 57–63.
20. EMINI, E. A., P. L. NARA, W. A. SCHLIEFF, *et al.* 1990. Antibody-mediated *in vitro* neutralization of human immunodeficiency virus type 1 abolishes infectivity for chimpanzees. J. Virol. **64:** 3674–3678.
21. BERMAN, P. W., T. J. GREGORY, L. RIDDLE, *et al.* 1990. Protection of chimpanzees from infection by HIV-1 after vaccination with recombinant glycoprotein gp120 but not gp160. Nature **345:** 622–625.
22. GIRARD, M., M.-P. KIENY, W. A. PINTER, *et al.* 1991. Immunization of chimpanzees confers protection against challenge with human immunodeficiency virus. Proc. Natl. Acad. Sci. USA **88:** 542–546.
23. PRINCE, A. M., B. HOROWITZ, L. BAKER, *et al.* 1988. Failure of a human immunodeficiency virus (HIV) immune globulin to protect chimpanzees against experimental challenge with HIV. Proc. Natl. Acad. Sci. USA **85:** 6944–6948.
24. REDFIELD, R. R., D. L. BIRX, N. KETTER, *et al.* 1991. A Phase I evaluation of the safety and immunogenicity of vaccination with recombinant gp160 in patients with early human immunodeficiency virus infection. N. Engl. J. Med. **324:** 1677–1684.
25. WINTSCH, J., C.-L. CHAIGNAT, D. G. BRAUN, *et al.* 1991. Safety and immunogenicity of a genetically engineered human immunodeficiency virus vaccine. J. Infect. Dis. **163:** 219–225.
26. CHERNOFF, D., F. SINANGIL, K. STEIMER & C. DEKKER. 1992. Safety and immunogenicity of vaccines containing denatured recombinant HIV gp120 (Env 2-3) combined with MF59 adjuvant emulsion in HIV seronegative subjects (abstr. 859, p. 253). Program and Abstracts: 32nd Interscience Conference on Antimicrobial Agents and Chemotherapy. American Society for Microbiology. Washington, D.C.
27. KAHN, J., D. CHERNOFF, F. SINANGIL, *et al.* 1992. Phase I study of an HIV-1 gp120 vaccine combined with the novel adjuvant emulsion, MF59/MTP-PE, in seronegative adults (abstr. 860, p. 254). Program and Abstracts: 32nd Interscience Conference on Antimicrobial Agents and Chemotherapy. American Society for Microbiology. Washington, D.C.
28. COONEY, E. L., A. C. COLLIER, P. D. GREENBERG, *et al.* 1991. Safety of an immunological response to a recombinant vaccinia virus vaccine expressing HIV envelope glycoprotein. Lancet **337:** 567–572.
29. LAROSA, G. J., J. P. DAVIDE, K. WEINHOLD, *et al.* 1990. Conserved sequence and structural elements in the HIV-1 principal neutralizing domain. Science **249:** 932–935.
30. CRYZ, S. J., JR., E. FÜRER, A. S. CROSS, A. WEGMANN, R. GERMANIER & J. C. SADOFF. 1987. Safety and immunogenicity of a *Pseudomonas aeruginosa* O-polysaccharide–toxin A conjugate vaccine in humans. J. Clin. Invest. **80:** 51–56.
31. CRYZ, S. J., JR., A. S. CROSS, J. C. SADOFF, A. WEGMANN, J. U. QUE & E. FÜRER. 1991. Safety and immunogenicity of *Escherichia coli* 018 O-polysaccharide–cholera toxin conjugate vaccines in humans. J. Infect. Dis. **163:** 1040–1045.
32. FREIS, L. F., D. M. GORDON, I. SCHNEIDER, *et al.* 1992. Safety, immunogenicity, and efficacy of a *Plasmodium falciparum* vaccine comprising a circumsporozoite protein repeat region peptide conjugated to *Pseudomonas aeruginosa* toxin A. Infect. Immun. **60:** 1834–1839.
33. SCHAAD, U. B., A. B. LANG, J. WEDGWOOD, A. RUEDEBERG, J. U. QUE, E. FÜRER & S. J. CRYZ, JR. 1991. Safety and immunogenicity of *Pseudomonas aeruginosa* conjugate A vaccine in cystic fibrosis. Lancet **338:** 1236–1237.

Tissue Culture Models of HIV-1 Infection[a]

WILLIAM D. LYMAN,[b] WILLIAM C. HATCH,[b] JORGE N. LAROCCA,[c] AND WILLIAM K. RASHBAUM[d]

[b] Department of Pathology
[c] Department of Neurology
[d] Department of Obstetrics & Gynecology
Albert Einstein College of Medicine
Bronx, New York 10461

INTRODUCTION

Many of the tissue culture models of HIV-1 infection, and especially those that have been developed for pediatric AIDS, focus on the effects that this virus has on the central nervous system (CNS). This is appropriate, because the number of children infected by HIV-1 and who develop AIDS with neurologic complications continues to increase.[1,2] When these observations are viewed in conjunction with the data that indicate that most of these children are infected by HIV-1 during gestation,[3,4] the use of human fetal tissue for these studies is supported and the need of *in vitro* models gains more importance.

Several *in vitro* models have been used to study the interactions of HIV-1 with the developing human CNS. Some studies have relied on the use of neoplastic cell lines derived from neural tissue or dissociated primary cells obtained from adult CNS.[5,6] These models, however, have problems related to the influence of aberrant gene expression in the transformed cells and terminally differentiated cells in the case of models based on the use of adult CNS.

Human fetal CNS has also been used to study the effects of HIV-1 on the nervous system. These studies have focused primarily on dissociated fetal CNS cell cultures,[7] the use of transfected cells,[8] reaggregated cultures,[9] and xenograft transplant[10] models, or peripheral nervous system tissue.[11] In each case, although indications about the mechanisms by which HIV-1 may affect CNS function have been described, each set of conclusions must be understood against the backdrop of significant differences between the tissue culture conditions and the CNS *in vivo*.

---

[a] This work was supported by United States Public Health Service Grants MH 46815 and MH 47667.

In contrast to these models, we have developed an organotypic tissue culture of the human fetal CNS.[12,13] This model has been designed to allow CNS tissue to grow in culture requiring no special conditions for cell growth, culture development, or differentiation. These cultures have been shown to contain all the major CNS cell types. Because the cultures are established from brain slices or spinal cord tissue, they maintain many of the cellular connections established *in vivo*.

MATERIALS AND METHODS

Source of Fetal Tissue

This study is part of an ongoing research protocol that has been approved by the Albert Einstein College of Medicine Committee on Clinical Investigation and the City of New York Health and Hospitals Corporation. Informed consent was obtained from all participants. Fetal tissues were obtained at the time of elective termination of intrauterine pregnancy from otherwise healthy women. Gestational age was determined by multiple parameters.[14] The tissues used in this study were obtained from 21- to 23-week-old fetuses.

Establishment and Testing of Organotypic CNS Tissue Cultures

The method involved in establishing and testing organotypic cultures is routine in our laboratories.[12,13] Explants of tissue obtained from frontal pole, germinal matrix, or the dorsal columns of lumbar spinal cord were dissected and placed into tissue culture. From each CNS sample, between 50 and 100 explants were placed into culture.

The growth and differentiation of cultures were monitored by brightfield microscopy. Only cultures observed to have significant outgrowth of processes were used, as previous experience has shown that this criterion indicates healthy cultures that are free of contamination.

Infection of Organotypic CNS Cultures

The HIV-1 isolates that were used for these studies were obtained from the AIDS Research and Reference Reagent Program and included JR-CSF, JR-FL, MN, and RF. The lymphocytotropic (L-tropic) isolates MN and RF were propagated in H9 cells. The monocytotropic (M-tropic) isolates JR-CSF and JR-FL were propagated by passage through adherent human fetal liver macrophages.

Organotypic cultures were exposed to either RF, MN, JR-FL, or JR-CSF isolates. At the time of HIV-1 exposure, growth medium was removed from each culture well and exchanged for HIV-1 inoculated medium. Controls consisted of mock infections with either growth medium, uninfected supernatants of the cell type used to propagate HIV-1, or heat-inactivated HIV-1. Cultures were maintained with virus or control media between 1 and 7 days, after which the virus or control medium was removed. Subsequently, the cultures were assayed for HIV-1 DNA, reverse transcriptase activity, p24 antigen concentration, and infectious virus by syncytium-forming assay. The cultures were repeatedly probed in this way for over 60 days.

Light and Electron Microscopy of Cultures

Organotypic cultures were sampled for microscopy every seven days. At each time point, the cultures were fixed, dehydrated, and flat-embedded in Araldite-Epon. One-micron sections were taken at desired orientations and stained with toluidine blue for light microscopy. Thin sections were examined by electron microscopy after contrasting with lead and uranium salts. These techniques are described in detail elsewhere.[15]

Immunocytochemical Staining of Cultures

In addition to morphological analyses of the cultures, immunocytochemical probes were used to identify different cell types. The primary antibodies were anti-glial fibrillary acidic protein (GFAP) for astrocytes; anti-neurofilament protein (NFP) and anti-nerve growth factor receptor (NGFr) for neurons; anti-EBM 11 and anti-HAM 56 antibodies and the lectin *Ricinus communis* agglutinin-1 (RCA-1) for microglia; and anti-myelin basic protein (MBP), anti-galactocerebroside (GC), and anti-HNK-1 for oligodendrocytes.

Immunocytochemical Studies for Viral Antigens

Because other studies showed that we can successfully detect HIV-1 specific proteins in fetal tissue sections using immunocytochemical methods at both the light and electron microscopic levels,[16,17] we examined HIV-exposed fetal CNS organotypic cultures for the presence of viral proteins in CNS parenchymal cells. In addition, antibodies that recognize CNS cell-type specific markers were used in double-label studies with antibodies to the HIV-1 protein gp41.

Nucleic Acid Hybridization

For HIV DNA analysis of the fetal CNS, 1 µg of tissue DNA was amplified for 30 cycles using the "gag" oligonucleotide primers SK38 and 39, the thermostable "Taq" polymerase (Perkin Elmer/Cetus), and the salt and Mg^{2+} optimization as described by the manufacturers.[18] Detection of the amplified sequences used liquid hybridization to the ^{32}P end-labeled internal probe SK19 and gel retardation to separate free from hybridized probe.[19,20]

For each amplification, we tested negative control DNA obtained from a blood donor who was without risk factors for HIV-1 infection and who had been determined to be HIV-1 seronegative. Included in each amplification was a positive control that consisted of 1 µg of HIV-1 negative DNA to which either known numbers of HIV-1 BH-10 plasmid DNA genome copies or measured numbers of whole-cell DNA equivalents from the 8E5-LAV cell, which is known to contain a single proviral copy of HIV-1, were added. All amplifications were done at least in duplicate.

Reverse Transcriptase Assay

Samples of supernatants from all cultures were assayed for HIV-associated reverse transcriptase (RT) activity using the standard method.[21]

p24 Antigen Capture Assay

Supernatants from HIV-infected cells were assayed using this method,[22] and a standard curve of p24 antigen concentration was established with respect to RT activity. This system allows a more accurate estimation of the HIV concentration of the supernatants analyzed above.

Syncytium-Forming Microassay

Because neither the RT nor p24 antigen capture assays indicate the ability of the detected HIV to infect susceptible cells, an infectious center assay was used that is routine in our laboratory.[23]

Muscarinic-Dependent Activation of the Phospholipase C

Organotypic cultures of fetal CNS were established from frontal pole tissue. The standard tissue culture medium was replaced with medium containing [^{3}H]inositol, and, after 16 to 20 hours, excess inositol was eliminated by washing the cultures. The organotypic cultures were incubated in the presence of 10 mM LiCl for 10 min, and this was followed by stimulation with 1 mM carbachol for 1 hour. When the effect of antagonist was tested, it was added 10 min before the addition of the agonist. The tissue slice suspensions were incubated, and the reaction was stopped by freezing the vials over ice and by adding 1 ml of 15% TCA.

Separation of the [^{3}H]Inositol Phosphates

The TCA-treated tissue suspension was extracted four times with equal volumes of ether. The mixture of [^{3}H]inositol phosphates was resolved by anion-exchange chromatography. To determine the incorporation of [^{32}P]phosphate or myo-[^{3}H]inositol into phosphoinositol lipids, the cultures were prelabeled with [^{32}P]phosphate (100 μCi/ml) for 1 hour or with [^{3}H]inositol for 2 hours. At the end of the incubation period, lipids were extracted with chloroform–methanol. Aliquots of these extracts were used for total lipid phosphorus determination and for separation of the phospholipids.

Effect of HIV-1 on Signal Transduction

Organotypic tissue culture samples were incubated in the presence of [^{3}H]inositol and exposed to HIV-1 and carbachol as described above. The cultures were then harvested and examined for alterations in carbachol stimulation of signal transduction pathways.

RESULTS

Viability of the Cultures

Organotypic cultures can be maintained for over 12 weeks *in vitro*.[12,13] During this time there is both proliferation and differentiation of distinct CNS cell types within the body of the explant and in the outgrowth area. Microscopic observations of fixed and sectioned cultures revealed a homogeneous distribution of different cell types in a rich neuropil with an absence of necrotic foci or other indications of pathologic change.

Electron Microscopy

Ultrastructural examination of the cultures reveals that all the major CNS cell types are present. In cultures derived from the dorsal columns of the lumbar spinal cord, compact and recently elaborated myelin are evident.[13] Additionally, the myelin is seen being organized into functional internodes.

Immunocytochemistry and Lectin Histochemistry

All CNS cell types were detected during the culture period using these techniques. Anti-GFAP labeled cells both within the body of the explant and in the outgrowth area, and these cells were reminiscent of both protoplasmic and fibrous astrocytes. As the outgrowth area increased, the relative percentage of astrocytes increased more rapidly than the other cell types.

Cells expressing NGFr and NFP epitopes were detected both within the explant body and in the outgrowth area. The cells that stained positively with anti-NGFr were predominantly bipolar and consistent with the size and morphology of neurons. NFP-positive cells were more numerous than NGFr-positive cells, possibly indicating the differential expression of these two neuron-specific proteins.

Microglia were also abundant within the culture upon initial isolation. These cells were detected by reactivity with both anti-EBM 11 and anti-HAM 56 antibodies. Although these antibodies were originally raised against alveolar macrophages, they are considered a reliable marker for microglia. Additional support for this belief is provided by the staining pattern seen using histochemistry techniques and RCA-1. Abundant evidence exists that this lectin labels both microglia and endothelial cells. Therefore, because of the similarity between the cell types stained with anti-EBM 11, anti-HAM 56, and RCA-1, the presence of microglia in the cultures is compelling. Although microglia were evenly distributed throughout the explant upon initial isolation, with time in culture they were seen to migrate first to the interface between the explant and the outgrowth area, and, subsequently, some cells migrated into the outgrowth area.

Oligodendrocytes were detected using the three cell-type-specific markers anti-MBP, anti-HNK-1, and anti-GC. Similar to the other CNS cell types, oligodendrocytes were observed in both the main body of the explant and in the outgrowth area throughout the entire culture period. The cells staining positive with these markers were small, round cells or others that had the general morphologic characteristics of "lacy" oligodendrocytes.

HIV-1 Infection of Organotypic CNS Cultures

Organotypic cultures were exposed to titrations of various cell-free HIV-1 isolates with no apparent cytopathology at the light microscopic level. Only rarely were cytomorphological changes detected, and these were in frontal cortex cultures only. These changes were manifest by what appeared to be microglia having formed multinucleated giant cells within these cultures, with a distinct area of clearing seen around these multinuclear cells. Electron microscopic examination of HIV-1 exposed CNS cultures has not detected the presence of any intact virions in these CNS-organotypic cultures.

Immunocytochemical Detection of HIV-1 Proteins

HIV-1 exposed CNS cultures were probed with anti-HIV gp41, p24, and gp120 antibodies to detect the presence of HIV-1 specific proteins. HIV-1 gp41 antigens were routinely detected in individual HIV-1 positive cells in the outgrowth area and to a lesser extent in the main body of the explant. At higher magnifications, the HIV-1 gp41 antigens appeared to be localized in the cytoplasm of individual cells, often spreading into the processes. The p24 antibody was slightly less sensitive than the gp41, possibly owing to the requirement for antibody to enter cytoplasm to localize the antigen. Detection of HIV-1 gp120 by immunocytochemistry was sensitive but prone to high backgrounds in these cultures probably because it is a sheep polyclonal. HIV-1 antigens were never detected in non-HIV-1 exposed control cultures.

In situ *Hybridization*

HIV-1 mRNA was detected in HIV-1 exposed cultures by *in situ* hybridization. Positive hybridizations have been detected in cells in both the explant body and in the outgrowth area. The alkaline phosphatase chromogen coupled to the DNA probe appeared to routinely localize in the cytoplasm of HIV-1 exposed CNS organotypic cultures. Unfortunately, this procedure involved the use of proteinases, which interfere with the identification of individual cells within these cultures. HIV-1 mRNA was never detected in non-HIV-1 exposed cultures.

Polymerase Chain Reaction

HIV-1 DNA was detected in HIV-1 exposed CNS organotypic cultures by the use of the polymerase chain reaction. Detection of HIV-1 DNA has routinely required a minimum of 1 μg of DNA extracted from CNS cultures exposed to either lymphotropic (RF or MN) or monocytotropic (JRCSF or JRFL) HIV-1 isolates. The presence of HIV-1 gag sequences was detected. HIV-1 DNA was never detected in non-HIV-1 exposed cultures.

Phenotypes of HIV-1 Infected Cells in Organotypic Cultures

To determine which cells are infected in CNS organotypic cultures, double-label immunocytochemistry was performed. Cell phenotypes were identified using a diaminobenzidine reaction and HIV-1 gp41 antigens were localized by an alkaline phosphatase reaction.

The most predominant HIV-1 positive cell types identified were HAM 56 staining microglia. The HIV-1 antigen was seen to localize in the cytoplasm around the nucleus in these cells. HIV-1 antigens were less frequently observed in cells identified as astrocytes by both morphology and GFAP positivity. In addition, astrocytes were only infected by HIV-1 in those CNS organotypic cultures exposed to the lymphocytotropic isolates MN and RF. HIV-1 antigens were not detected in oligodendrocytes or neurons in cultures in which HIV-1 infected microglia and astrocytes.

Detection of Multinucleated Cells

HIV-1 antigens detected by immunocytochemistry were occasionally seen to localize in clusters of three or more cells. Counter-staining of nuclei with propidium iodide and observation under fluorescent microscopy demonstrated that single cells within these HIV-1 positive clusters appeared to contain multiple nuclei. These clusters of multinucleated cells were never detected in non-HIV-1 exposed cultures.

Effect of HIV-1 Infection on Signal Transduction

To test the effect of HIV-1 infection on signal transduction, organotypic cultures were infected with the RF isolate of HIV-1 at a multiplicity of infection (MOI) of 4.3×10^5 syncytial forming units. The cultures were exposed for 5 days and tested for infection using a number of techniques including immunocytochemistry for HIV-1 proteins (e.g. gp41) in combination with cell-type specific markers (e.g., antibodies to glial fibrillary acidic protein). These experiments showed that, after 5 days of exposure to the virus, both microglia and astrocytes were positive for HIV-1 associated antigens. Additionally, these cultures did now show evidence of cytopathology (cell death), although multinucleated cells were seen.

To determine if there was an effect on muscarinic receptors linked to phospholipase C in the presence of virus, some cultures were labeled with [^{3}H]inositol as described above and stimulated with 1 mM carbachol in the presence of 10 mM LiCl. In parallel, control experiments were performed with tissue cultures obtained from the same brain without exposure to virus. In these experiments, a significant increase in carbachol stimulation was observed in the infected tissue but not in the nonstimulated control cultures. We are presently conducting experiments to determine how the amount of time that cultures are infected and the viral titer affect these observations. Additionally, because different brain areas probably contain different populations of cells (both phenotype and stage of differentiation), current plans include an examination of how these variables may affect the observed results.

DISCUSSION

Cultures of human fetal CNS tissue have been established as a model of the developing nervous system. These cultures have been characterized by immunocytochemistry and Western blot to contain all major cell types of the CNS, including astrocytes, neurons, microglia, oligodendrocytes, and endothelial cells. These cultures have also been exposed to HIV-1 isolates and determined to be infected by detecting HIV-1 proteins by immunocytochemistry, RNA by *in situ* hybridization, and DNA by PCR. Double-label experiments have identified microglia as the predominant cell type infected regardless of HIV-1 tropism. Astrocytes are infected to a lesser extent and only by lymphocytotropic HIV-1 isolates. Exposure to HIV-1 and infection results in little cytopathology other than the formation of multinucleated cells in these CNS cultures. The parameters of infection were examined by titration experiments that determined that the minimum inoculum capable of infecting CNS cultures is partly due to the virus isolate and partly due to the titer of input virus. The *in vitro* age of CNS culture before infection did not appear to act as a factor in their susceptibility to HIV-1 infection. CNS cultures were determined to be infected productively as long as 67 days post infection by experiments that isolated HIV-1 from supernatants of HIV-1 exposed cultures. These data suggest that, while HIV-1 is capable of infecting cells of the developing CNS, this virus and its components may not be directly responsible for the neuropathology seen in pediatric AIDS patients. Furthermore, these results and evidence from animal models support the role of HIV-1 infected macrophages/microglia and their release of inflammatory cytokines, and give them greater credibility in the development of AIDS dementia.

Of major interest are the observations that HIV-1 exposure of organotypic CNS cultures is associated with alterations in signal transduction. Although the present results only report our findings with the muscarinic neurotransmitter receptor, we believe that this effect may be more general and not restricted to a particular receptor or pathway. Additionally, although we have not as yet confirmed the belief that CNS cells are infected by replication competent HIV-1 in this model system, the observations of alterations in signal transduction stimulate provocative speculations about the underlying mechanisms. For instance, these alterations may not require infection of cells but rather may be dependent on the "toxic" effects that HIV-1 proteins or the degradation products of the same have on cell surface molecules. Alternatively, there may be endocytosis of viral proteins, and this then becomes the substrate for altered cellular metabolism resulting in disturbed cell function. Whatever the final outcome of these studies demonstrates in terms of the precise mechanisms associated with HIV-1-mediated alterations in signal transduction, this effect may in fact be the biological substrate for the neurologic dysfunction witnessed during the course of AIDS.

Despite these findings, the results also indicate that it is important that we develop additional biochemical measures of change in these CNS organotypic cultures. Because the biochemical parameters of AIDS dementia are unknown, we can only guess whether the parameters we measured are relevant to the *in vivo* situation. Future experiments to determine if HIV-1 infection alters protein expression will focus on obtaining a quantitative measure of CNS protein changes by Western blot, which will increase the sensitivity of protein detection. Although tissue culture models are important, they also demonstrate the importance for parallel experiments in animal systems.

Because this model does not contain a blood–brain barrier, it cannot be used to address the mechanism of viral entry into CNS. Related questions, such as whether blood–brain barrier endothelial cells are infected by HIV-1, the passage of HIV-1 infected macrophages through vessel walls, or the role of HIV-1 infected perivascular microglia in virus transmission, will have to be answered using other culture systems. HIV-1, cytokines, and lymphoid cells may also have an effect on CNS homeostasis through the blood–brain barrier.

This work, using organotypic cultures of human fetal CNS tissue, has demonstrated that HIV-1 infection of microglial cells, and to a lesser extent of astrocytes, and the presence of viral proteins are not sufficient to induce significant cytopathology. This suggests, as reported previously, that cytopathology and probably dementia are due to a combination of factors. The role of neurotoxins produced by HIV-1 infected macrophages has been questioned as being the result of mycoplasma contamination. This may, however, be relevant to the *in vivo* situation since many HIV-1 infected person are coinfected with mycoplasma. Cytokines are thought to play a role in normal CNS homeostasis and may, in abnormal concentrations or combinations, act to contribute to dementia. These cytokines and/or viral glycoproteins may alter neural cell functions either directly or indirectly as a result of altered astrocyte functions.

In conclusion, the model of human fetal neurodevelopment presented in this report may provide the necessary laboratory model to answer many questions related to normal human nervous tissue differentiation and pathologic conditions.

ACKNOWLEDGMENTS

We thank Barbara Shea for her excellent secretarial assistance. We also want to acknowledge cooperation from New York City Health and Hospitals Corporation and the Bronx Municipal Hospital Center with its excellent nursing staffs at Van Etten and Jacobi Hospitals.

REFERENCES

1. CENTERS FOR DISEASE CONTROL. 1991. HIV/AIDS Surveillance Report, January: 1–22.
2. REPORT OF A CONSENSUS WORKSHOP, ITALY. 1992. Maternal factors involved in mother-to-child transmission of HIV-1. J. Acq. Immune Def. Syn. **5:** 1019–1029.
3. CORUGNAUD, V., F. LAURE, A. BROSSARD, et al. 1991. Frequent and early in utero HIV-1 infection. AIDS Res. Hum. Retrovir. **7:** 337–341.
4. SOEIRO, R., A. RUBINSTEIN, W. K. RASHBAUM & W. D. LYMAN. 1992. Maternofetal transmission of AIDS: Frequency of nucleic acid sequences in human fetal tissue DNA. J. Infect. Dis. **166:** 699–703.
5. CHENG-MAYER, C., J. T. RUTKA, M. L. ROSENBLUM, T. MCHUGH, D. P. STITES & J. A. LEVY. 1987. Human immunodeficiency virus can productively infect cultured human glial cells. Proc. Natl. Acad. Sci. USA **84:** 3526–3530.
6. WATKINS, B. A., H. H. DORN, W. B. KELLY, R. C. ARMSTRONG, B. J. BOTTS, F. MICHAELS, C. V. KUFTA & M. DUBOIS-DALCQ. 1990. Specific tropism of HIV-1 for microglial cells in primary human brain cultures. Science **249:** 549–552.
7. KUNSCH, C., H. HARTLE & B. WIGDAHL. 1989. Infection of human fetal dorsal root ganglion glial cells with human immunodeficiency virus type 1 involves an entry mechanism independent of the CD4A epitope. J. Virol. **63:** 5054–5061.
8. TORNATORE, C., A. NATH, K. AMEMIYA & E. O. MAJOR. 1991. Persistent human immunodeficiency virus type 1 infection in human fetal glial cells reactivated by T-cell factor(s) or by the cytokines tumor necrosis factor-α and interleukin-β. J. Virol. **65:** 6094–6100.
9. PULLIAM, L., B. G. HERNDIER, N. M. TANG & M. S. MCGRATH. 1991. Human immunodeficiency virus-infected macrophages produce soluble factors that cause histological and neurochemical alterations in cultured human brains. J. Clin. Invest. **87:** 503–512.
10. CVETKOVICH, T. A., E. LAZAR, B. M. BLUMBERG, Y. SAITO, T. ESKIN, R. REICHMAN, D. A. BARAM, C. DEL CERRO, H. E. GENDELMAN, M. DEL CERRO & L. G. EPSTEIN. 1992. Human immunodeficiency virus type 1 infection of neural xenografts. Proc. Natl. Acad Sci. USA **89:** 5162–5166.
11. KUNSCH, C. & B. WIGDAHL. 1989. Transient expression of human immunodeficiency virus type 1 genome results in a nonproductive infection in human fetal dorsal root ganglia glial cells. Virology **173:** 715–722.
12. LYMAN, W. D., M. TRICOCHE, W. C. HATCH, Y. KRESS, F. C. CHIU & W. K. RASHBAUM. 1991. Human fetal central nervous system organotypic cultures. Dev. Brain Res. **60:** 155–160.
13. LYMAN, W. D., W. C. HATCH, E. POUSADA, G. STEPHNEY, W. K. RASHBAUM & K. M. WEIDENHEIM. 1992. Human fetal myelinated organotypic cultures. Brain Res. **599:** 34–44.
14. KALOUSEK, D. K., V. J. BALDWIN, J. E. DIMMICK, M. G. NORMAN, N. CIMOLAI, A. ANDREWS & B. PARADICE. 1992. Embryofetal perinatal autopsy and placental examination. In Developmental Pathology of the Embryo and Fetus. J. Dimmick & D. Kalousek, Eds.: 799–824. Lippincott. Philadelphia.
15. RAINE C. C. 1973. Ultrastructural applications of cultured nervous system tissue to neuropathology. In Progress in Neuropathology. H. M. Zimmerman, Ed. Vol. **2:** 27–68. Grune and Stratton. New York.
16. LYMAN, W. D., Y. KRESS, W. K. RASHBAUM, T. A. CALVELLI, E. STEINHAUER, J. M. KASHKIN, C. E. HENDERSON & A. RUBINSTEIN. 1988. An AIDS virus-associated antigen localized in human fetal brain. In Advances in Neuroimmunology. Ann. New York Acad. Sci. **540:** 628–629.
17. LYMAN, W. D., Y. KRESS, A. RUBINSTEIN, S. UDEM, T. A. CALCELLI, E. STEINHAUER, J. M. KASHKIN, C. E. HENDERSON, W. K. RASHBAUM & R. SOEIRO. 1988. Evidence of human immunodeficiency virus infection in human fetal tissues. In Impact on the Fetus of Parental Sexually Transmitted Disease. Ann. N. Y. Acad. Sci. **549:** 258–259.
18. KELLOGG, D. E. & S. KWOK. 1990. Detection of human immunodeficiency virus. In PCR Protocols: A Guide to Methods and Application. M. A. Innis, D. H. Felfand, J. J. Sninsky & T. J. White, Eds.: 337–347. Academic Press. San Diego.

19. SHAW, G. S., B. H. HAHN, S. K. SYRA, et al. 1984. Molecular characterization of human T-cell leukemia (lymphotropic) virus type III in the acquired immune deficiency syndrome. Science **226:** 1165–1171.
20. FOLKS, T. M., D. POWELL, M. LIGHTFOOTE, et al. 1986. Biological and biochemical characterization of a cloned leu-3' cell surviving infection with the acquired immune deficiency syndrome retrovirus. J. Exp. Med. **164:** 280–290.
21. HOFFMAN, A. D., B. BANAPOUR & J. A. LEVY. 1985. Characterization of the AIDS-associated retrovirus reverse transcriptase and optimal conditions for its detection in virions. Virology **147:** 326–335.
22. NARA, P. L., W. C. HATCH, N. M. DUNLOP, W. G. ROBEY & P. J. FISCHINGER. 1989. Simple, rapid, quantitative micro-syncytium forming assay for the detection of neutralizing antibody against infectious HTLV-III/LAV. AIDS Res. Hum. Retrovir. **3:** 283–302.
23. NARA, P. L. & P. J. FISCHINGER. 1988. Quantitative infectivity assay for HIV-1 and -2. Nature **332:** 469–470.

Animal Models for Perinatal Transmission of Pathogenic Viruses[a]

R. M. RUPRECHT,[b,c,d] C. FRATAZZI,[b,d] P. L. SHARMA,[b,e]
M. F. GREENE,[f] D. PENNINCK,[g] AND M. WYAND[h]

MATERNAL TRANSMISSION OF RETROVIRUSES

Maternal Transmission of HIV-1

Maternal transmission of the human immunodeficiency virus type 1 (HIV-1) represents an increasing public health problem worldwide. In the United States, the number of women of child-bearing age infected with HIV-1 is rising. On January 13, 1988, the *New York Times* reported that 1 in 61 babies born in the New York City area carried antibodies to HIV-1, implying an infection rate of 1 in 61 among parturient women in this metropolitan region. Given that a pregnant woman infected with HIV-1 has a 20 to 30% chance of passing the virus to her infant,[1] this translates into a neonatal infection rate of approximately 1 in 200 to 300. Since then, however, the prevalence of HIV-1 in young women in inner-city areas has increased. A World Health Organization study estimated that currently 8 to 10 million persons are infected worldwide. By the year 2,000, a total of 25 to 30 million may be infected, including 10 million children. These staggering projections make it clear that methods of preventing HIV-1 transmission from an infected woman to her infant need to be developed.

---

[a] Supported in part by AmFAR Grants 500033-7-PG and 500110-9-PGR and NIH Grant #R01-AI-32330 to RMR for the primate work and by NIH Contract N01-AI-72664 and NIH Grant #R01-AI25715 for the murine experiments. RMR is the recipient of a Faculty Research Award from the American Cancer Society. We also acknowledge the Center for AIDS Research (CFAR) Core Grant #IP30 28691-01 awarded to the Dana-Farber Cancer Institute as support for the Institute's AIDS research efforts.

[b] Address for correspondence: Dr. Ruth M. Ruprecht, Dana-Farber Cancer Institute, 44 Binney Street, Boston, MA 02115.

[c] Laboratory of Viral Pathogenesis, Dana-Farber Cancer Institute, Boston, Massachusetts 02115.

[d] Department of Medicine, Harvard Medical School, Boston, Massachusetts 02115.

[e] Department of Biological Chemistry and Molecular Pharmacology, Harvard Medical School, Boston, Massachusetts 02115.

[f] Department of Obstetrics and Gynecology, Harvard Medical School, Boston, Massachusetts 02115.

[g] Department of Surgery, Tufts University School of Veterinary Medicine, North Grafton, Massachusetts 01536.

[h] TSI Mason Laboratories, Worcester, Massachusetts 01608.

Infection of human fetuses has been documented at as early as 15 to 20 weeks of gestation, using *in situ* techniques.[2-4] Nevertheless, most infants seem to acquire HIV-1 infection shortly before or during delivery, according to newer studies involving the polymerase chain reaction (PCR).[5,6] Intrapartum HIV-1 transmission is implied also by the discordance of infection seen in twins.[7] The first-born baby was more than twice as likely to be infected than the second born. Infection through milk has been documented in several cases involving postpartum transfusion of the mother.[8-10]

Maternal Transmission of SIV

Maternal transmission of pathogenic retroviruses has been studied in some animal species in relative detail. In viremic rhesus monkeys *(Macaca mulatta)*, no transplacental fetal infection was seen with the simian immunodeficiency virus (SIV) in a study reported by Davison-Fairburn *et al.*[11] In a later experiment, a 25% vertical transmission rate has been recorded for SIV,[12] but the infants were most likely infected through contaminated milk and not across the placenta. In a third primate study,[13] however, transplacental passage of SIV was documented. One out of three pregnant *M. nemestrina* inoculated with SIV during the third trimester delivered an infected infant. Thus far, this is the only instance of documented transplacental passage of SIV. A 33% transmission rate, however, will not permit studies of SIV pathogenesis during ontogeny because the high rate of negative events will render them too costly. Likewise, this low transmission rate will render prophylactic studies too difficult and expensive.

Maternal Transmission of Pathogenic Retroviruses in Mice

Vertical transmission of murine leukemia viruses (MuLVs) and mouse mammary tumor viruses (MMTVs) occurs primarily, if not exclusively, through infected milk.[14-16] In mice, transplacental and intrapartum retroviral infections are rare, if they occur at all.

POTENTIAL STRATEGIES FOR PROPHYLAXIS TO PREVENT MATERNAL VIRUS TRANSMISSION

Treatment strategies potentially useful in preventing vertical HIV-1 transmission are listed in TABLE 1. First, a pregnant woman could be treated with antiviral

TABLE 1. Prophylactic Treatment Strategies to Prevent Maternal Virus Transmission

- Drug prophylaxis given to pregnant women
- Prophylaxis with neutralizing anti-HIV antibodies during gestation
- Cleansing of birth canal with topical virucidal agents
- Active vaccination of HIV-1-infected pregnant women
- Post-exposure prophylaxis of newborns
- Avoid breast feeding (if infant formula is readily available and sanitary conditions are adequate for bottle feeding)

drug(s), not only in the hope of stemming viremia and delaying the development of AIDS in the woman herself, but also with the aim of preventing infection of the fetus. Such a strategy would be potentially successful with a drug that can interfere with HIV-1 replication during early steps in the viral life cycle, steps preceding viral integration into host chromosomal DNA. To be effective, such drug therapy must ultimately prevent proviral integration in fetal target cells, either directly or indirectly. Thus, the drug(s) must be able to cross the placenta, yield therapeutic levels in the fetus, and, most importantly, they must be nontoxic to the mother, fetus, and placenta.

Further prophylactic treatments might include passive immunotherapy with neutralizing anti-HIV-1 antibodies administered to the mother toward the end of gestation. These antibodies must be of the IgG subtype. From the onset of the third trimester, IgG antibodies can cross the placenta, and maternal IgG levels in the fetus increase steadily up to delivery. Passive immunoprophylaxis with neutralizing antibodies is expected to be most promising if vertical HIV-1 transmission occurs through cell-free virus, as opposed to infected maternal cells.

If HIV-1 is passed from mother to infant primarily during delivery, a relatively noninvasive prophylactic approach could consist of simple cleansing and sterilization of the birth canal with topical virucidal agents. Intrapartum infection implies that the fetus is likely to become infected through skin and mucous membrane contact when it is exposed to virus-shedding mucosal surfaces. The application of topical agents may be able to decrease significantly the number of infectious virus particles released from birth canal surfaces.

Active vaccination of HIV-1 infected women could represent a therapeutic option if it induces neutralizing antibodies of the IgG subtype. The mother could benefit directly by a decrease in her virus burden. Vaccination may also increase her chances of delivering an uninfected baby if virus shedding from mucosal surfaces can be reduced significantly and/or if the fetus has therapeutic levels of neutralizing IgG at the time of virus exposure.

Post-exposure prophylaxis of newborn babies might be successful, especially if the time span between virus contact and onset of therapy is short. Post-exposure prophylaxis, while unproven in humans, has been shown to be successful in several animal models,[17,18] including HIV-1 infection in chimeric SCID mice transplanted with human fetal tissues.[19]

The problem of perinatal HIV-1 infection through contaminated milk is difficult to address in a generalized approach. For the U.S. and other industrialized countries, infant formula is readily available, and breast feeding by HIV-1-positive women should be discouraged. In contrast, avoidance of breast feeding in the developing world may jeopardize more infants because of malnutrition or poor hygienic conditions than would be imperiled by HIV-1 infection. Thus, the issue of breast feeding should be decided after careful consideration of environmental factors.

MURINE MODELS FOR PERINATAL RETROVIRAL INFECTION AND PROPHYLAXIS

We wished to test whether some prophylactic strategies could be successful in protecting offspring from maternal retroviruses. When our work was initiated, only murine model systems were available for study. Unfortunately, natural vertical transmission of MuLVs differs from maternal HIV-1 transmission because of a lack of transplacental and intrapartum virus passage, as mentioned above. MuLVs are primarily passed to the offspring via contaminated milk.[14-16] Therefore, high rates of congenital MuLV infection had to be achieved experimentally through (1) direct surgical infection of fetuses and (2) the use of transgenic mice that activate an infectious MuLVs during gestation.

Surgical Infection of Mouse Embryos with the Neurotropic Cas-Br-E Virus[20]

The virus used in this study,[20] Cas-Br-E, was first isolated by Gardner et al.[21] from wild mice trapped in the Lake Casitas area in California. This population of mice had a 20% incidence of spontaneous lymphoma and paralysis at two years of age. Initial virus isolates consisted of a mixture of ecotropic, xenotropic, and amphotropic viruses, which were cloned biologically.[22] The development of hindlimb paralysis was associated only with the ecotropic murine leukemia virus, Cas-Br-E (for review, see Gardner[23]). Inoculation of neonatal mice with this virus isolate led to 100% incidence of hind-limb paralysis in susceptible strains of laboratory mice, with an incubation time of 3 to 5 months. Infection of adult mice did not induce disease. Neonatally infected mice became immune tolerant to the virus, thus allowing unrestricted virus replication. Like HIV-1, Cas-Br-E is transmissible sexually and through contaminated milk. Initially, the virus replicates in the peripheral blood and lymphoid organs. The virus appears to be B-cell tropic, and infection of the central nervous system (CNS) is a secondary event. Clinically, the mice first develop hind-limb tremors, followed by foot drop, and finally complete spastic paralysis between 3 and 6 months of life. The hallmark of Cas-Br-E-induced CNS pathology is spongiform polioencephalomyelopathy. Virus-induced lesions are found in the anterior horns of the spinal cord, in the brain stem, and in the dentate nucleus of the cerebellum. The white matter is involved to a lesser degree than gray matter. The lesions are associated with marked astroglial proliferation, but no inflammatory reaction is seen. These neuropathological lesions resemble HIV-1 induced lesions in the spinal cord, in which also no inflammatory reaction is seen.[24-28]

The experimental approach for direct surgical fetal infection is depicted in FIGURE 1. Between embryonic days 8.75 and 9.0,[29] pregnant females were anesthetized and subjected to laparotomy. The bicornuate uterus was exteriorized to allow visualization of each individual embryonic sac under the dissecting microscope. Instead of injecting cell-free virus, virus-producing cells were injected into each individual embryonic sac to ensure infection. Subsequently, the uterus was replaced, and the abdominal cavity was sutured. This surgical approach was used to ask the following questions:

1. What is the interaction between the virus and the developing nervous system?
2. Does the extent of the disease change? Or, is the paralysis still limited to the hind limbs?
3. Can prenatal infection be used to study transplacental antiviral therapy?

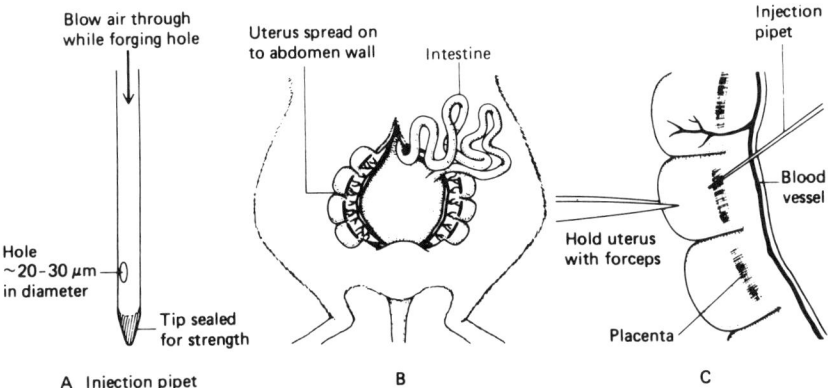

FIGURE 1. Method for *in utero* injection of viruses and/or cells. **A:** the proper injection pipet used for this technique; **B:** during laparotomy, the intestines are exteriorized and the uterus visualized; **C:** viruses and/or cells are microinjected into each individual amniotic sac. (Reprinted from *Manipulating the Mouse Embryo*; E. Lacy, F. Constantini, and B. Hogan, Eds. with permission from Cold Spring Harbor Press, Cold Spring Harbor, NY).

To address the last point, the pharmacokinetics of 3′-azido-3′-deoxythymidine (AZT, zidovudine) were investigated. AZT was absorbed well orally by pregnant females, and it penetrated the blood–brain and placental barriers effectively. Embryonic tissue levels were found to equal maternal serum levels, and AZT was also excreted very effectively into milk, resulting in high levels.[20,30] On the basis of these results, AZT was administered according to the following schedule. After surgical infection of individual embryos, the pregnant females were given a 12-hr postoperative recovery time. They then received AZT via drinking water until birth. Subsequently, oral AZT therapy was given to lactating females, and after weaning, infected offspring were treated via drinking water directly.

Perinatal AZT therapy was very successful.[20] Untreated, infected mice first showed tremors with a median time of onset of 13 days (FIG. 2). About a week later, the pups were fully paralyzed (median time, 20 days). In contrast, mice given AZT (0.2 mg/ml in drinking water) developed tremors with a median time of onset of 50 days. Full paralysis did not develop until 4 to 6 months of age. Thus, AZT therapy not only delayed the onset of disease, but also it slowed disease progression considerably. The therapeutic benefit was lost when therapy started only after birth. AZT therapy was also evaluated in mice injected as newborns.[20] Cell-free virus was inoculated intraperitoneally on postnatal days 1 or 2. Four hours later, oral AZT (dissolved in drinking water) was given to lactating females, and after weaning, the offspring were treated directly. In these mice, AZT also delayed the onset of disease and slowed disease progression significantly. In summary, transplacental AZT therapy ameliorated the neurologic disease in mice infected *in utero;* it was only effective when started during gestation, but not when initiated only after birth. Mice infected as newborns improved on AZT therapy; life-long treatment was superior to therapy given only during the 3 weeks of lactation.

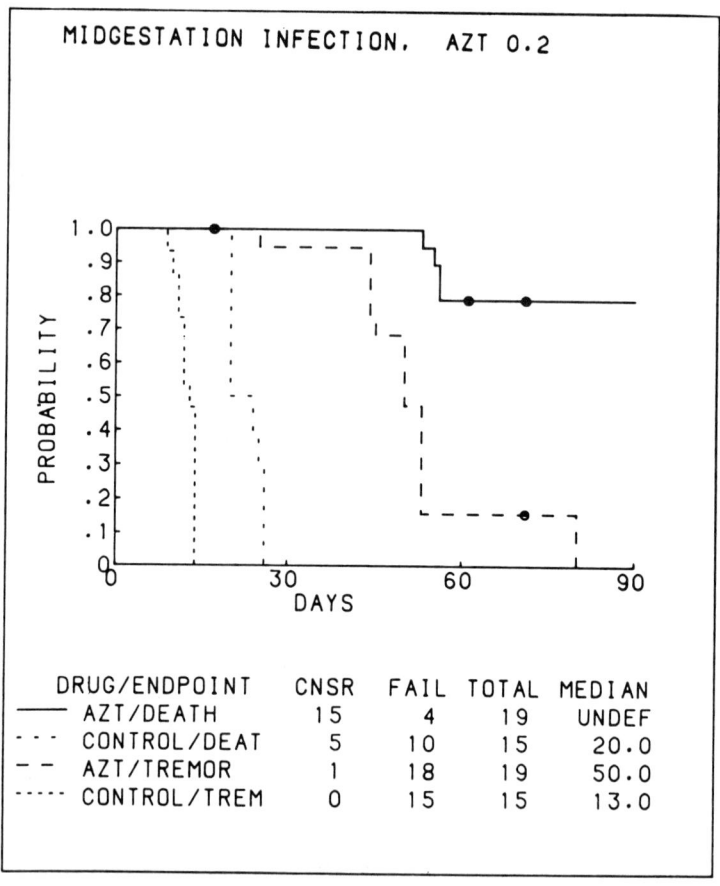

FIGURE 2. Kaplan-Meier plot showing the probability of an adverse event for mouse offspring infected *in utero* with Cas-Br-E virus-producing cells. *Solid line* (AZT, DEATH): the probability of death for mice treated with 0.2 mg/ml of AZT; *dashed line* (CONTROL/ DEATH): probability of death for infected, untreated control mice; *broken line with long dashes* (AZT/TREMOR): probability of developing tremor for mice treated with 0.2 mg/ml of AZT; *dotted line* (CONTROL/TREM): probability of developing tremor for infected, untreated control mice. CNSR: censored at the time of final analysis; FAIL: mice that had developed tremor or had died at the time of final analysis; TOTAL: number of mice enrolled in analysis; MEDIAN: median time (in days) for onset of tremor or death for the mice in a given study group.

Transgenic Mice as Models for Perinatal Retrovirus Infection and Prophylaxis[31]

This series of experiments was carried out with the T-cell Moloney murine leukemia virus (MoMuLV). Like Cas-Br-E, MoMuLV causes disease only when mice are inoculated during the neonatal period. With an incubation time of 3 to 6 months, T-cell leukemia or lymphoma develops.[32] Several strains of mice that carry the MoMuLV provirus as a transgene have been developed by Jaenisch and coworkers.[31,33–37]

Our studies revealed that the transgenic strain Mov 14 is of particular interest for evaluating antiviral prophylaxis during gestation.[31] Mov 14 mice were created by microinjection of cloned proviral MoMuLV DNA into the zygote of a C57/BL mouse. In transgenic offspring, the provirus is integrated on the X-chromosome. Proviral sequences are activated in a few fetal cells during gestation on embryonic day 14, rendering the developing fetus viremic, which leads to exogenous infection of sensitive target cells. Malignant transformation ensues, and the mice die eventually of T-cell leukemia/lymphoma at 3 to 6 months of age. We postulated that AZT could prevent the exogenous infection of viral target cells and thus ultimately protect the animals against disease. However, we did not expect the animals to be completely free of virus since they were genetically programmed to release a predetermined amount of virus on embryonic day 14 (FIG. 3).

To avoid potential problems with infectious virus passing through milk, Mov 14 strain males were bred with uninfected congenic females.[31] Only female offspring were infected, but male mice were enrolled in the experiments as uninfected controls. Control mice received no therapy, whereas experimental animals were given oral AZT during gestation, the lactating period, and in some cases, throughout life. Similar experimental protocols, using AZT administration through the

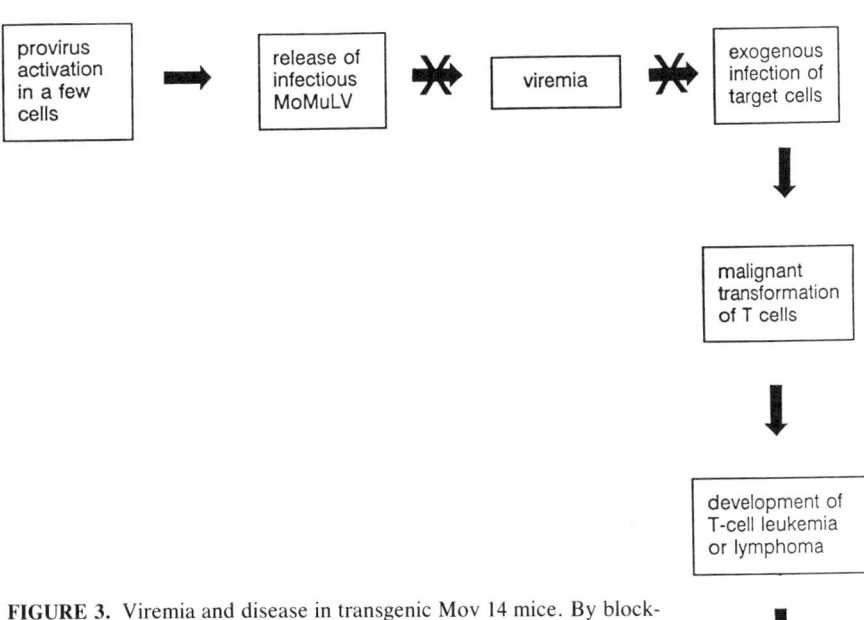

FIGURE 3. Viremia and disease in transgenic Mov 14 mice. By blocking secondary virus spread, AZT suppresses viremia and exogenous infection of target cells, thus preventing malignant transformation (X). (Reprinted with permission from the American Association for Cancer Research, Inc. Ruprecht et al. 1990. Murine models for evaluating antiretroviral therapy. Cancer Res. (Suppl.) 50: 5618s–5627s.)

TABLE 2. Effects of Continuous AZT Therapy in Mov 14 Animals[a]

Viremia at (months)	AZT (mg/ml)		
	0	0.2	0.4
1	6/6	1/10	0/6
6	dead	4/6	0/3
10	—	4/6	1/3
16	—	4/5	2/3

[a] Viremia was assessed by RIA for p30 at one month of age. The number of viremic mice/number mice alive is shown.

drinking water, were used as described above for Cas-Br-E infection.[20] At one month of age, Mov 14 offspring were analyzed for viremia by radio immunoassay (RIA). All untreated animals were viremic at one month of age, whereas only one out of 10 mice given 0.2 mg/ml, and none of 6 mice given 0.4 mg/ml of AZT were viremic. Subsequently, virus-free mice were segregated into two experimental groups: Group 1 was continued on AZT, whereas therapy was discontinued in group 2. All animals were assessed for long-term survival and development of viremia. The effects of continuous AZT therapy in infected female Mov 14 animals are shown in TABLE 2. The proportion of viremic mice gradually increased with time in the treated group. Nevertheless, most animals survived, whereas all untreated animals were dead by six months. The protective AZT effect was only seen when therapy was started during gestation. Delaying the onset of therapy until after birth had some effect on viremia but very little effect on survival (TABLE 3); 9 out of 11 mice receiving AZT at 0.2 mg/ml were viremic as well as 19 out of 20 receiving 0.4 mg/ml.

In a later study,[38] Mov 14 mice were used to analyze 9-(2-phosphonylmethoxyethyl)-adenine (PMEA) as a potential antiviral agent during gestation. Unlike AZT, PMEA was found to be selectively toxic to developing embryos, but not to the mothers exposed to the same dosage.[38] In summary, Mov 14 mice represent a practical model for studying the effects of transplacental drug therapy. Chronic AZT therapy started before virus activation led to a dramatic decrease of viremia at one month of age. Despite lifelong AZT therapy, most animals eventually became viremic later. Nevertheless, short-term as well as long-term AZT therapy resulted in highly significant survival gains. Neither embryotoxicity nor developmental abnormalities were observed in animals exposed to AZT during gestation. Our data show that AZT was able to protect MoMuLV target cells during the critical

TABLE 3. Effect of Starting AZT Therapy after Birth in Mov 14 Animals[a]

AZT Start	AZT (mg/ml)		
	0	0.2	0.4
Embyonic day 10	6/6	3/21	5/22
	6/6	1/10	0/6
After birth		9/11	19/20

[a] The number of viremic mice/total mice is given. Viremia was assessed by RIA for p30.

window of time during which they are susceptible to malignant transformation by the virus. Mov 14 mice thus can be used as models for studying therapeutic approaches to restrict intrauterine retroviral infection.

Prevention of Natural Vertical Retrovirus Transmission in Mice[39]

Most MuLVs are passed vertically through contaminated milk, as mentioned above. To test whether AZT could prevent this natural maternal virus transmission, female BALB/c mice were inoculated at birth with MoMuLV and bred with normal, uninfected males (FIG. 4).[39] Pregnant females were assigned to two groups: Group 1 received no therapy, whereas group 2 was given AZT (via drinking water) starting on embryonic day 16. AZT treatment of viremic mothers did not depress the virus titer in the milk (data not shown). To test whether AZT therapy had protected the offspring, all pups were analyzed for the presence of virus by

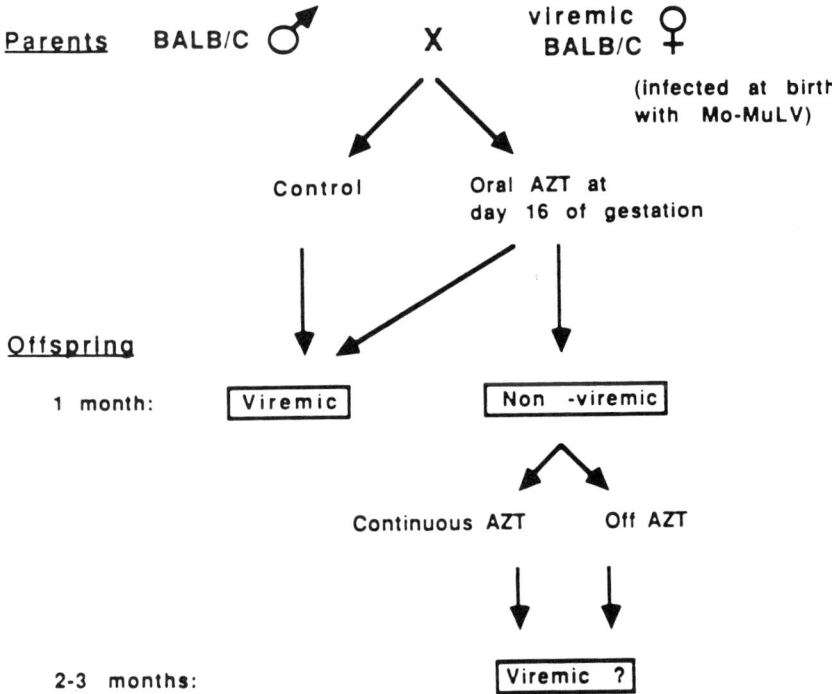

FIGURE 4. Evaluation of AZT effects on natural, vertical transmission of Mo-MuLV via milk. Females identified as viremic were mated with nonviremic males, beginning at 5 to 6 weeks of age. The day a vaginal plug was found was counted as day 1 of gestation. Oral AZT was administered in the drinking water as described. At 1 month of age, offspring were bled, and their sera were tested for viremia by RIA for p30. Some of the mice were removed from AZT therapy at this time. All mice were bled again and tested for viremia 1 to 2 months later. (Reprinted from Sharpe et al.,[39] with permission from the American Society for Microbiology.)

TABLE 4. Infectious Centers in Thymus of AZT-Treated Offspring of Viremic Mothers[a]

AZT Treatment (mg/ml) (no. of animals)	Thymus	
	Percent Positive	PFU/Number of Cells
None (9)	100	All cells
0.2 (9)	66	$2/10^5 - 7/10^2$
0.4 (8)	25	$3/10^7 - 2/10^5$

[a] Offspring were tested for evidence of infection by the XC Infectious Center Assay.[40] The percent of mice with infected thymuses is shown (middle column), as well as the frequency of infectious cells per given cell number for affected animals.

RIA at one month of age. Most treated pups were virus free, but all untreated offspring were viremic. Nonviremic pups were then divided into two groups: Group 1 was continued on AZT therapy, whereas therapy was stopped in group 2 to test for evidence of low-grade infection. None of the animals continued on AZT therapy (0.2 or 0.4 mg/ml) had evidence of viremia at age 3 months. In contrast, a fraction of the mice taken off therapy at one month of age developed viremia 2 months later.

To investigate whether any virus was transmitted in the presence of AZT, a more sensitive assay, the XC infectious center assay,[40] was carried out in offspring of viremic mothers. All thymic cells of mice given no therapy produced virus. In contrast, only 66% of the mice given 0.2 mg/ml of AZT and 25% of animals given 0.4 mg/ml of AZT had evidence of thymic infection. Interestingly, the number of virus-producing cells was markedly decreased in AZT-treated animals with evidence of infection as compared to untreated controls (TABLE 4). In conclusion, 50% of AZT-treated offspring were protected from infection overall, 75% at the highest dose of AZT. In infected offspring, AZT therapy markedly reduced the virus load. No AZT-treated offspring developed malignancies during several months of follow-up, in contrast to untreated animals. This, while AZT therapy did not prevent viremia in all treated offspring, disease was prevented nevertheless with 100% efficiency. Again, no toxic effects were noted in this experimental series.

The three studies[20,31,39] reported were all carried out with MuLVs, type C retroviruses that lack the regulatory genes present in primate lentiviruses. Although our studies have yielded important information regarding the use of AZT during gestation, the model systems have serious drawbacks: Pharmacological agents targeted at lentiviral regulatory genes cannot be evaluated.[41] Furthermore, it would be advantageous to carry out teratogenicity studies in primates as opposed to rodents. For these reasons, we have developed a primate model for congenital infection.[42]

HIGH RATE OF SIV INFECTION OF RHESUS MONKEY FETUSES VIA AMNIOTIC FLUID: A MODEL TO STUDY IMMUNOPATHOGENESIS AND PROPHYLAXIS[42]

As mentioned previously, vertical SIV transmission in captive rhesus monkeys occurred with a very low frequency. In *M. nemestrina,* a 33% transmission rate has been reported in a small number of experimental animals.[13] Studies of immunopathogenesis as well as prophylaxis need to be carried out in a system that yields a high rate of fetal infection. To accomplish this, direct inoculation of fetal compartments was chosen, based on our experience in murine models. Our first approach was intravenous injection of rhesus monkey fetuses with a high dose of SIV. Although we were successful in infecting all fetuses inoculated with SIV, too many fetuses were lost due to either obstetrical complications or an excessively high virus inoculum. Thus, a less invasive approach was developed, using ultrasound-guided inoculation of the amniotic fluid.[42]

Random-bred rhesus monkeys were enrolled in the studies. First, the fetal age was determined by measuring biparietal diameters and femur lengths on transabdominal ultrasound scans. For virus inoculations, pregnant rhesus monkeys were anesthetized during the second or third trimester of gestation. Under ultrasound guidance, a few milliliters of clear amniotic fluid were withdrawn. Subsequently, 200 animal infectious doses of the biological isolate SIV_{mac251} were injected into the amniotic cavity. There was no evidence of bleeding; all procedures were nontraumatic. The first two animals were inoculated on gestational days 136 and 140 (gestation is approximately 165 days) (TABLE 5). Normal spontaneous vaginal deliveries occurred 30 and 19 days postinoculation, respectively. Both mothers became SIV positive a few days before delivery. Both infants were born with congenital SIV infection, as documented both by cocultivation of blood obtained by peripheral venipuncture as well as by PCR. The next two animals were inoculated on gestational days 134 and 124, respectively. Both animals were delivered by cesarean section, in an attempt to analyze placental tissues for the presence of SIV. Both infants, which appeared healthy, were sacrificed at birth in order

TABLE 5. Intra–Amniotic Fluid Inoculation with SIV: Outcome[a]

Animal Number	Gestational Day of SIV Inoculation	Delivery Gestational Day	Delivery Day Post-Inoculation	Delivery Mode V or C	Birth Weight (g)	First SIV$^+$ Culture (days p.i.)
RC 51, mother	136	166	30	V		28
91-1, ♂ infant					465	30
CH 690, mother	140	159	19	V		16
91-6, ♀ infant					333	19
CH 682, mother	134	148	14	C		14
91-7, ♂ infant					438	Uninfected
419 T, mother	124	152	28	C		Uninfected
91-9, ♂ infant					NA	28
CH 790, mother	120	151	31	C		27
92-1, ♀ infant					398	31
CH 922, mother	117	148	31	C		27
92-2, ♂ infant					324	31
RQ 042, mother	96	146	50	C		25
92-3, ♀ infant					298	50

[a] Pregnant mothers were infected via the amniotic fluid route at the gestational days indicated. In *M. mulatta*, normal gestation is 165 days. The gestational day on which delivery occurred and the day post-inoculation (p.i.) are given. V, vaginal delivery; C, cesarian section. The normal birth weight for a full-term *M. mulatta* is 472 ± 72 g.

TABLE 6. SIV Status after Amniotic Fluid Inoculation[a]

Mother/Infant Pairs	Mother	Placenta	Offspring	Culture Positive (days p.i.)		First Negative Culture (day p.i.)
				First	Last	
RC51	+			28	35	42
91-1		NA	+	30	210	390
CH690	+			16	19	26
91-6		NA	+	19	120	300
CH682	+			14	14	21
91-7		+	−	−	sac.	
419T	−			−	−	
91-9		−	+	28	sac.	
CH790	+			27	27	34
92-1		NA	+	31	still+	still+
CH922	+			27	27	34
92-2		NA	+	31	still+	still+
RQ042	+			25	still+	pend.
92-3		+	+	50	still+	pend.

[a] Mothers and infants were followed at regular intervals by cocultivation. The days postinoculation (p.i.) of the first and last positive and of the first negative culture are given. (Reprinted with permission from Raven Press, Ltd., New York; Fazely et al.[42] with permission from the *Journal of the Acquired Immune Deficiency Syndrome*.)

to determine SIV tissue distribution. Both mother–infant pairs were discordant for SIV infection (TABLE 6). In the first case, mother CH682 and placenta were infected, whereas the infant 91-7 was negative by cocultivation and PCR of all organ tissues. In the second case, mother 419T and placenta were negative, whereas the infant 91-9 was positive by cocultivation only. PCR of all tissues remained negative. Cultures became positive only after 3 and 4 weeks of culture, respectively. Apparently, this infant had a very low SIV load at the time of birth. Because both mother and placenta were negative, the virus most likely infected this fetus through skin or mucous membrane contact.

The next three pregnant animals underwent intra-amniotic fluid SIV inoculation earlier, on gestational days 120, 117, and 96 (TABLE 5). All mothers became viremic before C-section delivery. All three animals had abnormally low birth weights, and all were born with congenital SIV infection. SIV infection was documented also by Western blot analysis. Discordance of anti-SIV antibody responses was noticed in a mother–infant pair. The mother developed antibodies to p27 on postpartum day 18, whereas her infant was born with antibody against p27. This differential response again documents that fetal infection was not secondary to maternal infection.[42]

Mother–infant pairs were followed clinically for development of disease. With follow-up times ranging from 1 to 17 months (mostly <6 months), no AIDS-related deaths have occurred. Infants with congenital SIV infection exhibited the following signs of disease (TABLE 7): low birth weights, weight loss, failure to thrive, transient lymphadenopathy, and rashes. All mother–infant pairs were followed by repeated cocultivation and PCR. All animals remained PCR-positive throughout the duration of the experiment. Virus could be isolated from most mothers

TABLE 7. Signs of Disease in Infants with Congenital SIV Infection[a]

Clinical Sign	Frequency
Low birth weight	3/5
Weight loss	1/6
Failure to thrive	1/6
Transient lymphadenopathy	2/6
Rash	1/6

[a] Six congenitally infected rhesus monkey infants were followed for 1 to 17 months. The number of affected infants per total number is shown. The birth weight was not available for one infant.

only once or twice, in contrast to their infants, which remained culture positive for prolonged periods of time. We postulated that this discrepancy in culture positivity may be attributed to protective cellular immune responses in infected adult animals. The cytotoxic T-cell (CTL) responses of mothers and their infants are being investigated.

SUMMARY

In earlier work, mouse models have been used to demonstrate the efficacy and lack of toxicity of transplacental and perinatal AZT therapy. These practical small animal models can be useful for evaluating antiviral drugs aimed at common retroviral functions only, since Type C MuLVs are used. A primate model for fetal infection with an immunosuppressive lentivirus, SIV, has been established using ultrasound-guided inoculation of the amniotic fluid. The infection rate was 86% overall and 100% if the fetal SIV exposure occurred at least 19 days before delivery. The suspected major route of vertical HIV-1 transmission, that is, virus entry through fetal mucous membranes or skin, is replicated by our approach. The high fetal infection rate will allow studies of SIV pathogenesis during various stages of fetal development. This model should be well suited to development and evaluation of therapeutic strategies for preventing fetal infection.

ACKNOWLEDGMENTS

We thank Dr. Norman Letvin (New England Regional Primate Research Center) for the gift of titrated SIV_{Mac251}, Dr. Dennis Panicali (Therion Inc., Cambridge, MA) for the recombinant vaccinia viruses, and Suzanne Ress for preparing this manuscript.

REFERENCES

1. OXTOBY, M. F. 1991. Perinatally acquired HIV infection. *In* Pediatric AIDS: The Challence of HIV Infection in Infants, Women and Adolescents. P. A. Pizzo, C. M. Wilfert, Eds.: 3–21. Baltimore: Williams & Wilkins.

2. COURGNAUD, V., F. LAURE, A. BROSSARD, C. BIGNOZZI, A. GOUDEAU, F. BARIN & C. BRECHOT. 1991. Frequent and early in utero HIV-1 infection. AIDS Res. Hum. Retroviruses **7**: 337–341.
3. SPRECHER, S., G. SOUMENKOFF, F. PUISSANT & M. DEGUELDRE. 1986. Vertical transmission of HIV in 15-week fetus (letter). Lancet **2**: 288–289.
4. JOVAISAS, E., M. A. KOCH, A. SCHAFER, M. STAUBER & D. LOWENTHAL. 1985. LAV/HTLV-II in 20-week fetus (letter). Lancet **2**: 1129.
5. EHRNST, A., S. LINDGREN, M. DICTOR, B. JOHANSSON, A. SONNERBORG, J. CZAJKOWSKI, G. SUNDIN & A. B. BOHLIN. 1991. HIV in pregnant women and their offspring: Evidence for late transmission. Lancet **338**: 203–207.
6. KRIVINE, A., G. FIRTION, L. CAO, C. FRANCOUAL, R. HENRION & P. LEBON. 1992. HIV replication during the first weeks of life. Lancet **339**: 1187–1189.
7. GOEDERT, J. J., A. M. DULIEGE, C. I. AMOS, S. FELTON & R. J. BIGGAR. 1991. High risk of HIV-1 infection for first-born twins. The International Registry of HIV-exposed Twins. Lancet **338**: 1471–1475.
8. THIRY, L., S. SPRECHER-GOLDBERGER, T. JONCKHEER, J. LEVY, P. VAN DE PERRE, P. HENRIVAUX, J. COGNIAUX-LECLERC & N. CLUMECK. 1985. Isolation of AIDS virus from cell-free breast milk of three healthy virus carriers. Lancet **2**: 891–892.
9. SENTURIA, Y. D., C. S. PECKHAM & A. E. ADES. 1987. Seronegativity and paediatric AIDS (letter). Lancet **1**: 1151–1153.
10. ZIEGLER, J. B., D. A. COOPER, R. O. JOHNSON & J. GOLD. 1985. Postnatal transmission of AIDS-associated retrovirus from mother to infant. Lancet **1**: 896–898.
11. DAVISON-FAIRBURN, B., J. BLANCHARD, F. S. HU, L. MARTIN, R. HARRISON, M. RATTERREE & M. MURPHEY-CORB. 1990. Experimental infection of timed-pregnant rhesus monkeys with simian immunodeficiency virus (SIV) during early, middle, and late gestation. J. Med. Primatol. **19**: 381–393.
12. MCCLURE, H. M., D. C. ANDERSON, P. N. FULTZ, A. A. ANSARI, T. JEHUDA-COHEN, F. VILLINGER, S. A. KLUMPP, W. SWITZER, E. LOCKWOOD & A. BRODIE, et al. 1991. Maternal transmission of SIVsmm in rhesus macaques. J. Med. Primatol. **20**: 182–187.
13. OCHS, H. D., W. R. MORTON, C. C. TSAI, M. E. THOULESS, Q. ZHU, L. D. KULLER, Y. P. WU & R. E. BENVENISTE. 1991. Maternal–fetal transmission of SIV in macaques: Disseminated adenovirus infection in an offspring with congenital SIV infection. J. Med. Primatol. **4**: 193–200.
14. BUFFET, R., J. GRACE & E. MIRAND. 1969. Vertical transmission of murine leukemia virus. Cancer Res. **29**: 588–595.
15. IDA, N., A. FUKUHARA & Y. OHBA. 1966. Several aspects of vertical transmission of Moloney virus. Natl. Cancer Inst. Monogr. **22**: 287–311.
16. LAW, L. W. 1966. Transmission studies of a leukemogenic virus, MLV, in mice. Natl. Cancer Inst. Monogr. **22**: 267–285.
17. RUPRECHT, R. M., L. G. O'BRIEN, L. D. ROSSONI & S. NUSINOFF-LEHRMANN. 1986. Suppression of mouse viraemia and retroviral disease by 3'-azido-3'-deoxythymidine. Nature **323**: 467–469.
18. TAVARES, L., C. RONEKER, K. JOHNSTON, S. N. LEHRMAN & F. DE NORONHA. 1987. 3'-Azido-3'-deoxythymidine in feline leukemia virus-infected cats: A model for therapy and prophylaxis of AIDS. Cancer Res. **47**: 3190–3194.
19. SHIH, C.-C., H. KANESHIMA, L. RABIN, R. NAMIKAWA, P. SAGER, J. MCGOWAN & J. M. MCCUNE. 1991. Postexposure prophylaxis with zidovudine suppresses human immunodeficiency virus type 1 infection in SCID-hu mice in a time-dependent manner. J. Infect. Dis. **163**: 625–627.
20. SHARPE, A. H., R. JAENISCH & R. M. RUPRECHT. 1987. In utero infection of mouse embryos: A rapid model for the study of retroviral neurovirulence and transplacental antiviral therapy of CNS disease. Science **236**: 1671–1674.
21. GARDNER, M. B., B. E. HENDERSON, J. E. OFFICER, R. W. RONGEY, J. C. PARKER, C. OLIVER, J. D. ESTES & R. J. HUEBNER. 1973. A spontaneous low motor neuron disease apparently caused by indigenous type-C RNA virus in wild mice. J. Natl. Cancer Inst. **51**: 1243–1253.

22. GARDNER, M. B. 1978. Type C viruses of wild mice: Characterization and natural history of amphotropic, ecotropic, and xenotropic MuLV. Curr. Top. Microbiol. Immunol. **79:** 215–259.
23. GARDNER, M. B. 1985. Retroviral spongiform polioencephalomyelopathy. Rev. Infect. Dis. **7:** 99–110.
24. PETITO, C. K., B. A. NAVIA, E. S. CHO, B. D. JORDAN, D. C. GEORGE & R. W. PRICE. 1985. Vacuolar myelopathy pathologically resembling subacute combined degeneration in patients with the acquired immunodeficiency syndrome. N. Engl. J. Med **312:** 874–879.
25. SWARZ, J. R., B. R. BROOKS & R. T. JOHNSON. 1981. Spongiform polioencephalomyelopathy caused by a murine retrovirus. II. Ultrastructural localization of virus replication and spongiform changes in the central nervous system. Neuropathol. Appl. Neurobiol. **7:** 365–380.
26. BROOKS, B. R., J. R. SWARZ & R. T. JOHNSON. 1980. Spongiform polioencephalomyelopathy caused by a murine retrovirus-I. Lab. Invest. **43:** 480–486.
27. OLDSTONE, M. B., F. JENSEN, F. J. DIXON & P. W. LAMPERT. 1980. Pathogenesis of the slow disease of the central nervous system associated with wild mouse virus. II. Role of virus and host gene products. Virology **107:** 180–193.
28. OLDSTONE, M. B., P. W. LAMPERT, S. LEE & F. J. DIXON. 1977. Pathogenesis of the slow disease of the central nervous system associated with WM 1504 E virus. I. Relationship of strain susceptibility and replication to disease. Am. J. Pathol. **88:** 193–212.
29. JAENISCH, R. 1980. Retroviruses and embryogenesis: Microinjection of Moloney leukemia virus into midgestation mouse embryos. Cell **19:** 181–188.
30. RUPRECHT, R. M., A. H. SHARPE, R. JAENISCH & D. TRITES. 1990. Analysis of 3′-azido-3′-deoxythymidine levels in tissues and milk by isocratic high-performance liquid chromatography. J. Chromatogr. **582:** 371–383.
31. SHARPE, A. H., J. J. HUNTER, R. M. RUPRECHT & R. JAENISCH. 1988. Maternal transmission of retroviral disease: Transgenic mice as a rapid test system for evaluating perinatal and transplacental antiretroviral therapy. Proc. Natl. Acad. Sci. USA **85:** 9792–9796.
32. WEISS, R., N. TEICH, H. VARMUS & J. COFFIN, eds. 1985. RNA Tumor viruses, 2nd edit. Cold Spring Harbor Press. Cold Spring Harbor, NY.
33. JAENISCH, R. 1976. Germ line integration and Mendelian transmission of the exogenous Moloney leukemia virus. Proc. Natl. Acad. Sci. USA **73:** 1260–1264.
34. JAHNER, D. & R. JAENISCH. 1980. Integration of Moloney leukaemia virus into the germ line of mice: correlation between site of integration and virus activation. Nature **287:** 456–458.
35. JAENISCH, R., D. JAHNER, P. NOBIS, I. SIMON, J. LOHLER, K. HARBERS & D. GROTKOPP. 1981. Chromosomal position and activation of retroviral genomes inserted into the germ line of mice. Cell **24:** 519–529.
36. STEWART, C., K. HARBERS, D. JAHNER & P. JAENISCH. 1983. X chromosome-linked transmission and expression of retroviral genomes microinjected into mouse zygotes. Science **221:** 760–762.
37. SORIANO, P. & R. JAENISCH. 1986. Retroviruses as probes for mammalian development: allocation of cells to the somatic and germ cell lineages. Cell **46:** 19–29.
38. LEE, J. S., S. MULLANEY, R. BRONSON, A. H. SHARPE, R. JAENISCH, J. BALZARINI, E. DE CLERCQ & R. M. RUPRECHT. 1991. Transplacental antiretroviral therapy with 9-(2-phosphonylmethoxyethyl)adenine is embryotoxic in transgenic mice. J. Acquir. Immune Defic. Syndr. **4:** 833–838.
39. SHARPE, A. H., J. J. HUNTER, R. M. RUPRECHT & R. JAENISCH. 1989. Maternal transmission of retroviral disease and strategies for preventing infection of the neonate. J. Virol. **63:** 1049–1053.
40. HARTLEY, J. A. & W. P. ROWE. 1975. Clonal cell lines from a feral mouse embryo which lack host-range restrictions for murine leukemia viruses. Virology **65:** 128–134.
41. RUPRECHT, R. M., J. A. KOCH, P. L. SHARMA & R. S. ARMANY. 1992. Development

of antiviral treatment strategies in murine models. AIDS Res. Hum. Retrovir. **8:** 997–1011.
42. FAZELY, F., P. L. SHARMA, C. FRATAZZI, M. F. GREENE, M. S. WYAND, M. A. MEMON, D. PENNINCK & R. M. RUPRECHT. 1993. Simian immunodeficiency virus infection via amniotic fluid: A model to study fetal immunopathogenesis and prophylaxis. J. Acquir. Immune Defic. Syndr. **6:** 107–114.
43. MILLER, M. D., C. I. LORD, V. STALLARD, G. P. MAZZARA & N. L. LETVIN. 1990. The *gag*-specific cytotoxic T lymphocytes in rhesus monkeys infected with the simian immunodeficiency virus of macaques. J. Immunol. **144:** 122–128.

AIDS and the Central Nervous System

Examining Pathobiology and Testing Therapeutic Strategies in the SIV-Infected Rhesus Monkey[a]

LEE E. EIDEN,[b,c] DIANNE M. RAUSCH,[b]
ANNA DA CUNHA,[b] ELISABETH A. MURRAY,[d]
MELVYN HEYES,[e] LEROY SHARER,[f] DONATUS NOHR,[g]
AND EBERHARD WEIHE[g]

[c] *Section on Molecular Neuroscience*
Laboratory of Cell Biology
[d] *Laboratory of Neuropsychology*
[e] *Laboratory of Clinical Science*
National Institute of Mental Health
National Institutes of Health
Bethesda, Maryland, 20892

[f] *Department of Laboratory Medicine and Pathology*
UMD New Jersey Medical School
Newark, New Jersey 07103

[g] *Department of Anatomy*
Johannes Gutenberg-University
Mainz, Germany

INTRODUCTION

Elucidating mechanisms of disease progression and preclinical testing of potential antiviral therapies in human acquired immunodeficiency syndrome (AIDS) are

---

[a] Support to E. W. and D. N. through the Volkswagenstiftung is gratefully acknowledged. Dr. da Cunha is a Pediatric AIDS Foundation Scholar.

[b] Address for correspondence: Building 36, Room 3A-17, NIMH, NIH, Bethesda, MD 20892.

interrelated goals that can be approached by studying rhesus monkeys experimentally infected with simian immunodeficiency virus (SIV). The central nervous system (CNS) is a target organ for immunodeficiency virus infection,[1-9] the results of which are manifested by motor and cognitive impairment, encephalopathy, and acquired microcephaly in the developing host.[10-12] The brain may also be a virus sanctuary that affords protection from immune clearance and allows the emergence of viral quasispecies with altered virulence in the course of immune disease.[13] The pathogenesis of CNS impairment and the role of the brain as a viral reservoir in immune disease can potentially be understood by studying the characteristics of virus that enters the brain and the neurochemical and cytopathological events that occur in the brain, early and late in the course of viral disease. Identification of early and reversible CNS events that occur in disease may allow intervention in both CNS dysfunction and immune disease progression.

Here we summarize recent studies on cellular and neurochemical events occurring in the CNS of rhesus monkeys experimentally infected with simian immunodeficiency virus (SIV), with an emphasis on staging of disease manifestations and their relationship to CNS function. Preliminary data on zidovudine (AZT) administration to animals infected with SIV within days of birth as a model for perinatal transmission of AIDS is described to illustrate the utility of experimental SIV infection in addressing treatments for human AIDS and AIDS encephalopathy in newborns.

CYTOPATHOLOGIC AND NEUROCHEMICAL CNS CORRELATES OF MOTOR/COGNITIVE IMPAIRMENT IN THE SIV-INFECTED RHESUS MONKEY

Several mechanisms can be proposed that link the observed leptomeningeal, viral encephalitic, and leukoencephalitic neuropathology of HIV/SIV disease[14,15] to both CNS dysfunction and progression of immune disease. Leptomeningeal infection and inflammation, which is an early event in SIV/HIV infection, may be completely unrelated to later events occurring in the brain parenchyma. On the other hand, it may contribute to CNS dysfunction indirectly through a virally induced immunopathogenic mechanism in which productive viral replication in the brain has little importance. Alternatively, it may directly contribute to CNS parenchymal changes that ultimately affect the function of the blood–brain barrier (BBB), thereby leading to increased virus infection of the brain and altered CNS function in late-stage AIDS. Alterations in brain neurochemistry and viral status following initial leptomeningeal infection can only be assessed as contributors to CNS dysfunction if motor and cognitive performance in the SIV-infected rhesus monkey can be continuously monitored and impairment quantitatively assessed.

SIV disease in monkeys, like HIV disease in humans, includes quantifiable impairment in motor and cognitive performance.[16] Results obtained in a cohort of rhesus macaques infected with a single virus strain, $SIV_{smm/B670}$, suggest that host as well as viral factors contribute to the variable penetrance of CNS dysfunction in primate immunodeficiency virus infection.[16] Experimental SIV infection of the rhesus monkey offers the opportunity for direct histochemical observation of the brain before the onset of motor/cognitive impairment, at the time of motor/cognitive impairment, and during end-stage AIDS.

The relationship between initial viral entry into the CNS and CNS dysfunction during disease is unknown. HIV is clearly present in cerebrospinal fluid (CSF) upon initial infection in humans,[2,3,17] and it has been correlated with aseptic meningitis accompanying seroconversion after HIV infection.[18,19] Leptomeningeal inflammation accompanied by lymphocytic and SIV-positive macrophage infiltration into the meninges is seen neuropathologically in the SIV model (FIG. 1)[20-22] and may correlate with acute and chronic meningitis observed clinically in man. Viral meningitis is infrequently observed on neuropathological examination in human AIDS brain,[5,23-27] in contrast to the SIV-infected rhesus macaque with AIDS. Either it does not occur early in human HIV disease or has resolved and is not detectable neuropathologically in the brain at end-stage AIDS. Evidence favoring the latter hypothesis is the finding of lymphocytic meningitis at autopsy in CNS of non-AIDS HIV-seropositive persons dead of drug overdose, compared to HIV-seronegative persons matched for age and cause of death.[28]

Infection of the monkey CNS parenchyma also occurs early following experimental SIV inoculation.[29-31] Viral RNA can be found in perivascular inflammatory infiltrates, consisting of macrophages and microglial nodules, as early as 7 days after intravenous inoculation of virus.[29] Nevertheless, the appearance of frequent multinucleated giant cells containing both viral RNA and protein seems to be a later event in SIV-induced CNS disease[30,31] (also, Rausch et al., in preparation). In one series of pediatric HIV encephalopathy cases, only a small percentage showed evidence of multinucleated giant cell formation and elevated viral burden in CNS, suggesting that in human pediatric AIDS as well increased expression of viral proteins and giant cell neuropathology are late events that do not necessarily precede functional impairment of the CNS.[32] Techniques to distinguish viral ge-

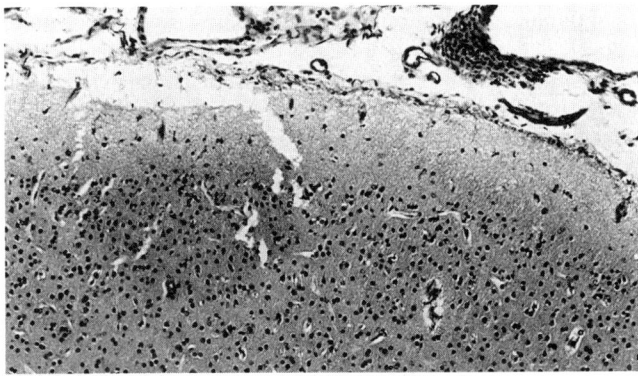

FIGURE 1. Lymphocytic infiltration of the leptomeninges is seen in the frontal cortex of an SIV-infected animal with motor and cognitive impairment (M023). Paraformaldehyde-perfused, formalin-fixed, and paraffin-embedded tissue sections were stained with hematoxylin and counterstained with eosin. Magnification: 100×.

nome from viral mRNA species generated from proviral genomes have not yet been employed to determine when activation of viral gene expression occurs in the brain of the SIV-infected rhesus macaque. This question has added significance with the report of latent viral infection and *nef* gene expression in astrocytes in the HIV-infected pediatric brain.[33]

White matter neuropathology, including pallor of myelin staining, loosening of brain substance, diffuse astrogliosis, angiocentric foci, and vacuolar encephalomyelopathy, has been considered the most pervasive neuropathological event occurring in human HIV disease.[5,23–27,34] White matter pallor with diffuse reactive astrogliosis has been reported in several cases of HIV-seropositive, non-AIDS accidental deaths, and thus appears to occur early in the disease.[35] HIV leukoencephalopathy is also proposed as the CNS neuropathological event most closely correlated with severity of AIDS dementia complex in end-stage AIDS.[34]

White matter neuropathology is perhaps the most divergent feature of pediatric human and juvenile macaque immunodeficiency virus encephalitides, in that its frequency is about 80% in pediatric AIDS autopsy, but less than 20% in SIV-infected macaques examined at various stages of SIV disease.[15,16,21] Differences may reflect (i) fundamental dissimilarities in the pathogenesis of human and monkey lentiviral disease, (ii) greater similarity between SIV and HIV-2 for which less neuropathological data is available, or (iii) decreased frequency of observation of some terminal manifestations of lentivirus infection in brains of experimentally infected rhesus monkeys euthanized when first noted as moribund, compared to those seen in human AIDS at autopsy when disease has been the actual cause of death. Early inflammation that has resolved in human brain by autopsy (see above) may be still in evidence in the rhesus brain, while cumulative insult to the CNS during the often more lengthy course of human disease resulting in severe white matter degeneration may frequently not reach detectable levels during the 6- to 18-month course of SIV disease. In any case, prominent white matter pathology was absent in most of the SIV-infected animals studied to date that also exhibited either mild or profound motor or cognitive impairment, suggesting that these particular neuropathological manifestations of disease are not relevant to the onset of motor/cognitive impairment in SIV disease and may be concommitant with end-stage AIDS, but not the onset of functional encephalopathy, in humans as well. In the study of Murray *et al.*,[16] one of four animals with AIDS at time of necropsy exhibited white matter pallor as well as multinucleated giant cells within the CNS (FIG. 2; Rausch *et al.*, in preparation), both frequently observed in end-stage AIDS brain but less frequently in early AIDS brain in humans.

As described above, a variety of neurochemical and cytological alterations, which may or may not be related to the onset of CNS dysfunction, are observed in the brain at autopsy in human HIV disease. White and gray matter neuropathology includes so-called myelin pallor (decreased staining with acidic dyes such as luxol fast blue), angiocentric microglial nodules, diffuse reactive astrogliosis, multinucleated giant cell formation, perivascular macrophage cuffing, vacuolar myelopathy, neuronal cell loss, and synaptic simplification.[14,36–40] Which of these alterations precede CNS dysfunction, and therefore potentially contribute to it, can be temporally resolved in the SIV model.

Cerebrocortical astrogliosis was observed in SIV-infected rhesus monkeys with

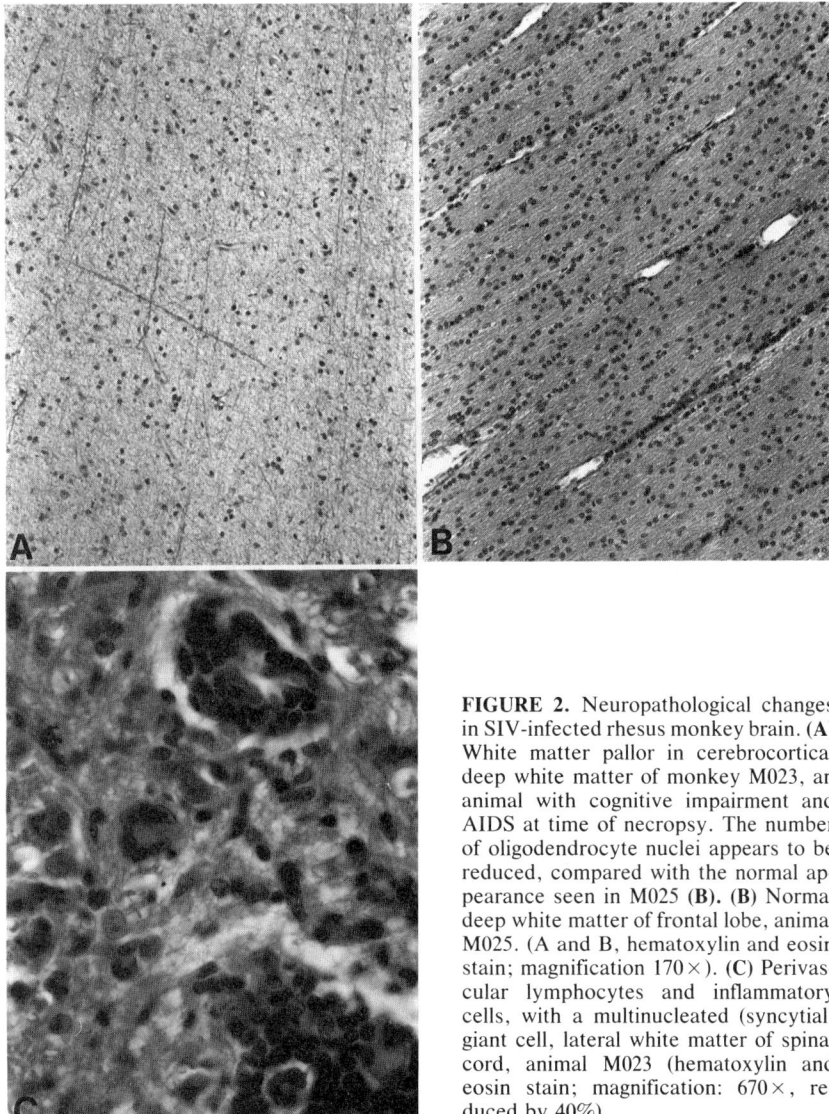

FIGURE 2. Neuropathological changes in SIV-infected rhesus monkey brain. **(A)** White matter pallor in cerebrocortical deep white matter of monkey M023, an animal with cognitive impairment and AIDS at time of necropsy. The number of oligodendrocyte nuclei appears to be reduced, compared with the normal appearance seen in M025 **(B)**. **(B)** Normal deep white matter of frontal lobe, animal M025. (A and B, hematoxylin and eosin stain; magnification 170×). **(C)** Perivascular lymphocytes and inflammatory cells, with a multinucleated (syncytial) giant cell, lateral white matter of spinal cord, animal M023 (hematoxylin and eosin stain; magnification: 670×, reduced by 40%).

motor or cognitive impairments whether or not these animals had developed signs of AIDS, including weight loss, opportunistic infection, or lymphoma (FIG. 3).[16,41] Among 15 animals examined to date in which motor and cognitive function was continuously monitored after productive experimental infection with $SIV_{smm/B670}$, this finding was absent at necropsy in a single animal that had demonstrated no signs of motor or cognitive impairment.[41] These data are consistent with the hy-

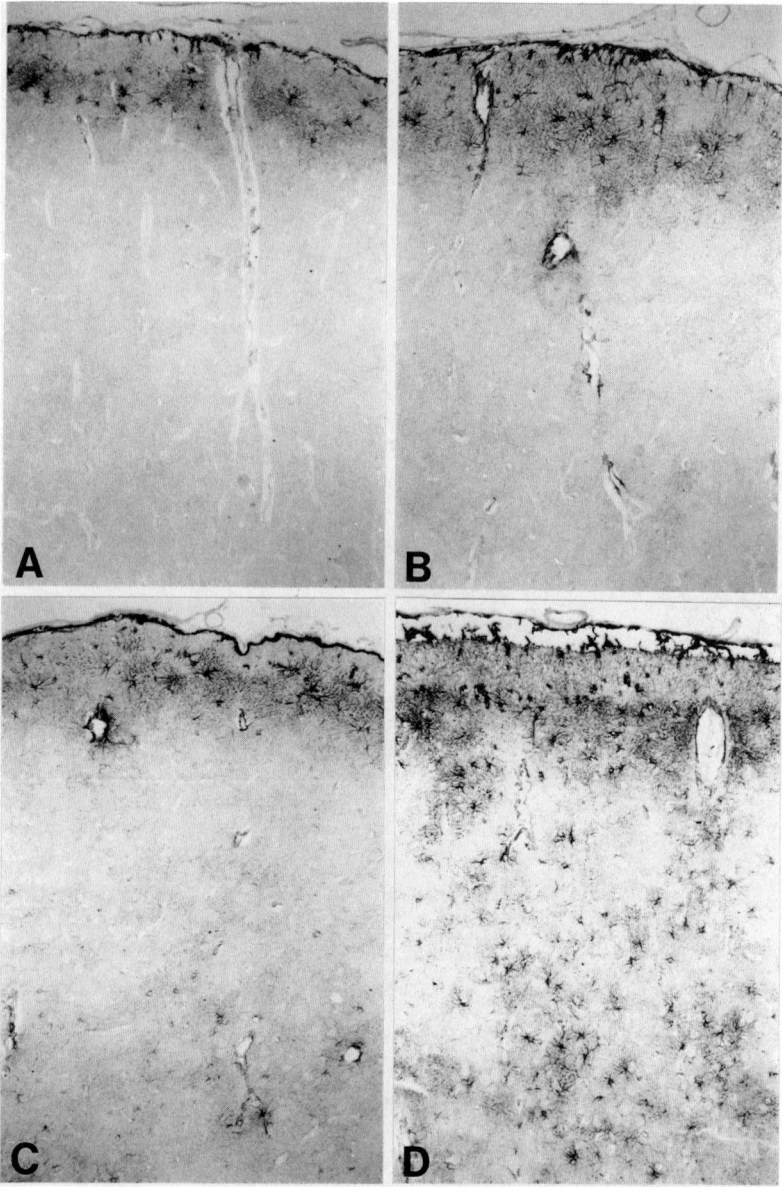

FIGURE 3. Cerebrocortical reactive astrogliosis, detected by staining for GFAP in **(A)** normal juvenile rhesus macaque cerebral cortex (M001) and in **(B)** an SIV-inoculated but uninfected rhesus monkey without motor/cognitive impairment or AIDS (M010), **(C)** an SIV-infected rhesus monkey with motor impairment but without AIDS (M030), and **(D)** an SIV-infected rhesus monkey with motor/cognitive impairment and AIDS (M023). Note pattern of GFAP immunoreactivity indicative of diffuse astrogliosis in layers 2 through 6 of cerebral cortex in C and D, but not A and B. Conditions of tissue preparation and staining as described.[41] Magnification: 50×; reduced by 30%.

pothesis that diffuse cerebrocortical astrogliosis precedes, or is concommitant with, the onset of motor/cognitive impairment.

Other early and persistent signs of immune activation of the brain include upregulation of expression of MHC Class I antigens on vascular endothelial cells, and MHC Class II antigens on vascular endothelial and putative microglial cells as well (FIG. 4). Upregulation of MHC Class II expression in brain has been noted as early as seven days after infection with SIV_{mac251}.[29] Upregulation of MHC-I expression on endothelial cells throughout the BBB is reminiscent of the increased endothelial cell expression of vascular cell adhesion molecule-1 (VCAM-I) observed throughout the brain following infection of rhesus macaques with a SIV_{mac} simian immunodeficiency virus isolate.[42] MHC antigens and cellular adhesion molecules may act together, perhaps with other molecules induced on endothelial cells by SIV infection, to promote recruitment of blood-borne mononuclear cells to and through the BBB.

The alterations of the BBB described above, as well as SIV-induced reactive astrocytosis within the CNS, may occur quite early in the course of disease, perhaps related to the early lymphocytic meningitis seen in both SIV and HIV infection.[28] The relationship of these changes to CNS impairment at any stage of immune disease and to the monocyte infiltration of the brain throughout the course of HIV/SIV disease that appears to culminate in increased viral burden and HIV encephalitis/leukoencephalitis in late-stage AIDS requires further elucidation in the SIV-infected rhesus monkey.

Increased cytokine expression has been noted in endothelial cells of both HIV- and SIV-infected brain[43] (FIG. 5). Interleukin-1 (IL-1) as well as other cytokines have been shown to induce major histocompatibility (MHC) antigen expression on capillary endothelial cells *in vitro*.[44,45] The presence of IL-1 immunoreactivity in the CNS of the SIV-infected rhesus macaque provides a plausible molecular mechanism for immune activation of the BBB. Sasseville *et al.* have suggested that changes in the cytokine microenvironment on either the brain or circulatory side of the BBB may be responsible for VCAM-1 upregulation in SIV encephalitis.[42] In any event, "inflammatory activation" reflected in global rather than focal reactive astrogliosis and upregulation of major histocompatibility antigen expression in the CNS occurs in the absence of abundant viral protein expression, that is, productive SIV infection, in brain. Determining the sequence of these changes will require their rigorous examination during progression of both immune and CNS disease, and CNS viral burden, in the SIV-infected rhesus monkey.

Mild cognitive impairment has been noted in some studies of asymptomatic HIV-seropositive persons, while data gathered from the Multicenter AIDS Cohort Study (MACS) and other studies indicate that overall cognitive decline leading to dementia may be precipitous rather than insidious in HIV disease.[46–49] Decline in performance on tasks with a motor component may be gradual, and precede intellectual decline.[12,50–53] Cognitive performance specifically requiring intact basal ganglia structures, as well as motor skill tasks, appears to be more frequently affected in SIV disease than cognitive performance associated with higher cortical neuroanatomical substrates.[16] Initial learning of "higher cortical" tasks may be more frequently affected in SIV disease than task performance following learning.[54] It is unclear precisely how closely motor and cognitive deficits observed in

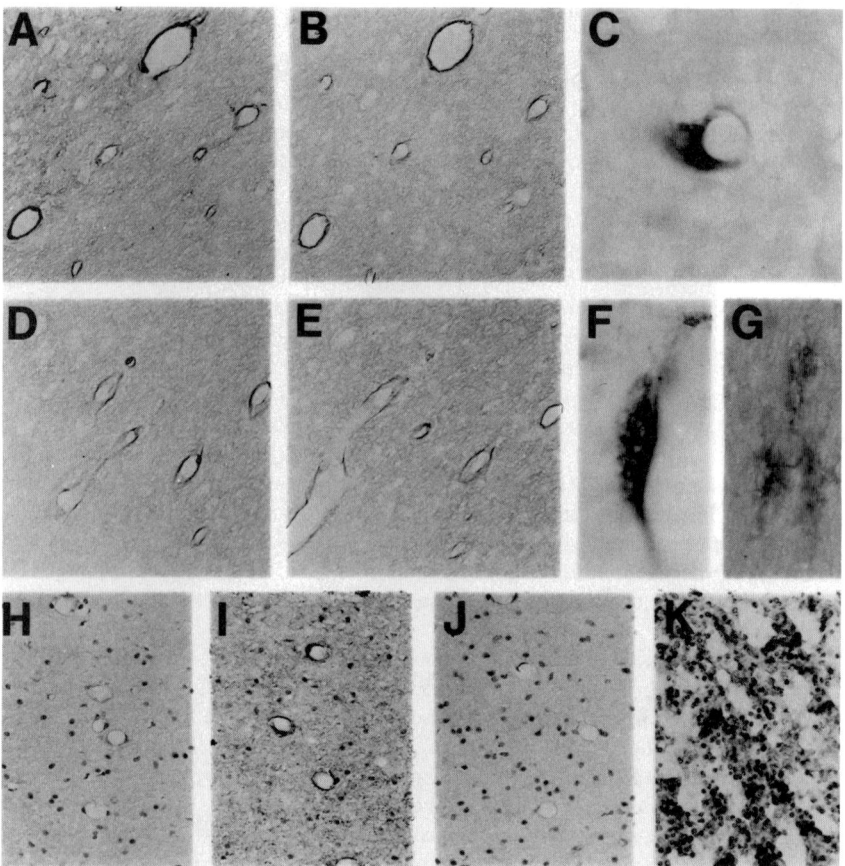

FIGURE 4. Localization of MHC Class I antigen (**A**) and MHC Class II antigen (**D**) serial to RCA-1 positive endothelial cells (**B,E**) in the frontal cortex of an SIV-infected animal with motor and cognitive impairments. MHC Class I and II immunoreactivity are present in endothelial cells (**C,F**). Less frequently, MHC Class II immunoreactivity is present in ramified microglia (**G**). In comparison, sections from an animal not infected with SIV have very scant MHC Class I (**H**) and MHC Class II (**J**) immunoreactivity, which colocalizes with RCA-1 positive endothelial cells (**I**). In contrast to normal brain, normal spleen (**K**) has MHC Class I expression in the vast majority of cells. Paraformaldehyde-perfused cryosections were incubated with a monoclonal antibody that reacts with monomorphic determinants on the HLA-A,B,C molecule (W6/32 IgG2a, ATCC, Rockville, MD) for detection of MHC Class I antigen; with a monoclonal antibody that reacts with nonpolymorphic HLA-DR (Ia-like) antigen (LN-3, ICN ImmunoBiologicals, Costa Mesa, CA) for detection of MHC Class II antigen; or with *Ricinus communis* aggultinin 1 (RCA-1, Vector Labs, Burlingame, CA) that binds endothelial and microglial cells. The reaction product in each section was detected with the immunoperoxidase technique. Sections H-K were counterstained with hemotoxylin to reveal nuclei. Magnification: 200×, except for C, F, and G (1000×); reduced by 35%.

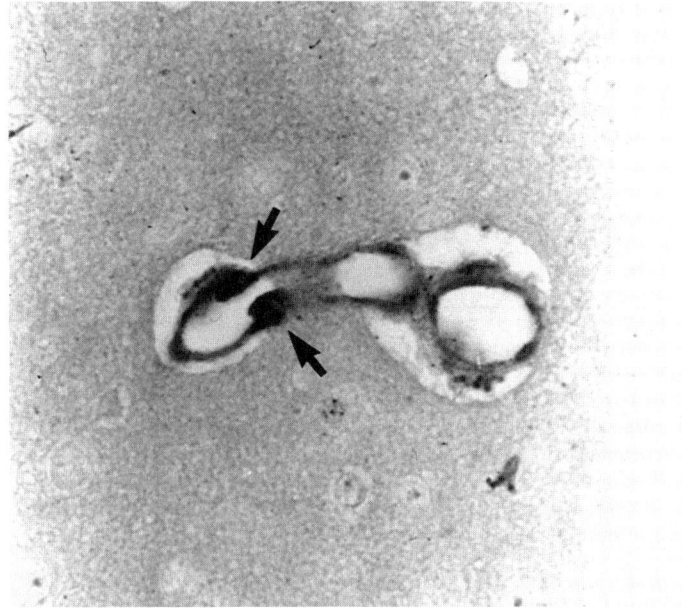

FIGURE 5. Photomicrograph of IL-1 *(arrows)* immunoreactivity in endothelial cells of a blood vessel in the frontal cortex of an SIV-infected animal with motor and cognitive impairments (M023). Formalin-fixed paraffin sections from a perfused animal were incubated with a polyclonal antibody that binds human and primate IL-1 (Endogen, Boston, MA). The reaction product was detected with alkaline phosphatase and the sections counterstained with nuclear fast red. Magnification: 1000×.

the SIV-infected rhesus monkey correspond to the motor and cognitive deficits observed in HIV-seropositive adults and children, and how early motor/cognitive impairment in HIV-seropositive persons relates to profound AIDS dementia complex, generally observed late in the course of immune disease.

Progressively increasing CSF quinolinic acid (QUIN) levels appear to be associated with progressive decline in motor performance in man and onset of motor impairment in the SIV-infected rhesus macaque[52,53] (Rausch *et al.*, submitted). Longitudinal examination of serum and CSF QUIN demonstrates a correlation between peak levels of CSF QUIN and onset of motor but not cognitive impairment, whereas peak levels of plasma QUIN are not associated with onset of either motor or cognitive impairment (TABLE 1; Rausch *et al.*, submitted). Elevated QUIN in the CSF of the SIV-infected rhesus monkey could be blood-borne, arising from systemic tissues and tissue macrophages, or could be generated in the CNS itself.[55–57] Within the CNS, infiltrating macrophages, especially in late-stage AIDS, are the strongest cellular candidates for generation of high levels of QUIN, since macrophages are the only cell type present in the infected brain that can convert L-tryptophan to QUIN.[58]

Relatively large increases in CSF QUIN were found in one animal with signs

TABLE 1. Correlation between Onset of Motor or Cognitive Impairment and Time at Which Peak CSF and Plasma QUIN Levels Occurred in SIV-Infected Rhesus Monkeys

Animal	Cognitive	Motor Skill	CSF-QUIN	Plasma-QUIN
M007	None	10	10	9
M008	None	10	10	4
M011	5	8	8	9
M014	None	4	6	8
M023	2	3	8	8
M025	2	None	5	10
M030	None	9	10	6
M031	None	10	9	9

NOTE: Numbers indicate the testing block (1 block ~1 month) following inoculation during which each animal showed onset of motor skill or cognitive impairment, and during which plasma and CSF QUIN levels reached their highest peak. Based on a statistical analysis using Spearman's rho, a measure of rank correlation, the onset of motor skill impairment is significantly correlated with highest measured value of CSF-QUIN, $r = 0.777$, $p < 0.05$, but onset of motor skill impairment does not correlate with peak levels of plasma-QUIN, $r = 0.097$. Although this statistical analysis cannot be applied to compare the onset of cognitive deficits with peak elevation of CSF or plasma QUIN because only three animals were so impaired, there appears to be no relationship between these parameters.

of late-stage SIV encephalitis (M023, see FIG. 2) and exhibiting both cognitive and motor impairment. MNGCs, white matter pallor, and increased CNS viral burden are signs of late-stage CNS viral disease in man accompanied by highly elevated QUIN, perhaps of CNS origin, and observed more frequently in patients with AIDS dementia complex than those without functional CNS complications of AIDS. A tentative hypothesis suggested by the limited but well-controlled data available from the rhesus monkey infected experimentally with SIV is that early motor impairments are associated with neurochemical, cytological, and immune changes that are insufficient to trigger gross neuropathological changes in the CNS. These set the stage for the CNS-associated events of late-stage AIDS that include profound cognitive impairment, increased number and viral expression of infected macrophages in the CNS, and grossly elevated levels of QUIN as well as the observable neuropathology of HIV/SIV encephalitis. If this is so, the major challenge to investigators of the experimentally infected rhesus macaque will be identification of those events in the pathogenic cascade leading to end-stage SIV encephalitis that can be reversed to effect, for both CNS dysfunction and potentially for the progress of immune disease. Specifically, it is necessary to determine if the diffuse astrogliosis and moderate elevation of CSF QUIN, which appear to accompany mild motor impairment, merely presage further inflammatory, viral, and cognitive events, or actually contribute to them. Further examination of SIV-infected animals sacrificed at various stages of CNS disease and AIDS will help elucidate these questions, as will preclinical testing of both anti-viral and CNS-active pharmacological treatments at various stages of both CNS and immune disease.

ZIDOVUDINE TREATMENT OF THE SIV-INFECTED NEONATE: IMPLICATIONS FOR PROGRESSION OF AIDS AND CNS DYSFUNCTION

In both pediatric AIDS and SIV infection of the juvenile rhesus monkey, a poor prognosis for survival of immune disease and severity of encephalopathy appear to be linked, underscoring the importance of the SIV model both for the study of disease pathogenesis and the relative efficacy of potential therapeutics at various stages of disease. This is especially critical for neonatal AIDS acquired via maternal transmission, in which equal opportunity for intervention before, during, and after infection may not exist in practice. Infection of infant rhesus monkeys within 24 to 48 hours of birth is a model for perinatal maternal–fetal transmission, which may represent a significant proportion of maternal–fetal infection events.[59–62] It is also a preclinical model for the relative risks and benefits of antiviral therapy in the immunodeficiency virus-infected newborn. Infant rhesus macaques of both sexes were inoculated i.v. with $SIV_{smm/B670}$ within 72 hours of birth and with zidovudine or saline administered s.c. for a six-month period. Serum chemistry, virus rescue from CSF and blood, and behavioral assessments were carried out during the six months of treatment and for an additional six months following cessation of AZT or saline. In all groups of animals, including the uninfected controls, CD4 counts decreased throughout the first year of life. Virus could be rescued from the serum of all infected animals throughout the first year of life regardless of treatment (TABLE 2). Virus rescue from CSF was significantly less frequent in zidovudine-treated animals at the time of cessation of AZT treatment. Frequency of CSF rescue of virus increased in the zidovudine-treated group

TABLE 2. Comparison between Virus-Inoculated, AZT-Treated Animals and Animals Inoculated and Not Treated (CON), with Respect to Clinical, Immunological, and Survival Status; Systemic and CNS Viral Burden; and Motor Impairments during the Period, and after the Cessation, of Treatment

	0–6 Months		6–12 Months		>12 Months	
	AZT[a]	CON	AZT	CON	AZT	CON
Virus, serum	8/8	5/5	8/8	3/3	7/7	3/3
Virus, CSF	NA	2/2 (necropsy)	2/8	3/3	3/7	3/3
CD4/CD8 <1	0/8	2/5	2/8	1/3	2/7	1/3
Clinical disease (AIDS)	0/8	2/5	1/8	0/3	0/7	3/3
Mortality	0/8	2/5	1/8	0/3	0/7	3/3
Antigenemia	5/8	5/5	8/8	3/3	7/7	3/3
Motor impairment	0/8	2/5	3/8	1/3	NA	NA

NOTE: The denominator in each category gives the number of animals alive at the beginning of the period indicated. CSF was considered positive if inoculation of PHA-stimulated human PBMCs (peripheral blood mononuclear cells) with CSF resulted in production of p26 for two successive months. A ratio <1 for CD4/CD8 surface antigens on T cells is reported when two successive samples (2–4 weeks apart) showed this ratio. An animal was considered antigenemic if any serum sample showed detectable p26 (ELISA, Coulter Corp.). Motor impairment was identified when (1) an animal's testing scores averaged below the 95% tolerance limit (a statistic based on the mean and standard deviation of the scores of controls, which indicates a range of scores within which a specified percentage of a statistical population can be expected to fall) for a week of testing before 6 months, or for a month of testing after 6 months; or (2) an animal showed a delay in learning resulting in a mean >2 SD (standard deviations) from the mean of the control, uninfected animals during the first six-month period

[a] AZT, animals inoculated with SIV and treated with AZT; CON, animals inoculated with SIV and not treated; NA, not applicable.

as a function of time following cessation of therapy. An initial spike in serum antigenemia occurred within the first two weeks after virus inoculation in untreated animals. The frequency and magnitude of detectable serum p26 in the first two weeks of life were lower in the AZT-treated than in untreated animals. This pattern of peak antigenemia within the first month of life has also been found in human infants thought to be infected perinatally, but not in those thought to be infected *in utero*, by the criterion of postpartum onset of PCR-detectable serum viremia.[61,62] Survival was significantly greater for zidovudine-treated monkeys than for untreated, SIV-infected monkeys during the first six months of life. Survival in the group of SIV-infected animals treated with AZT was also higher during the first seventeen months of life in this group, although AZT treatment was discontinued in the sixth month of life (TABLE 2). Two of the infected and untreated animals, and none of the AZT-treated animals, exhibited motor skill testing scores more than two SD lower than the control mean (five uninfected and untreated infants) during the first six months of life, whereas decrements in motor skill performance were noted in 3/8 of the initially AZT-treated animals during the six-month period following cessation of drug treatment (TABLE 2). The animals treated as infants with AZT are currently being followed to determine if onset of motor or cognitive impairment is predictive of the emergence of either CSF virus rescue or signs of immunodeficiency disease. These studies provide a basis for further examination of the variable efficacy of AZT treatment depending on duration after infection, as well as of AZT treatment at variable intervals after perinatal infection in the infant rhesus monkey.

SUMMARY, CONCLUSIONS, AND FUTURE DIRECTIONS

Leptomeningeal inflammation, MHC-I and MHC-II upregulation, and diffuse astrogliosis are early events in SIV infection, while white matter pallor and MNGC formation appear to occur much later in immune disease. Expression of other components of the immune system and BBB, including cytokines, occurs in the SIV-infected CNS, but its course relative to CNS impairment is not known. In the experimentally infected macaque, a single defined strain of SIV can be used, groups can be balanced for behavioral parameters, and baselines can be clearly established before infection. This offers a remarkable opportunity to temporally stage the events leading to viral entry into the brain, CNS impairment, and changes in the state of viral replication in the brain that may have an impact on the course of both CNS and immune disease. It is not clear if immunopathogenic or direct viral insult governs CNS damage and dysfunction, or whether early/mild motor and cognitive impairment is part of a continuum leading to profound motor/cognitive impairment. If inflammation leads to dysfunction and only later to viral reinfection of the brain, for example, an "anti-cytokine strategy" may be effective. If latent virus established early in infection in brain leads to inflammation, dysfunction, and is later "reactivated," a different therapeutic strategy, dependent on penetration of anti-viral or CNS-specific therapeutic agents to the brain, may be appropriate. These issues can best be addressed by careful longitudinal and serial sacrifice studies that examine viral DNA, RNA, and protein burden in the course of SIV disease in which immune and CNS disease parameters are carefully and continuously monitored.

ACKNOWLEDGMENTS

The authors wish to thank Dr. Karen Pettigrew (NIMH) for expert assistance with statistical analyses; Russ Byrum and Dr. Tom Moskal (Bioqual, Inc.) for assistance in animal husbandry, behavioral testing, tissue preparation, and veterinary support and consultation; and Dr. Jerrold Ward (FCRDC) for veterinary pathology consultation.

REFERENCES

1. EPSTEIN, L. G., L. R. SCHARER, E.-S. CHO & M. MYENHOFER. 1985. HTVL-III/LAV-like retrovirus particles in the brains of patients with AIDS encephalopathy. AIDS Res. **1**: 447–454.
2. HO, D. D., T. R. ROTA, R. T. SCHOOLEY, J. C. KAPLAN, J. D. ALLAN, J. E. GROOPMAN, L. RESNICK, D. FELSENSTEIN, C. A. ANDREWS & M. S. HIRSCH. 1985. Isolation of HTLV-III from cerebrospinal fluid and neural tissues of patients with neurologic syndromes related to the acquired immunodeficiency syndrome. N. Engl. J. Med. **313**: 1493–1497.
3. RESNICK, L., F. DIMARZO-VERONESE, J. SCHUPBACH, W. W. TOURTELLOTTE, D. D. HO, F. MULLER, P. SHAPSHAK, M. VOGT, J. E. GROOPMAN, P. D. MARKHAM & R. C. GALLO. 1985. Intra-blood–brain-barrier synthesis of HTLV-III-specific IgG in patients with neurologic symptoms associated with AIDS or AIDS-related complex. N. Engl. J. Med. **313**: 1498–1504.
4. SHAW, G. M., M. E. HARPER, B. H. HAHN, L. G. EPSTEIN, D. C. DAJDUSEK, R. W. PRICE, B. A. NAVIA, C. K. PETITO, C. J. O'HARA, J. E. GROOPMAN, E.-S. CHO, J. M. OLESKE, F. WONG-STAAL & R. C. GALLO. HTLV-III infection in brains of children and adults with AIDS encephalopathy. Science **227**: 177–181.
5. SHARER, L. R., L. G. EPSTEIN, E.-S. CHO, V. V. JOSHI, M. F. MEYENHOFER, L. F. RANKIN & C. K. PETITO. 1986. Pathologic features of AIDS encephalopathy in children: evidence for LAV/HTLV-III infection of brain. Hum. Pathol. **17**: 271–284.
6. KOENIG, S., H. E. GENDELMAN, J. M. ORENSTEIN, M. C. D. CANTO, G. H. PEZESHKPOUR, M. HUNGBLUTH, F. JANOTTA, A. AKSAMIT, M. A. MARTIN & A. S. FAUCI. 1981. Detection of AIDS virus in macrophages in brain tissue from AIDS patients with encephalopathy. Science **233**: 1089–1093.
7. WILEY, C. A., R. D. SCHRIER, J. A. NELSON, P. W. LAMPERT & M. B. A. OLDSTONE. 1986. Cellular localization of human immunodeficiency virus infection within the brains of acquired immune deficiency syndrome patients. Proc. Natl. Acad. Sci. USA **83**: 7989–7093.
8. DELAMONTE, S. M., D. D. HO, R. T. SCHOOLEY, M. S. HIRSCH & E. P. J. RICHARDSON. 1987. Subacute encephalomyelitis of AIDS and its relation to HTLV-III infection. Neurology **37**: 562–569.
9. SHARER, L. R. 1992. Pathology of HIV-1 infection of the central nervous system. J. Neuropathol. Exp. Neurol. **51**: 1–9.
10. EPSTEIN, L. G., L. R. SHARER, J. M. OLESKE, E. M. CONNOR, J. GOUDSMIT, L. BAGDON, M. ROBERT-GUROFF & M. R. KOENIGSBERGER. 1986. Neurologic manifestations of human immunodeficiency virus infection in children. Pediatrics **78**: 678–687.
11. NAVIA, B. A., B. D. JORDAN & R. W. PRICE. 1986. The AIDS dementia complex. I. Clinical features. Ann. Neural. **19**: 517–524.
12. BELMAN, A. L., G. DIAMOND, D. DICKSON, D. HOROUPIAN, J. ILENA, G. LANTOS &

A. RUBINSTEIN. 1988. Pediatric acquired immunodeficiency syndrome. Neurologic syndromes. Am. J. Dis Child. **142:** 29–35.
13. EPSTEIN, L. G., C. KUIKEN, B. M. BLUMBERG, S. HARTMAN, L. R. SHARER, M. CLEMENT & J. GOUDSMIT. 1991. HIV-1 V3 domain variation in brain and spleen of children with AIDS: Tissue-specific evolution within host-determined quasispecies. Virology **180:** 583–590.
14. BUDKA, H., C. A. WILEY, P. KLEIHUES, J. ARTIGAS, A. K. ASBURY, E.-S. CHO, D. R. CORNBLATH, M. C. D. CANTO, U. DEGIROLAMI, D. DICKSON, L. G. EPSTEIN, M. M. ESIRI, F. GIANGASPERO, G. GOSZTONYI, F. GRAY, J. W. GRIFFIN, D. HENIN, Y. IWASAKI, R. S. JANSSEN, R. T. JOHNSON, P. L. LANTOS, W. D. LYMAN, J. C. MCARTHUR, K. NAGASHIMA, N. PERESS, C. K. PETITO, R. W. PRICE, R. H. RHODES, M. ROSENBLUM, G. SAID, F. SCARAVILLI, L. R. SHARER & H. V. VINTERS. 1991. HIV-associated disease of the nervous system: Review of nomenclature and proposal for neuropathology-based terminology. Brain Pathol. **1:** 143–152.
15. SHARER, L. R. 1993. Neuropathology and pathogenesis of SIV infection of the central nervous system. J. Neuropathol. Exp. Neurol. In press.
16. MURRAY, E. A., D. M. RAUSCH, J. LENDVAY, L. R. SHARER & L. E. EIDEN. 1992. Cognitive and motor impairments associated with SIV infection in rhesus monkeys. Science **255:** 1246–1249.
17. RESNICK, L., J. R. BERGER, P. SHAPSHAK & W. W. TOURTELLOTTE. 1988. Early penetration of the blood–brain barrier by HIV. Neurology **38:** 9–14.
18. CARNE, C. A., R. S. TEDDER, A. SMITH, S. SUTHERLAND, S. G. ELKINGTON, H. DALY, F. E. PRESTON & J. CRASKE. 1985. Acute encephalopathy coincident with seroconversion for anti-HTLV-III. Lancet **i:** 537–540.
19. HOLLANDER, H. & S. STRINGARI. 1987. Human immunodeficiency virus-associated meningitis. Clinical course and correlations. Am. J. Med. **83:** 813–816.
20. BASKIN, G. B., M. MURPHEY-CORB, E. A. WATSON & L. N. MARTIN. 1988. Necropsy findings in rhesus monkeys experimentally infected with cultured simian immunodeficiency virus (SIV)/Delta. Vet. Pathol. **25:** 456–467.
21. SHARER, L. R., G. B. BASKIN, E. CHO, M. MURPHEY-CORB, B. M. BLUMBERG & L. G. EPSTEIN. 1988. Comparison of simian immunodeficiency virus and human immunodeficiency virus encephalitides in the immature host. Ann. Neurol. **23(Suppl):** S108–S112.
22. BASKIN, G. B., M. MURPHEY-CORB, E. D. ROBERTS, P. J. DIDIER & L. N. MARTIN. 1992. Correlates of SIV encephalitis in rhesus monkeys. J. Med. Primatol. **21:** 59–63.
23. NAVIA, B. A., E.-S. CHO, C. K. PETITO AND R. W. PRICE. 1986. The AIDS dementia complex: II. Neuropathology. Ann. Neurol. **19:** 525–535.
24. BUDKA, H., G. COSTANZI, S. CRISTINA, A. LECHI, C. PARRAVICINI, R. TRABATTONI & L. VAGO. 1987. Brain pathology induced by infection with the human immunodeficiency virus (HIV). A histological, immunocytochemical, and electron microscopical study of 100 autopsy cases. Acta Neuropathol. **75:** 185–198.
25. RHODES, R. H. 1987. Histopathology of the central nervous system in the acquired immunodeficiency syndrome. Hum. Pathol. **18:** 637–643.
26. GRAY, F., R. GHERARDI, C. KEOHANE, M. FAVOLINI, A. SOBEL & J. POIRIER. 1988. Pathology of the central nervous system in 40 cases of acquired immune deficiency syndrome (AIDS). Neuropathol. Appl. Neurobiol. **14:** 365–380.
27. LANG, W., J. MIKLOSSY, J. P. DERUAZ, G. P. PIZZOLATO, A. BROBST, T. SCHAFFNER, E. GASSAGA & P. KLEIHUES. 1989. Neuropathology of the acquired immune deficiency syndrome (AIDS): A report of 135 consecutive autopsy cases from Switzerland. Acta Neuropathol. **77:** 379–390.
28. GRAY, F., M.-C. LESCS, C. KEOHANE, F. PARAIRE, B. MARC, M. DURIGON & R. GHERARDI. 1992. Early brain changes in HIV infection: Neuropathological study of 11 HIV seropositive, non-AIDS cases. J. Neuropathol. Exp. Neurol. **51:** 177–185.
29. CHAKRABARTI, L., M. HURTREL, M.-A. MAIRE, R. VAZEUX, D. DORMONT, L. MONTAGNIER & B. HURTREL. 1991. Early viral replication in the brain of SIV-infected rhesus monkeys. Am. J. Pathol. **139:** 1273–1280.

30. HURTREL, B., L. CHAKRABARTI, M. HURTREL, M. A. MAIRE, D. DORMONT & L. MONTAGNIER. 1991. Early SIV encephalopathy. J. Med. Primatol. **20:** 159–166.
31. SHARER, L. R., J. MICHAELS, M. MURPHEY-CORB, F.-S. HU, D. J. KUEBLER, L. N. MARTIN & G. B. BASKIN. 1991. Serial pathogenesis study of SIV brain infection. J. Med. Primatol. **20:** 211–217.
32. VAZEUX, R., C. LACROIX-CIAUDO, S. BLANCHE, M.-C. CUMONT, D. HENIN, F. GRAY, L. BOCCON-GIBOD & M. TARDIEU. 1992. Low levels of human immunodeficiency virus replication in the brain tissue of children with severe acquired immunodeficiency syndrome encephalopathy. Am. J. Pathol. **140:** 137–144.
33. TORNATORE, C., R. CHANDRA & E. O. MAJOR. 1993. HIV-1 infection of subcortical astrocytes in the pediatric central nervous system. Neurology, in press.
34. SCHMIDBAUER, M., M. HUEMER, S. CRISTINA, G. R. TRABATTONI & H. BUDKA. 1992. Morphological spectrum, distribution and clinical correlation of white matter lesions in AIDS brains. Neuropathol. Appl. Neurobiol. **18:** 489–501.
35. LENHARDT, T. M., M. A. SUPER & C. A. WILEY. 1988. Neuropathological changes in an asymptomatic HIV seropositive man. Ann. Neurol. **23:** 209–210.
36. CIARDI, A., E. SINCLAIR, F. SCARAVILLI, N. J. HARCOURT-WEBSTER & S. LUCAS. 1990. The involvement of the cerebral cortex in human immunodeficiency virus encephalopathy: A morphological and immunohistochemical study. Acta Neuropathol. **81:** 51–59.
37. EVERALL, I. P., P. J. LUTHERT & P. L. LANTOS. 1991. Neuronal loss in the frontal cortex in HIV infection. Lancet **337:** 1119–1121.
38. WILEY, C. A., E. MASLIAH, M. MOREY, C. LEMERE, R. DETERESA, M. GRAFE, L. HANSEN & R. TERRY. 1991. Neocortical damage during HIV infection. Ann. Neurol. **29:** 651–657.
39. MASLIAH, E., C. L. ACHIM, N. GE, R. DETERESA, R. D. TERRY & C. A. WILEY. 1992. Spectrum of human immunodeficiency virus-associated neocortical damage. Ann. Neurol. **32:** 321–329.
40. MASLIAH, E., N. GE, C. L. ACHIM, L. A. HANSEN & C. A. WILEY. 1992. Selective neuronal vulnerability in HIV encephalitis. J. Neuropathol. Exp. Neurol. **51:** 585–592.
41. WEIHE, E., D. NOHR, L. SHARER, E. MURRAY, D. RAUSCH & L. EIDEN. 1993. Cortical astrocytosis in juvenile rhesus monkeys infected with simian immunodeficiency virus. NeuroReport, **4:** 263–266.
42. SASSEVILLE, V. G., W. A. NEWMAN, A. A. LACKNER, M. O. SMITH, N. C. G. LAUSEN, D. BEALL & D. J. RINGLER. 1992. Elevated vascular cell adhesion molecule-1 in AIDS encephalitis induced by simian immunodeficiency virus. Am. J. Pathol. **141:** 1021–1030.
43. TYOR, W. R., J. D. GLASS, J. W. GRIFFIN, P. S. BECKER, J. C. MCARTHUR, L. BEZMAN & D. E. GRIFFIN. 1992. Cytokine expression in the brain during the acquired immunodeficiency syndrome. Ann. Neurol. **31:** 349–360.
44. COTRAN, R. 1987. New roles for the endothelium in inflammation and immunity. Am. J. Pathol. **129:** 407–413.
45. MALE, D., G. PRYCE & J. RAHMAN. 1990. Comparison of the immunological properties of rat cerebral and aortic endothelium. J. Neuroimmunol. **30:** 161–168.
46. GRANT I., J. H. ATKINSON, J. R. HESSELINK, C. J. KENNEDY, D. D. RICHMAN, S. A. SPECTOR & J. A. MCCUTCHAN. 1987. Evidence for early central nervous system involvement in the acquired immunodeficiency syndrome (AIDS) and other human immunodeficiency virus (HIV) infections. Ann. Int. Med. **107:** 828–836.
47. PRICE, R. W. & J. J. SIDTIS. 1990. Early HIV infection and the AIDS dementia complex. Neurology **40:** 323–326.
48. SELNES, O. A., J. C. MCARTHUR, B. GORDON, E. N. MILLER, J. H. MCARTHUR & A. SAAH. 1991. Patterns of cognitive decline in incident HIV-dementia: Longitudinal observations from the multicenter AIDS cohort study. Neurology **41(Suppl. 1):** 252.
49. SELNES, O. A. & E. N. MILLER. 1992. Cognitive impairment of HIV infection. AIDS **6:** 602–604.
50. COBURN, K. L., N. C. MOORE, H. P. KATNER, K. A. TUCKER, W. S. PRITCHARD & D.

W. DUKE. 1992. HIV and the brain: Evidence of early involvement and progressive damage. NeuroReport **3:** 539–541.
51. DUNBAR, N., M. PERDICES, A. GRUNSEIT & D. A. COOPER. 1992. Changes in neuropsychological performance of AIDS-related complex patients who progress to AIDS. AIDS **6:** 691–700.
52. MARTIN, A., M. P. HEYES, A. M. SALAZAR, W. A. LAW & J. WILLIAMS. 1993. Impaired motor-skill learning, slowed reaction time, and elevated cerebrospinal fluid quinolinic acid in a subgroup of HIV-infected individuals. Neuropsychology **7:** 149–157.
53. MARTIN, A., M. P. HEYES, A. M. SALAZAR, M. S. KAMPEN, J. WILLIAMS, W. A. LAW, M. E. COATS & S. P. MARKEY. 1992. Progressive slowing of reaction time and increasing cerebrospinal fluid concentrations of quinolinic acid on HIV-infected individuals. J. Neupsychiatr. Clin. Neurosci. **4:** 270–279.
54. EIDEN, L. E., D. M. RAUSCH & E. A. MURRAY. 1993. In Neuropsychology of HIV Infection. I. Grant & A. Martin, Eds. Oxford University Press. Oxford, England. In press.
55. HEYES, M. P., D. P. RUBINOW, C. LANE & S. P. MARKEY. 1989. Cerebrospinal fluid quinolinic acid concentrations are increased in acquired immune deficiency syndrome. Ann. Neurol. **26:** 275–277.
56. HEYES, M., B. J. BREW, A. MARTIN, R. W. PRICE, A. M. SALAZAR, J. J. SIDTIS, J. A. YERGEY, M. M. MOURADIAN, A. E. SADLER, J. KEILP, D. RUBINOW & S. P. MARKEY. 1991. Quinolinic acid in cerebrospinal fluid and serum in HIV infection: Relationship to clinical and neurologic status. Ann. Neurol. **29:** 202–209.
57. HEYES, M. P., E. K. JORDAN, K. LEE, K. SAITO, J. A. FRANK, P. J. SNOY, S. P. MARKLEY & M. GRAVELL. 1992. Relationship of neurologic status in macaques infected with the simian immunodeficiency virus to cerebrospinal fluid quinolinic acid and kynurenic acid. Brain Res. **570:** 237–250.
58. SAITO, K., C. Y. CHEN, M. MASANA, J. S. CROWLEY, S. P. MARKEY & M. P. HEYES. 1993. 4-Chloro-3-hydroxyanthranilate, 6-chlorotryptophan and norharmane attenuate quinolinic acid formation by interferon-gamma stimulated monocytes (THP-1 cells). Biochem. J. In press.
59. DULIEGE, A. M., S. FELTON, J. J. GOEDERT & THE INTERNATIONAL REGISTRY OF HIV-INFECTED TWINS. 1992. High risk of HIV-1 infection for first-born twins VIII International Conference on AIDS, July 19–24, Amsterdam, the Netherlands. Abstract no. p. We56.
60. GOEDERT, J. J., A. M. DULIEGE, C. I. AMOS, S. FELTON, R. J. BIGGAR & THE INTERNATIONAL REGISTRY OF HIV-INFECTED TWINS. 1991. High risk of HIV-1 infection for first-born twins. Lancet **338:** 1471–1475.
61. ALIMENTI, A., K. LUZURIAGA, B. STECHENBERG & J. L. SULLIVAN. 1991. Quantitation of human immunodeficiency virus in vertically infected infants and children. J. Pediatr. **119:** 225–229.
62. BRYSON, Y. J., K. LUZURIAGA, J. L. SULLIVAN & D. W. WARA. 1992. Proposed definitions for in utero versus intrapartum transmission of HIV-1. N. Engl. J. Med. **327:** 1246–1247.

Maternal Drug Use in Perinatal HIV Studies

The Women and Infants Transmission Study[a]

EVELYN M. RODRIGUEZ,[b] HERMANN MENDEZ,[c]
KENNETH RICH,[d] AMY SHEON,[b] HAROLD FOX,[e]
KAREN GREEN,[f] CLEMENTE DIAZ,[g]
DONALD BRAMBILLA,[h] AND LYNNE MOFENSON[i]

A history of current or past drug use is common among women with human immunodeficiency virus (HIV) infection. Injecting drug use (IDU) is reported by half of the (12,844) women with AIDS reported to the Centers for Disease Control.[1]

Use of alcohol and other drugs of abuse during pregnancy is documented to be associated with poor fetal outcome.[2] However, self-reported history of maternal drug use has neither proven reliable nor sensitive as a detection method.[2] Self-reported drug use in one large cohort study has been demonstrated to lead to a misclassification bias in the direction of identifying no differences between two study groups when, in fact, a difference might exist (bias toward the null hypothesis).[3] Cohort studies of perinatal HIV transmission and HIV natural history have thus far found inconsistent associations between maternal HIV status and adverse neonatal outcome.[4–6]

The Women and Infants Transmission Study (WITS), which began in 1987, is an ongoing natural history study of factors related to maternal–infant HIV transmission. It is cosponsored by NIAID and NICHD and has enrolled approxi-

---

[a] This work was sponsored by the National Institute of Allergy and Infectious Disease and the National Institute of Child Health and Human Development.

[b] Division of AIDS, National Institute of Allergy and Infectious Disease, National Institutes of Health, Bethesda, Maryland 20892.

[c] State University of New York—Health Sciences Center at Brooklyn, Brooklyn, New York 11203.

[d] Department of Pediatrics, Associate Professor of Pediatrics, University of Illinois—Chicago, Chicago, Illinois 60612.

[e] Department of Obstetrics and Gynecology, Columbia University College of Physicians and Surgeons, New York, New York 10032.

[f] Department of Obstetrics and Gynecology, University of Massachusetts Medical School, Worcester, Massachusetts 01605.

[g] Department of Pediatrics, University of Puerto Rico Medical Sciences Campus, San Juan, Puerto Rico 00936.

[h] New England Research Institute, Watertown, Massachusetts 02172.

[i] NICHD, Pediatric, Adolescent, and Maternal AIDS Branch, Rockville, Maryland 20852.

mately 600 HIV-infected pregnant women at sites in Boston-Worcester, New York City, Chicago, and San Juan.

The objectives of this report from the WITS are (1) to determine the prevalence of maternal drug use among HIV-infected pregnant women, (2) to compare maternal self-reported and urine toxicology assessments, and (3) to determine the association of maternal drug use with infant outcome, including HIV infection, among infants born to HIV-infected women in the WITS cohort.

METHODS

Two hundred and three HIV-infected pregnant women who had both self-report and urine toxicology drug use data available were evaluated. Maternal self reports of drug use during pregnancy were assessed at the time of enrollment using a standardized questionnaire. Urine toxicology was assessed at enrollment and throughout pregnancy.

Independent variables used in these analyses were maternal drug use, smoking, alcohol use, maternal AZT use, CD4 positive lymphocyte count (cells/mm^3), maternal age, and maternal race/ethnicity. Neonatal outcomes included gestational age (GA) by obstetrical evaluation and birth weight (BW) head circumference (HC), birth length (BL), and infant HIV infection. Univariate and multivariate analyses were performed using SAS. Logistic regression and linear modeling were performed as indicated.

Interim definitions for infant HIV infection status were used. HIV-infected infants were defined as those with at least two positive peripheral (non-umbilical cord) HIV cultures. HIV-uninfected infants were those in whom all peripheral (non-umbilical cord) HIV cultures were negative (at least two cultures, one of which was obtained $\geq$ 6 months of age).

RESULTS

The prevalence of maternal drug use by self report and urine toxicology are presented in TABLE 1. Overall, 49% of HIV-infected women in the WITS were found to use drugs during pregnancy based on combined report and urine toxicol-

TABLE 1. Prevalence of Maternal Drug Use Among HIV-Infected Women

	Self-Report at Enrollment	Self-Report + Urine Toxicology at Enrollment	Self-Report All Urine Toxicology During Pregnancy
Cocaine/crack (C)	44/202 = 22%	67/198 = 34%	70/200 = 35%
Heroin (H)	25/202 = 12%	34/191 = 18%	41/189 = 22%
Methadone (ME)	21/202 = 10%	23/200 = 12%	23/200 = 12%
Marijuana (MA)	30/202 = 15%	34/199 = 17%	35/201 = 17%
C/H/ or ME	56/202 = 28%	79/201 = 39%	86/202 = 43%
C/H/ME or MA	70/202 = 35%	92/201 = 46%	99/202 = 49%

TABLE 2. Multivariate Linear Model of Infant Outcomes

Outcome Variable		Effect Estimate[a]	p	R-Square
Gestational age (Mean = 38.6 wks)	CD4+ cells (<200)	−1.5 wks	0.06	0.32
	Infant HIV infected	−1.5 wks	<0.01	
	C/H or ME use	−1.7 wks	<0.01	
Birth weight (Mean = 3050 g)	CD4+ cells (<200)	−187 g	0.33	0.34
	Infant HIV infected	−297 g	<0.03	
	C/H or ME use	−579 g	<0.01	
Head circumference (Mean = 33.7 cm)	CD4+ cells (<200)	−1.4 cm	<0.02	0.32
	Infant HIV infected	−0.6 cm	0.14	
	C/H or ME use	−1.5 cm	<0.01	
Birth length (Mean = 48.9 cm)	CD4+ cells (<200)	−1.5 cm	0.20	0.36
	Infant HIV infected	−0.7 cm	0.38	
	C/H or ME use	−4.6 cm	<0.01	

[a] Excluding outliers.
NOTE: Controlling for smoking, alcohol use, maternal AZT use, maternal race/ethnicity, maternal age category, (<20, 20–29, 30+).

TABLE 3. Logistic Regression Model of Infant HIV Status

A. The Model before Backward Elimination					
Term	Coefficient	SE	Odds Ratio	95% C.I. of Odds Ratio	
Gestational age	0.5105	0.708	1.7	0.41	6.8
C/H or ME use	1.064	0.561	2.9	0.95	8.8
AZT	−0.3905	0.766	0.7	0.15	3.1
CD4+ cells	1.335	0.841	3.8	0.71	20.2
Constant	−1.911	0.418	0.15	0.06	0.34
B. The Final Model					
Term	Coefficient	SE	Odds Ratio	95% C.I. of Odds Ratio	
C/H or ME use	1.173	0.536	3.23	1.11	9.38
Constant	−1.771	0.382	0.17	0.08	0.364

Step No.	Term Removed	p
0		
1	AZT	0.602
2	Gestational age	0.481
3	CD4+ cells	0.094

NOTE: Maternal use of AZT during pregnancy (yes/no), maternal CD4+ cell count at delivery (CD4: <200 vs. >200), and gestational age (<37 vs. >37 wks). All predictors are binary (1 vs. 0) with a code of 1 indicating drug use, AZT use, low CD4+ cells, or premature birth.

ogy data. Nevertheless, 29 out of 99 (29%) women who used drugs did not self-report this use. Multivariate technique was used to control for possible confounding variables (TABLE 2). In these analyses, maternal CD4-positive lymphocyte count <200 cells/mm^3 was associated with decreased HC; infant HIV infection was associated with decreased GA and BW; and maternal drug use was associated with prematurity, decreased BW, decreased HC, and decreased BL.

The logistic regression model of infant HIV infection status is presented in TABLE 3. In this model, maternal drug use of cocaine/crack, heroin, or methadone was associated with increased odds for infant HIV infection compared to mothers who did not take drugs.

DISCUSSION

Almost half of women enrolled in the WITS cohort used cocaine/crack, heroin, methadone, or marijuana. Overall, women underreported drug use by 30%. As found in other studies,[2] maternal drug use is associated with prematurity, decreased BW, decreased HC, and decreased BL. Another important finding was that infants subsequently found to be HIV infected had significantly lower BW than uninfected infants after controlling for maternal factors. These data underscore the need to confirm maternal drug use by toxicology to accurately assess its association with neonatal outcomes among HIV-infected women.

REFERENCES

1. CENTERS FOR DISEASE CONTROL AND PREVENTION. 1992. October HIV/AIDS Surveillance Report. Oct.: 1–18.
2. RODRIGUEZ, E. M., & S. H. VERMUND. 1992. Maternal Drug Use and Pediatric HIV Infection: A Methodologic Review. Pediatr. AIDS HIV Infect. Fetus to Adolesc. **2:** 107–122.
3. ZUCKERMAN, B., D. A. FRANK, R. HINGSON, et al. 1989. Effects of maternal marijuana and cocaine use on fetal growth. N. Engl. J. Med. **320:** 762–768.
4. EUROPEAN COLLABORATIVE STUDY GROUP. 1988. Mother-to-child transmission of HIV infection. The European Collaborative Study. Lancet **2(8619):** 1039–1043.
5. SCOTT, G. B., C. HUTTO, R. W. MAKUCH, et al. 1989. Survival in children with perinatally acquired human immunodeficiency virus type 1 infection. N. Engl. J. Med. **321:** 1791–1796.
6. ROGERS, M. F., C. Y. OU, M. RAYFIELD, et al. 1989. Use of the polymerase chain reaction for early detection of the proviral sequences of human immunodeficiency virus in infants born to seropositive mothers. New York City Collaborative Study of Maternal HIV Transmission Study Group. N. Engl. J. Med. **320:** 1649–1654.
7. BLANCHE, S., C. ROUZIOUX, M. L. MOSCATO, et al. 1989. A prospective study of infants born to women seropositive for human immunodeficiency virus type 1. HIV Infection in Newborns French Collaborative Study Group. N. Engl. J. Med. **320:** 1643–1648.
8. ANDIMAN, W. A., B. J. SIMPSON, B. OLSON, et al. 1990. Rate of transmission of human immunodeficiency virus type 1 infection from mother to child and short-term outcome of neonatal infection. Results of a prospective cohort study. Am. J. Dis. Child. **144:** 758–766.
9. EUROPEAN COLLABORATIVE STUDY GROUP. 1991. Children born to women with HIV-1 infection: Natural history and risk of transmission. Lancet **337:** 253–260.

A Controlled Study of Cognitive and Language Function in School-Aged HIV-Infected Children[a]

J. HAVENS, A. WHITAKER, J. FELDMAN,
L. ALVARADO, AND A. EHRHARDT

*New York State Psychiatric Institute
New York, New York 10032*

This study compares psychiatric and cognitive function in older children (ages 5 to 12) who are HIV-positive to that in a group of seroreverted and nonexposed children of similar background. Almost all of HIV-exposed children were exposed to maternal drug use *in utero*, and control children were selected who were born to a substance-abusing mother. All three groups of children are in foster care, eliminating the potential contribution of ongoing parental drug use to behavioral morbidity.

SUBJECTS AND METHODS

All children were between 5 and 12 years old and were recruited from an agency specializing in the foster placement of HIV-infected children. This sample consists of 26 HIV-positive children and 14 seroreverted children. Thirty-seven out of forty of the children had a documented history of prenatal substance exposure (primarily opiates and/or cocaine). Although HIV-positive children were in varying stages of illness associated with HIV infection, all were healthy and had no hospitalizations three months before testing.

HIV-positive children were matched for age, sex, and race with children from an affiliated foster placement program. Control children either had a documented history of prenatal drug exposure or were removed from biological parents because of substance abuse. There was no known history of HIV exposure in control children. Twenty control children were evaluated. The mean age of the sample was 7 years, 4 months; and the sample was 34% female and 66% male and 67% African-American, 30% Hispanic, and 3% Caucasian.

The cognitive evaluation included the Stanford-Binet: Fourth Edition, including subtests of Verbal Reasoning, Abstract Visual Reasoning, Quantitative Reasoning,

---

[a] This research supported by the Aaron Diamond Foundation.

Short Term Memory, and the Test Composite. Language evaluation consisted of the Gardner One Word Picture Vocabulary Tests of Receptive and Expressive Language. Cognitive and language evaluation were done by an examiner blind to the child's serostatus.

Parents completed diagnostic psychiatric evaluations that had also been completed by a child psychiatrist aware of the child's serostatus. This evaluation was done with the Diagnostic Interview Schedule for Children—Parent Version (DISC-P-2.1), a structured psychiatric interview of the child's primary caretaker based on DSM-III-R diagnostic criteria. Medical history, T-cell counts, and information regarding antiviral treatment was collected on HIV^+ children.

RESULTS

Results are reported for the three groups: HIV^+ children ($n = 26$), seroreverted children ($n = 14$), and control children ($n = 20$).

1. Intelligence (Stanford Binet: Fourth Edition): When comparing HIV^+ children to HIV^- children (seroreverters plus controls), HIV^+ scored significantly lower on the Short Term Memory subtest. When comparing HIV^+ children to control children, HIV^+ children scored lower on Quantitative Reasoning, Short Term Memory, and the Test Composite subtests.

2. Language (Gardner One Word Vocabulary Tests of Receptive and Expressive Language): Scores on both Receptive and Expressive Language were in the low average range, with no difference between HIV^+, seroreverted, and control children.

3. Psychiatric Disorder (DISC-P-2.1): Rates of psychiatric disorder were high in all three groups, with no significant differences between the groups in rates of disorder. The most frequently occurring diagnoses were disruptive behavior disorders. Fifty-eight percent of HIV^+ children, 50% of seroreverted children, and 55% of control children met DSM-III-R criteria for attentional deficit hyperactivity disorder; 25% percent of HIV^+ children, 14% of seroreverted children, and 15% of control children met DSM-III-R criteria for oppositional defiant disorder.

CONCLUSIONS

Older HIV^+ children show deficits in short-term memory and quantitative reasoning relative to control children selected for the high-risk background common to HIV infection in children. When HIV^+ children were compared to all HIV^- children (seroreverters plus control), their only cognitive deficit was in the area of short-term memory. The language function in this sample of school-aged HIV^+ children is in the low-average range and is not different than that of their HIV^- peers.

Of particular concern are the very high rates of disruptive behavior disorders in all three groups. The comparability across groups speaks against a direct etiological role of HIV infection. Rather, genetic factors and/or background factors common to this high-risk group, such as prenatal drug exposure, may be more important influences. These data suggest that behavior problems in HIV-infected children with a concurrent history of prenatal drug exposure deserve careful assessment and should not be routinely attributed to the effects of HIV infection.

Elective Pregnancy Terminations and HIV-1[a]

WILLIAM K. RASHBAUM AND WILLIAM D. LYMAN

Department of Obstetrics & Gynecology and
Department of Pathology
Albert Einstein College of Medicine
Bronx, New York 10461

The number of women of childbearing age at risk for infection by the human immunodeficiency virus type-1 (HIV-1) continues to increase.[1] Recent reports indicate that a significant percentage of these women have been exposed to HIV-1 through heterosexual contact, whereas the previous means of exposure in this patient population was predominantly intravenous drug use.[2,3] We report data that support this conclusion and, in addition, indicate that the average gestational age at which these women elect to terminate their pregnancies is increasing.

Our GYN Day Hospital, which provides abortion services, is located at the Bronx Municipal Hospital Center and serves a poor and working-class, mixed racial and ethnic population. Of the women presenting at our clinic, risk factors for HIV-1 infection involve either direct intravenous use of drugs, a history of multiple sexually transmitted diseases, or a sexual liaison with an HIV-seropositive male known to be either bisexual or an intravenous drug user (IVDU). Before the pregnancy termination, and after the patient's independent decision to abort, informed consent was obtained from all patients after the nature of the circumstances and the possible consequences of this study had been fully explained. The consent forms and procedures used in this study were reviewed and approved by the Committee on Clinical Investigation of the Albert Einstein College of Medicine and the Health and Hospitals Corporation of the City of New York.

The serostatus of the women enrolled in this study was determined using standard HIV-1 testing techniques including ELISA and Western blot. Each sample was tested, and the results compared to a panel of sera obtained from known AIDS patients (positive control) and normal individuals (negative control). Multiple parameters were used to determine the length of pregnancy. The date of the last menstrual period by history, uterine size by bimanual and abdominal examination, ultrasonography using predominantly the maximum biparietal diameter, and, post-abortally, measurement of fetal foot length.[4]

---

[a] This work was supported by United States Public Health Service Grants MH 46815 and MH 47667.

TABLE 1. Study Population

	1987	1988	1989	1990	1991
Number studied	12	40	50	68	76
IVDU-associated risk[a]	12	33	34	39	30
Heterosexual risk[b]	0	7	16	29	46
HIV seropositive[c]	8	12	14	23	32
HIV seronegative	4	28	36	45	44
Mean gestational age[d]	14.7	16.8	18.5	19.8	19.1

[a] Patient's personal use of drugs.
[b] Sex partner HIV-seropositive.
[c] Patient positive by Elisa and Western blot.
[d] Determined by foot length.

The results of this five-year study are shown in TABLE 1. From the beginning of 1987 to December 1991, the number of HIV-1 seropositive women and others at risk for infection requesting abortions has increased on a yearly basis. In 1987, 12 women who were either HIV seropositive or at risk for infection elected to terminate their pregnancies, while in 1991 76 women in these categories entered our study. Of these women, eight were HIV seropositive in 1987 and 32 were positive in 1991. Furthermore, the absolute number of IVDUs in the study population has not changed significantly since 1988, while the number of heterosexual females at risk or seropositive has increased from none in 1987 to 46 in 1991. Of the HIV-seropositive patients, heterosexual risk increased significantly ($p < 0.05$), inasmuch as it was associated with infection in 1 of 12 women in 1988, 4 of 14 in 1989, 12 of 23 in 1990, and 17 of 32 in 1991. This confirms the findings of Gabiano et al. who reported heterosexual transmission increasing from 5.8% in 1985 to 28.5% in 1990.[5] Additionally, the average gestational age of the abortuses has increased significantly ($p < 0.002$), from 14.7 weeks in 1987 to 19.1 in 1991.

Although the data we report here may, in part, be the result of an expanding referral network, we conclude that the population of HIV-seropositive or at-risk women desiring pregnancy terminations is increasing and that a growing percentage of these women were infected via heterosexual contact. Furthermore, this population appears not to be adequately assisted by existing prenatal- and abortion-counseling services because of the increased gestational age of patients being seen at our hospitals in contrast to the decreasing gestational age of patients presenting themselves for pregnancy termination nationally.[6,7]

REFERENCES

1. CENTERS FOR DISEASE CONTROL. 1991. HIV/AIDS Surveillance Report, January: 1–22.
2. PAPPAIOANOU, M., J. R. GEORGE, W. H. HANNON, M. GWINN, T. J. DONDERO, G. F. GRADY, R. HOFF, A. D. WILLOUGHBY, A. WRIGHT, A. C. NOVELLO & J. W. CURRAN. 1990. HIV seroprevalence surveys of childbearing women—objectives, methods, and uses of the data. Public Health Rep. **105:** 147–152.
3. GWINN, M., J. R. GEORGE, W. H. HANNON, R. HOFF, M. PAPPAIOANOU & A. C. NOVELLO. 1990. Estimates of HIV seroprevalance in childbearing women and incidence of infection in infants, United States. (Abstract F.C. 43) Sixth International AIDS Conference, San Francisco, June 20–24, 1990.

4. HERN, W. M. 1984. Correlation of fetal age and measurement between 10 and 26 weeks of gestation. Obstet. Gynecol. **63:** 26–32.
5. GABIANO, C., P. TOVO, M. DE MARTINO, *et al.* 1992. Mother-to-child transmission of human immunodeficiency virus type-1: Risk of infection and correlates of transmission. Pediatrics **90:** 369–374.
6. HENSHAW, S. K., L. M. KOONIN, & J. C. SMITH. 1991. Characteristics of U.S. women having abortions, 1987. Family Plan. Persp. **23:** 75–81.
7. HENSHAW, S. K. Alan Guttmacher Institute, New York, NY. Personal communication.

Use of PCR for Detection of HIV-1 Sequences in Babies Born to Seropositive Mothers

MARK M. MANAK, JAMES V. SNIDER,
DAVID PETERSEN, WINSTON FREDERICK,
SANDRA BARNES, AND DAO-PEI HUANG

Biotech Research Labs
3 Taft Court
Rockville, Maryland 20850

A microtiter well format for the detection of PCR products was used to evaluate the significance of PCR-based tests for diagnosing HIV-1 infections in babies born to seropositive mothers. Standard serological tests (ELISA, Western Blot, RIPA) for HIV-1 are not useful indicators of actual virus infection since all these babies are initially seropositive owing to the presence of maternal antibodies. Yet the majority of these babies are not actually infected with the virus and become seronegative by 9 to 12 months of age.

The presence of viral nucleic acid in a sample, on the other hand, is a more direct indicator of the actual presence of virus. PCR-based assays may provide sufficient sensitivity to detect the extremely low levels of virus that may be expected in actual clinical samples. The microtiter-based assay for the detection of PCR products described here provides a standardized, semiquantitative, nonradioactive format that permits amplification and detection to be carried out in a single day. This format is compatible with available plate-processing equipment and can be conveniently used for the detection of HIV-1 in clinical samples.

MATERIALS AND METHODS

Peripheral blood lymphocytes (PBLs) were isolated from whole blood on Leukoprep gradients. The cells were digested with SDS/proteinase K and extracted with phenol:chloroform. Two-microgram DNA samples were adjusted to PCR buffer (70 mM Tris, pH 8.8; 4 mM $MgCl_2$; 20 mM $(NH_4)_2SO_4$; 100 µg/ml BSA; 6 mM DTT; 10% DMSO; 0.5 mM each dNTP; 0.5 µM each biotin-labeled primer) in a final volume of 100 µl. The reaction was denatured at 95°C for 7 min, cooled to room temperature, and 4 units of *Thermus aquaticus* (Taq) DNA polymerase

(Cetus) were added. The reaction was incubated for 30 cycles of alternating temperatures with each cycle consisting of 92°C for 1 min, 55°C for 1 min, and 72°C for 1 min. Duplicate samples were amplified with primers for β globin and analyzed on β-globin capture plates to verify DNA integrity in each sample.

DNA extracted from lymphocytes was amplified by PCR using the biotin-labeled primers for HIV-1. The product of the reaction was analyzed on agarose gels, transferred to nylon filters, hybridized with ^{32}P-labeled pBH10, and autoradiographed. The amplified product represents a 191-bp region of HIV-1 *gag*.

Capture hybridization assays were performed as previously described.[1] A 10-μl aliquot of the PCR product was heat denatured, adjusted to 1× hybridization buffer, and hybridized in the capture wells at 42°C for 2 hours. After hybridization and washing, the plates were blocked for 10 min in 200 μl/well of 3% BSA in wash buffer, and incubated for 10 min with 1 μg/ml streptavidin–peroxidase conjugate diluted in the same buffer. The plates were washed with the wash buffer and developed with 100 μl of a 1:1 mixture of TMB:hydrogen peroxide. Following a 30-min development in the dark, the reaction was stopped by the addition of 100 μl of 2N H_2SO_4. The optical density at 450 nm was read using an automatic plate reader.

RESULTS AND CONCLUSIONS

To evaluate the early predictive value of this assay, babies were tested within the first few months of birth and during follow-up studies. All babies examined were initially seropositive owing to the presence of maternal antibodies. Of 43 babies examined in this study, 15 (35%) were PCR positive, and 29 (65%) were PCR negative on initial testing. Significantly, all babies who were initially PCR negative remained PCR negative in subsequent bleeds, whereas all PCR-positive babies remained positive. Thus far, 9 of 15 PCR-positive babies developed symptoms of AIDS or ARC, while the others remain seropositive, but asymptomatic. None of the PCR-negative babies, on the other hand, have thus far developed symptoms of ARC or AIDS. Of 27 PCR-negative babies examined after one year of age, all but one has now become seronegative. These results suggest that PCR-

TABLE 1. Summary of PCR Results on Samples from Babies Born to HIV-1-Seropositive Mothers[a]

	PCR +	PCR −
AIDS/ARC	9 21%	0 0%
Seropositive/Asymptomatic	6* 14%	5** 12%
Seronegative	0 0%	23 53%
Total	15 35%	28 65%

[a] Number lost to follow-up: * 2/6 (11, 43); ** 4/5 (3, 4, 13, 15). Age in months at last test given in parentheses.

based assays may provide valuable tools for the early diagnosis of actual HIV-1 infection in babies born to seropositive mothers. The results are summarized in TABLE 1.

REFERENCE

1. KELLER, G. *et al.* 1990. J. Clin. Microbiol. **28:** 1411–1416.

Diagnosis and Quantitation of HIV-1 Infection in Infants and Children by Whole-Blood Culture[a]

WILLIAM V. RASZKA, JR.,[b] MERLIN L. ROBB,[c,d]
ARNOLD K. FOWLER,[e] CHESTER R. ROBERTS,[c]
NORMAN J. WAECKER,[f] DAVID P. ASCHER,[b,g] RICHARD
A. MORIARTY,[b,h] DAVID GOLDBERG,[b] AND
GERALD W. FISCHER[b]

Recent data have suggested that human immunodeficiency virus type 1 (HIV-1) cultures may be useful in quantifying viral burden in children.[1] We have evaluated a whole-blood culture method as a means of both diagnosing infection and quantitating viral burden in infants as young as 2 months of age.

METHODS

Patients evaluated were Department of Defense beneficiaries less than 13 years of age cared for at military medical facilities and enrolled in a pediatric HIV-1 natural history study. Informed consent was obtained from the guardians of all patients. HIV-1 infected patients were classified as asymptomatic (P1; 14 patients) or symptomatic (P2; 20 patients) according to the 1987 CDC classification system.[2]

Whole-blood (WB) cultures were performed by serially diluting 100 µl of heparinized WB in interleukin-2-supplemented complete medium to yield WB concentrations of 10.0, 3.1, 1.0, 0.31, and 0.1 µl/200 µl of medium. Six replicates of each

---

[a] The views expressed herein are the private views of the authors and do not necessarily reflect the opinions of the Department of Defense.

[b] Department of Pediatrics, Uniformed Services University of Health Sciences, Bethesda, MD 20814.

[c] Department of Retroviral Research, Walter Reed Army Institute of Research, Rockville, MD 29850.

[d] Address all correspondence to Merlin Robb, Department of Retroviral Research, Walter Reed Army Institute of Research, 13 Taft Court, Suite 200, Rockville, MD 29850.

[e] SRA Laboratories, Rockville, MD 29850.

[f] Department of Pediatrics, San Diego Naval Medical Center, San Diego, CA 92134.

[g] Department of Pediatrics, Wilford Hall Air Force Medical Center, San Antonio, TX 78236.

[h] Department of Pediatrics, National Naval Medical Center, Bethesda, MD 20889-5000.

dilution were seeded into 96-well plates containing 2.5×10^5 (50 μl) phytohemagglutinin-stimulated donor cells. Eighty percent of the medium was replaced every three days. Fresh, stimulated target cells were added every seven days. A positive culture was defined by the presence of greater than 59 pg/ml of p24 antigen in any well at day 28. Viral titer expressed as infectious doses per milliliter of blood was calculated by endpoint dilution. On occasion, the distribution of negative wells in a culture assay failed to represent a titration response. Therefore, the median tissue culture infectious dose per milliliter ($TCID_{50}$/ml WB) was calculated according to the method of Spearman-Karber.[3] To represent the viral titer in proportion to the $CD4^+$ T cell content, the median TCID was divided by the patient's $CD4^+$ cell count and expressed as $TCID_{50}/10^3$ $CD4^+$ cells. Data were log transformed and analyzed using a two-tailed Student's t test.

RESULTS

101 cultures from 34 HIV-1 infected children were analyzed. The mean age at the time of the first culture was 76 months with a range of 1.7 to 154 months. Risk factors for infection included perinatal exposure (21), transfusions (7), and

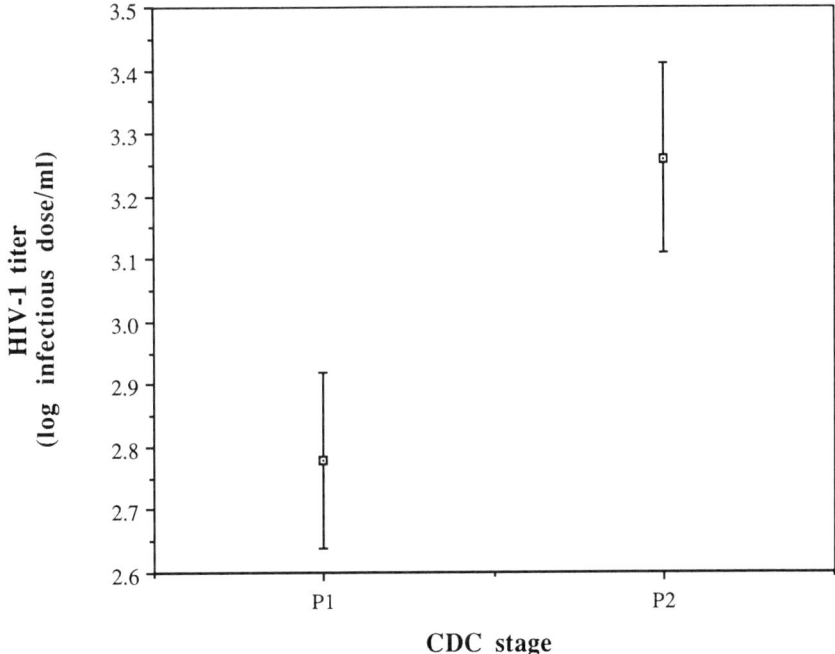

FIGURE 1. A comparison of the log mean HIV-1 titers, calculated by endpoint dilution, between CDC stages P1 and P2 and graphed with the standard error of the mean (P1 = 2.78; P2 = 3.26; $p < 0.025$).

TABLE 1. Mean log $TCID_{50}/10^3$ $CD4^+$ Cells in Three Patient Cohorts[a]

Cohort	P1 (SEM)	P2 (SEM)	p (t test)
All patients	0.14 (0.11)	0.62 (0.14)	<0.002
No therapy	0.12 (0.18)	1.16 (0.49)	0.02
On therapy	0.16 (0.13)	0.62 (0.14)	0.02

[a] SEM is the standard error of the mean.

hemophilia (6). The overall viral recovery rate was 83.7%. The sensitivity in patients not on antiretroviral therapy was 87.3%. The specificity was 100%.

As shown in FIGURE 1, patients with symptomatic disease had significantly higher mean viral titers, as determined by endpoint dilution, than did asymptomatic patients (P2 = 3.26; P1 = 2.78; $p < 0.025$, t test). Controlling for antiretroviral use revealed that a difference in mean viral titers between symptomatic and asymptomatic patients reached significance only in the cohort of patients receiving antiretroviral therapy (R_x group: P2 = 3.16; P1 = 2.52; $p < 0.05$, t test. No R_x group: P2 = 3.75; P1 = 3.04; $p = 0.12$). When viral titers were corrected for patient $CD4^+$ cell counts ($TCID_{50}/10^3$ $CD4^+$ cells), symptomatic patients had significantly higher mean viral titers than did asymptomatic patients (P2 = 0.62; P1 = 0.14; $p < 0.002$, t test), regardless of medical therapy (TABLE 1).

Viral titers, whether expressed as log infectious doses per milliliter or corrected for patient $CD4^+$ cell counts, varied by as much as two logs in individual patients over time and were not necessarily related to individual declines in $CD4^+$ count or percentage. The mean range of titers (expressed as log $TCID_{50}/10^3$ $CD4^+$ cells) in patients who had four or more cultures was -0.507 to 1.044. Viral titers, as determined by endpoint dilution, did not correlate with serum p24 antigen levels, $CD4^+$ number, or $CD4^+$ percentage.

DISCUSSION

The advantages of whole-blood HIV-1 cultures are that small volumes of blood are required, and the total viral burden (cellular and plasma) in a patient's peripheral circulation is measured. The whole-blood culture method described here is modestly less sensitive than previously published results.[1] This may reflect the very small volumes of blood tested (82 μl) and the impact of antiviral therapy. In some patients, the predicted total number of $CD4^+$ cells/culture was as low as 82. Despite this limitation, symptomatic patients had approximately one-half log greater mean HIV-1 titers, as determined by endpoint dilution, than did asymptomatic patients ($p = 0.025$). The difference in mean viral titers between symptomatic and asymptomatic patients was even greater if viral titers were corrected for the patient's $CD4^+$ cell count and expressed as log mean $TCID_{50}/10^3$ $CD4^+$ cells ($p < 0.002$). This significant difference persisted after correction for antiretroviral use.

Although the data are encouraging, limitations of this method include the observation that 20% of cultures in patients on antiretroviral therapy were negative.

No correlation was observed between HIV-1 titers (expressed as log infectious doses/ml of WB) and serum p24 antigen levels, absolute $CD4^+$ number or $CD4^+$ percentage. Furthermore, there was a wide range of titers among patients with similar disease stage and in the same patients over time. This effect was not secondary to antiretroviral use as patients both on and off medication had viral titers that fluctuated over time. Our data implies that total viral burden, as measured in the peripheral circulation, is neither constant nor does it appear to have a linear relationship with a known, measured laboratory value. The predictive value of a single viral titer in a patient is likely to be small.

These data suggest that further modifications in this microculture whole-blood technique will be required if it is to provide more clinically useful information regarding disease progression or response to antiretroviral therapy. The fluctuation, however, in viral titer in the peripheral blood lymphocyte compartment measured by this method may reflect biologically meaningful events. Determination of factors influencing these fluctuations, as measured by whole-blood culture titration, may merit further investigation.

REFERENCES

1. ALIMENTI, A., M. O'NEILL, J. L. SULLIVAN & LUZURIAGA. 1992. Diagnosis of vertical human immunodeficiency virus type 1 infection by whole-blood culture. J. Infect. Dis. 166: 1146–1148.
2. CENTERS FOR DISEASE CONTROL. 1987. Classification system for human immunodeficiency virus (HIV) infection in children under 13 years of age. 36: 225–236.
3. CHOU, T. C. & P. TALALAY. 1984. Quantitative analysis of dose–effect relationships: The combined effects of multiple drugs or enzyme inhibitors. Adv. Enzyme Regul. 22: 27–55.

HIV-Specific IgG3 in Cord Blood

Predictive Value for Seroreversion

D. CASELLI,[a] M. MARCONI,[a] A. MACCABRUNI,[b]
G. BOSSI,[a] G. PASINETTI,[d] M. STRONATI,[c] AND
M. ARICÒ[a]

[a] Department of Pediatrics
[b] Department of Infectious Disease
[c] Department of Neonatology
IRCCS Policlinico San Matteo
University of Pavia
27100 Pavia, Italy

[d] Department of Neonatology
Osp. Bergamo, Italy

Early identification of HIV infection in children is a central issue not only for the identification of infected children, but also for the precocious screening of uninfected ones that otherwise would undergo many unnecessary and expensive diagnostic procedures.

We previously reported the use of an assay based on detection of serum HIV-specific IgG3 for early diagnosis of HIV infection in children.[1] Our results suggest that the clearance of IgG3 antibodies predict seroreversion in non-HIV-infected, passive antibody carrier children.

On the basis of this evidence, we started a prospective study of HIV-seropositive newborns.

METHODS AND PATIENTS

The test was performed using a commercial kit (Bio Rad, Richmond, California) modified with overnight incubation of strips with patient serum and FBS and then matched with IgG-specific monoclonal antibodies (Immunotech, Marseille, France). Anti-mouse monoclonal antibody IgG alkaline phosphatase conjugate was finally used.

We tested cord blood serum from 22 consecutive newborns of HIV-infected mothers.

RESULTS

HIV-specific IgG3 were found in 15 of the 22 newborns. In the follow-up, 11 of the 15 IgG3-positive children seroreverted, one was lost, and in all the three persistently IgG3-positive children HIV infection was documented by PCR and virus isolation. Of the seven IgG3-negative newborns, six seroreverted; one had a very aggressive course, developed AIDS, and died of PCP at 2 months.

CONCLUSION

The present study confirms our previous observation that this simple and relatively inexpensive test predicted seroreversion in 6 out of 22 children at birth. The predictive power of a negative IgG3 test was 85.8%.

REFERENCE

1. ARICÒ, M., D. CASELLI, M. MARCONI, A. M. AVANZINI, A. COLOMBO, G. PASINETTI, A. MACCABRUNI, E. G. RONDANELLI & G. R. BURGIO. 1991. Immunoglobulin G3-specific antibodies as a marker for early diagnosis of HIV infection in children. AIDS **5:** 1315–1318.

A Rapid, Sensitive, PCR-Based Method for Detection of HIV-1 Specific Nucleic Acid in the Culture Supernatant of Infected Cells

INDIRA K. HEWLETT, BHARAT JOSHI, GARY RIORDAN, LAURIE POLLOCK, AND JAY S. EPSTEIN

Laboratory of Retrovirology
Center for Biologics Evaluation and Research
Food and Drug Administration
Bethesda, Maryland 20892

Several procedures using the polymerase chain reaction (PCR) have been developed for the early and direct detection of HIV-1 nucleic acid in infected specimens.[1] Viral markers currently being used for evaluation of HIV infection in patients include serum p24 antigen, reverse transcriptase (RT) activity, and p24 antigen levels in supernatants of cocultures of patients' peripheral blood mononuclear cells. In this study, we analyzed viral DNA and RNA in culture supernatants and evaluated their use as early markers for monitoring virus production in infected cell cultures. Briefly, H9 and U937 cells were infected with HIV-1 (100 ng

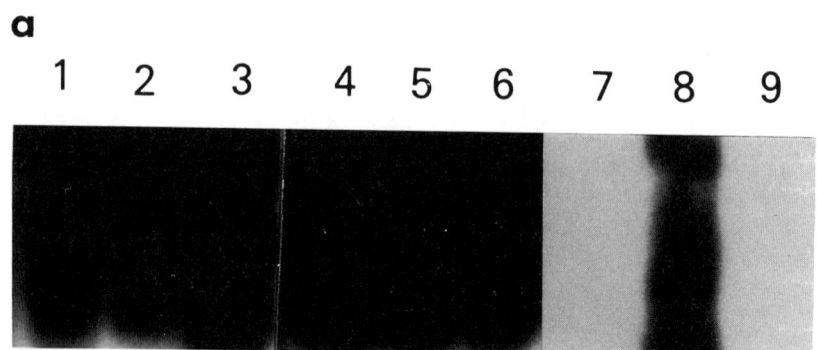

FIGURE 1. (a) Detection of viral DNA in the culture supernatant of H9 (lanes 1–3) and U937 (lanes 4–6) cells at days 1, 2, and 3 post infection using the SK 38/39 primers. Lanes 7 and 9 represent negative and lane 8 positive controls, respectively.

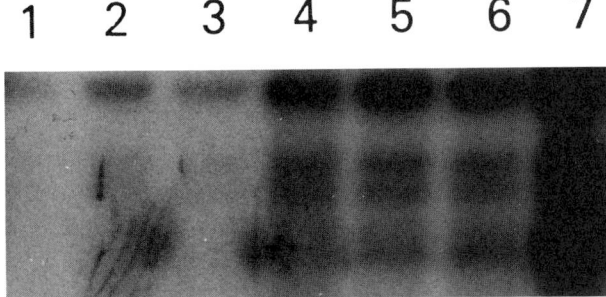

FIGURE 1. (b) Viral RNA in supernatant of infected U937 cells detected with SK 38/39 primers. Lanes 1–7 represent days 1–7.

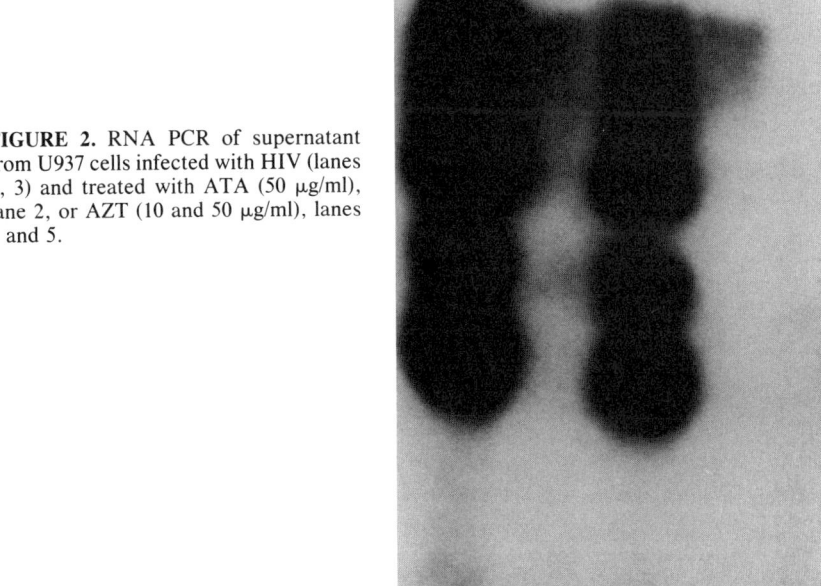

FIGURE 2. RNA PCR of supernatant from U937 cells infected with HIV (lanes 1, 3) and treated with ATA (50 μg/ml), lane 2, or AZT (10 and 50 μg/ml), lanes 4 and 5.

of p24 per 100 × 10⁶, IIIB strain). Culture supernatants were harvested on a daily basis for up to 7 days and monitored for p24 antigen production (Coulter Immunology). For analysis of DNA, supernatants were treated with 0.25 to 0.5% NP40 and heated to 75°C for analysis of DNA. RNA was isolated from 0.4 ml of serum using a guanidinium isothiocyanate extraction method. Viral DNA was detected in the culture supernatant one day post infection. Weak signals due to viral RNA, which increased in intensity with time, were observed at the same time (FIG. 1). Significant levels of viral p24 antigen were detected between 3 and 4 days post infection (data not shown). No viral RNA was detected in supernatants from H9 cells treated with AZT or ATA (FIG. 2) or with a combination of ddC and IFN (data not shown).

The sensitivity of viral DNA and RNA detection was investigated by infecting H9 and U937 cells with different doses of virus. Viral DNA, RNA, and antigen levels were measured at daily intervals. At day 7, an input of 500 pg of viral p24

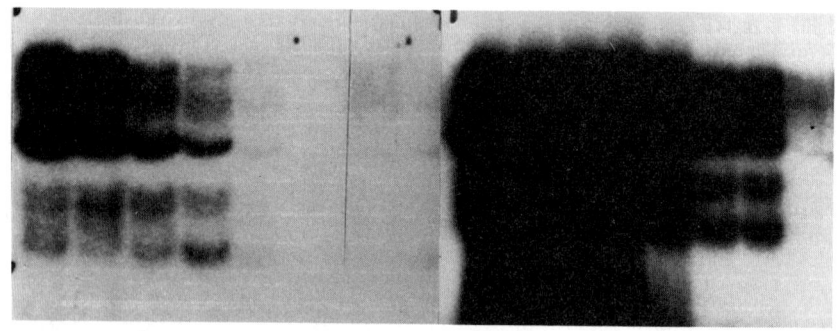

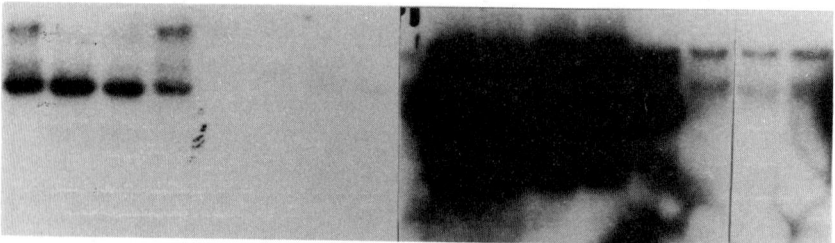

FIGURE 3. (a) Detection of viral DNA in the supernatant of U937 cells infected with varying amounts of virus at 3 (*lanes 1–8*) and 7 (*lanes 9–16*) days post infection. (b) Viral RNA in the same supernatants at day 3 (*lanes 1–8*) and day 7 (*lanes 9–16*).

antigen could be detected by the antigen assay. DNA and RNA PCR allowed the detection of 2.5 ng of p24 antigen at 4 days post infection (FIG. 3). Incubation of cultures for longer periods of time permitted the detection of 25 pg of input viral antigen at day 7 by PCR. Results from spiking experiments showed that 1 to 10 copies of viral DNA (BH10 plasmid) and an equivalent of 5 to 10 fg of viral antigen could be detected by PCR (data not shown) under these extraction and amplification conditions. In conclusion, simple, rapid, and sensitive PCR-based procedures have been developed for the detection of HIV-1 DNA and RNA in culture supernatants of infected cells. Because of their enhanced sensitivity relative to antigen detection, cell-free viral DNA and RNA may be useful markers for monitoring cocultures of PBMCs from patients in studies on disease progression and to analyze the *in vivo* and *in vitro* activity of therapeutic agents by similar methods.

REFERENCES

1. SCHOCHETMAN, G., C. Y. OU & W. K. JONES. 1988. Polymerase chain reaction. J. Infect. Dis. **158:** 1154–1157.
2. CHOMCZYNSKI, P. & N. SACCHI. 1987. Single-step method of RNA isolation by acid guanidinium thiocyanate-phenol-chloroform extraction. Anal. Biochem. **162:** 156–159.
3. MITSUYA, H., K. J. WEINHOLD, P. A. FURMAN, *et al.* 1985. 3'-Azido-3'-deoxythymidine (BW A509U): An antiviral agent that inhibits the infectivity and cytopathic effect of human T-lymphocytotropic virus type III/lymphadenopathy virus *in vitro*. Proc. Natl. Acad. Sci. USA **82:** 7096–7100.

HIV-1 Specific IgG Capture Enzyme Immunoassay to Study the Dynamics of HIV-1 Antibody and to Diagnose HIV-1 Infection in Infants

BHARAT PAREKH,[a,b] N. SHAFFER,[b] G. SCHOCHETMAN,[b]
R. T. COUGHLIN,[c] C.-H. HUNG,[c] J. R. GEORGE,[b] AND
NYC PERINATAL HIV TRANSMISSION COLLABORATIVE
STUDY GROUP

[b] *Centers for Disease Control*
Atlanta, Georgia 30333

[c]*Cambridge Biotech*
Worcester, Massachusetts 01605

Conventional commercial assays are unable to diagnose HIV-1 infection in infants born to seropositive women owing to their inability to distinguish between maternal IgG and the infant's own immune response.[1] Persistence of maternal IgG for up to 18 months of age is common in spite of a reported half-life ($T_{1/2}$) for IgG of only 23 to 26 days.[2] On the basis of this $T_{1/2}$, more than 99% of maternal antibodies would be lost by 6 months of age (7 $T_{1/2}$). We have used an HIV-1 specific IgG capture enzyme immunoassay (IgG-CEIA) to study the dynamics of the synthesis and decay of HIV-1 antibodies in infants. A total of 239 coded serum specimens from 77 infants (seroreverters [$n = 41$], HIV-1 infected [$n = 26$] and infants born to seronegative women [$n = 10$]) were analyzed by IgG-CEIA and by two conventional EIAs. With the IgG-CEIA, IgG in the serum was captured by an anti-human IgG mAb (3C8) reactive with all subclasses. The capture of HIV-1 *specific* IgG was detected by a recombinant HIV-1 envelope protein (CBre3)-peroxidase conjugate. The conventional EIAs, a viral lysate-based EIA (Organon Teknika Corp., OTC-EIA) and CBre3-EIA, were performed as described by the manufacturers' instructions.

The results with IgG-CEIA (FIG. 1A) showed a rapid, exponential decay of maternal antibodies in seroreverting infants after 2 months, reaching background

---

[a] Address for correspondence: Bharat S. Parekh, Ph.D., Division of HIV/AIDS, Mailstop D12, CDC/NCID, 1600 Clifton Road, Atlanta, GA 30333.

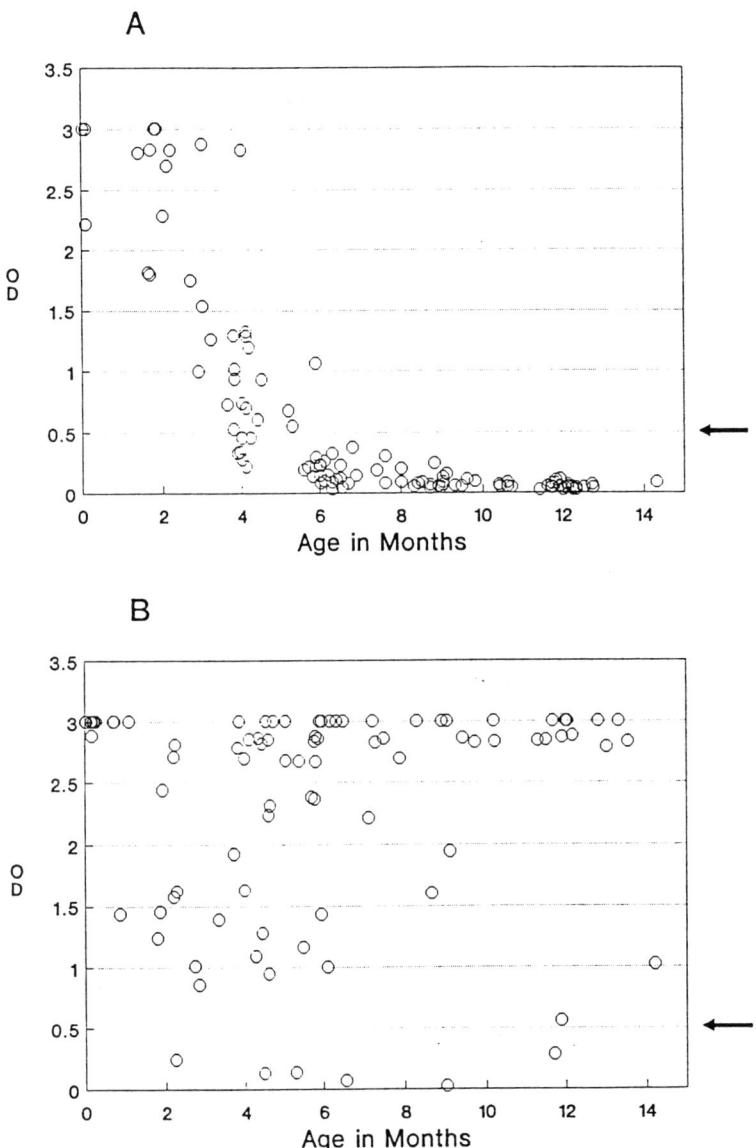

FIGURE 1. Results of IgG-CEIA. Optical density (OD) value for each specimen is plotted versus age of the infant when the specimen was collected. *Panel A* = uninfected, seroreverting infants; *panel B* = HIV-1 infected infants. Specimens up to 15 months of age are shown. Arrows indicate cut-off value.

levels by 6 months ($T_{1/2}$ = 28 to 30 days). Thus, all 69 sera collected from 39 seroreverting infants between the ages of 6 and 15 months were negative. In infected infants, however, (panel B) 39 of 43 (90.7%), sera collected after 6 months or 20 of 22 (90.9%) infants were positive. The two infants that were negative by IgG-CEIA were also negative by OTC-EIA and CBr3-EIA. The observed differences between the two groups of infants after 6 months of age by IgG-CEIA provides a simple method of diagnosing HIV-1 infection in infants that has a sensitivity >90% and specificity of 100%. In contrast, OTC-EIA and CBre3-EIA showed a slower decline of maternal antibodies in seroreverting infants (data not shown) with 49/69 (71%) and 30/69 (43.5%) of sera between 6 and 15 months being positive, respectively.

To determine trends in antibody syntheseis and decay, mean IgG-CEIA values were calculated for each group of sera collected at a given month of age and plotted against mean age (FIG. 2). In seroreverting infants, there was a rapid decline of HIV-1 antibodies, reaching background levels by 6 months. HIV-1 infected infants showed a similar decline for a period of two months, but thereafter there was an upward trend. By subtracting the mean EIA values of uninfected infants from those of infected infants in corresponding age groups, a curve was generated to represent mean antibody synthesis in HIV-1 infected infants. The results suggest that significant HIV-1 antibody synthesis begins between 3 and 4

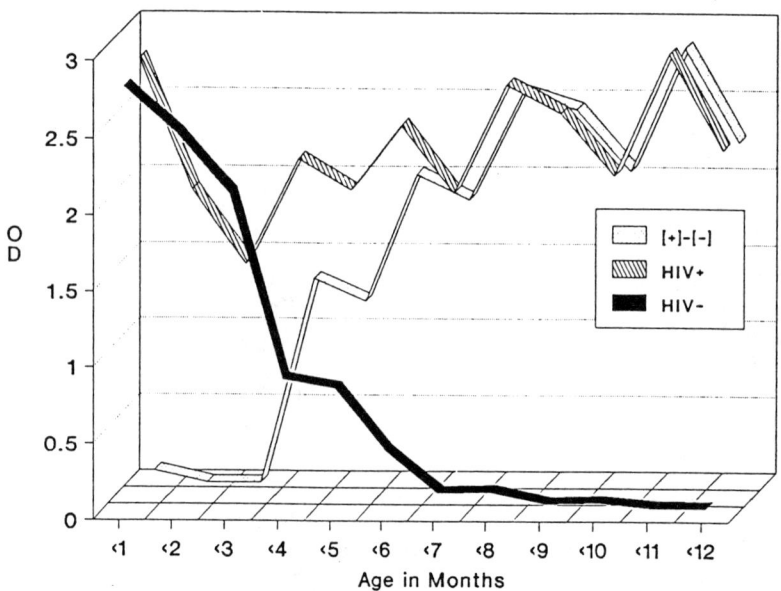

FIGURE 2. Dynamics of HIV-1 specific IgG antibodies in infants born to seropositive mothers. For each group, mean IgG-CEIA OD values for specimens collected in a given month are plotted. *Closed line,* uninfected infants; *shaded line,* HIV-1 infected infants; *open line,* mean model of seroconversion in infected infants (OD values of seroreverting infants subtracted from those of HIV-1 infected infants in corresponding age group).

months after birth. Thus, IgG-CEIA has provided valuable information about the rate of decay of maternal antibody and *de novo* synthesis of antibodies by the infant. IgG-CEIA also permits serologic diagnosis of HIV-1 infection after 6 months of age.

REFERENCES

1. ROGERS, M. F. et al. 1991. The challenge of HIV infection in infants, children and adolescents. *In* Pediatric AIDS. P. A. Pizzo & C. M. Wilfert, Eds.: 159–174. Williams & Wilkins. Baltimore, MD.
2. COLE, F. S. 1991. *In* Shaffer and Avery's Diseases of the Newborn. H. W. Taeusch, R. W. Ballard & M. E. Avery, Eds.: 305. W. B. Saunders. St. Louis, MO.

Detection of HIV-1 IgA by an IgA Capture Enzyme Immunoassay for Early Diagnosis in Infants

J. RICHARD GEORGE,[a,b] B. S. PAREKH,[b] N. SHAFFER,[b]
R. T. COUGHLIN,[c] C.-H. HUNG,[c] M. ROGERS,[b]
G. SCHOCHETMAN,[b] AND NYC PERINATAL HIV
TRANSMISSION COLLABORATIVE STUDY GROUP

[b] *Centers for Disease Control*
Atlanta, Georgia 30333

[c] *Cambridge Biotech*
Worcester, Massachusetts

HIV-1 specific IgA is an important serological marker for early diagnosis of HIV-1 infection in infants.[1] The assay procedure as described requires removal of competing HIV-1 IgG by adsorption with protein G, followed by a mini-Western blot.[1–3] As an alternative to this expensive and laborious procedure, we have evaluated an IgA capture enzyme immunoassay (IgA-CEIA) to detect HIV-1 IgA. The results were compared to IgA–Western blot (IgA-WB). A total of 232 coded serum specimens from 70 infants (23 HIV-1 infected, 37 seroreverters, and 10 infants born to seronegative mothers) were tested by both methods. In IgA-CEIA, IgA in the specimen was captured by a mAb 2E12. HIV-1 *specific* IgA was detected by a recombinant envelope protein (CBre3)-peroxidase conjugate. IgA-WB was performed as reported earlier[1] after three successive adsorptions with protein G sepharose beads to remove all IgG.

Of the specimens obtained from HIV-1 infected infants, IgA-CEIA was positive in 58 of 96 (60.4%) specimens, and IgA-WB was positive in 60 of 96 (62.5%) specimens. There was good agreement between the two methods, with 50 specimens testing positive and 28 specimens testing negative [78/96 (81.3%)] by both methods. Agewise analysis of the results (FIG. 1) indicated that below 2 months of age IgA-CEIA was less sensitive than IgA-WB (17.6% versus 41.2%). After two months of age, however, IgA-CEIA was better than or equivalent to IgA-WB, with sensitivity increasing from 65% to 83%. Two of 23 (8.7%) infected

---

[a] Address for correspondence: J. Richard George, Ph.D., Division of HIV/AIDS, Mailstop D12, CDC/NCID, 1600 Clifton Road, Atlanta, GA 30333.

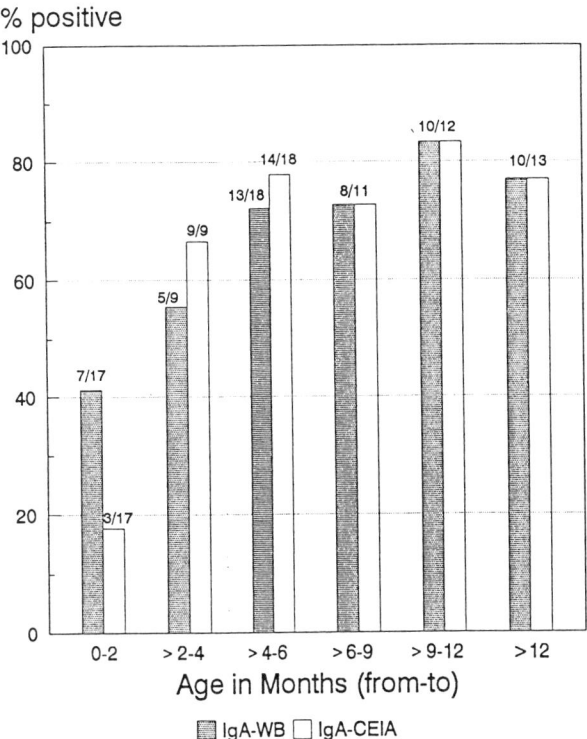

FIGURE 1. Comparative performance of IgA–Western blot and IgA-CEIA in detecting HIV-infected infants in different age groups. Number of infants positive per total number tested in each age group are shown above each bar.

infants, with early immunodeficiency, clinical AIDS, and death before 18 months of age, were IgA negative at all time-points tested by both assays.

To obtain quantitative information on IgA synthesis and relative levels of HIV-1 IgA in infants, optical density (OD) values of IgA-CEIA were plotted versus age of the infant when the specimen was collected (FIG. 2). Panel A represents results of uninfected, seroreverting population and indicates that none of them had detectable HIV-1 IgA. Results of HIV-1 infected infants (panel B) suggest that although some infants do have detectable HIV-1 IgA before two months of age, significant IgA synthesis in response to HIV-1 infection appears to begin after 2 months of age. These results suggest that most infants mount their humoral immune response after 2 to 3 months in response to the antigenic stimulation resulting from the viremia that has been reported to occur in the first few weeks of life.[4]

Thus, IgA-CEIA is a simple, inexpensive, and rapid assay for early diagnosis of HIV infection in infants. Sensitivity of the assay was age dependent, reaching

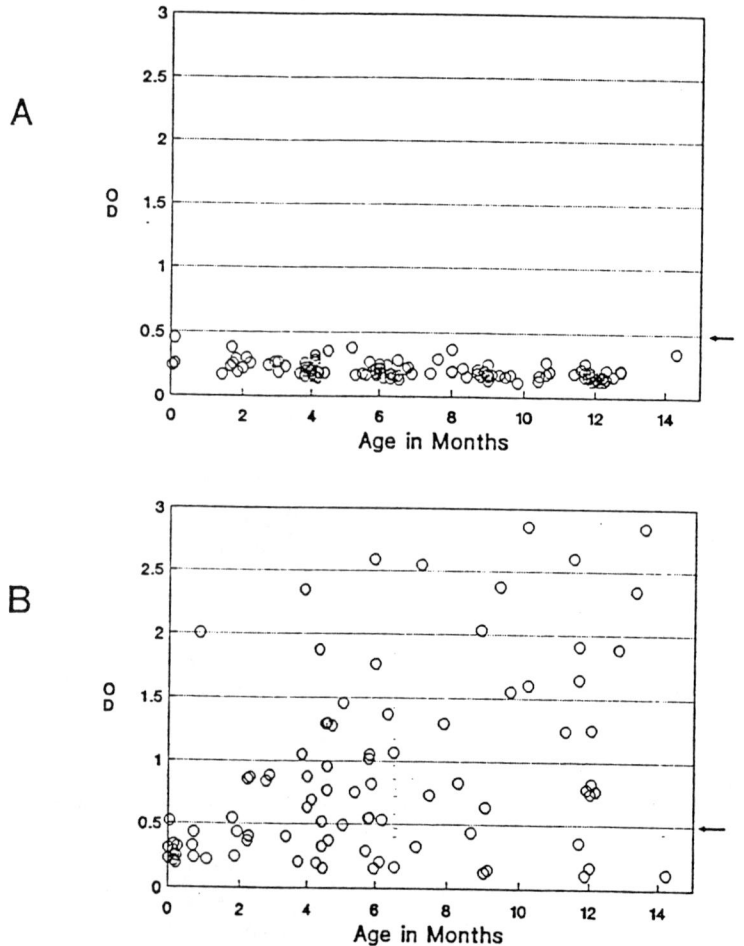

FIGURE 2. IgA-CEIA results for seroconverters **(panel A)** and HIV-infected **(panel B)** infants with respect to age. Specimen information up to 15 months of age is shown. Arrows indicate cut-off value of 0.5 OD.

a maximum of about 83% with a specificity of 100%. In addition, it provided quantitative information about IgA synthesis in response to HIV-1 infection.

REFERENCES

1. WEIBLEN, B., et al. 1990. Lancet **i:** 988–990.
2. LANDESMAN, S., et al. 1991. JAMA **266:** 3443–3446.
3. QUINN, T. C., et al. 1991. JAMA **266:** 3439–3442.
4. KRIVINE, A., et al. 1992. Lancet **339:** 1187–1189.

Indeterminate Western Blot in Children Who Serorevert for HIV

D. CASELLI,[a] A. MACCABRUNI,[b] A. DEICAS,[b] G. BOSSI,[a]
M. DEGIOANNI,[b] G. ACHILLI,[b] AND M. ARICÒ[a]

[a] *Department of Pediatrics*
and
[b] *Department of Infectious Diseases*
IRCCS Policlinico San Matteo
University of Pavia
27100 Pavia, Italy

The current laboratory confirmatory test for the diagnosis of HIV infection, Western blot (WB), detects antibodies to specific denatured HIV-1 proteins. Reactivity to viral proteins, however, is well documented in samples of uninfected adults,[1] and when the test's results do not meet CDC criteria for WB positivity, they are labeled indeterminate.[2] Indeterminate WB tests are reported in 10 to 20% of low-risk adults[3] and are considered secondary to one of the following: (a) antibody production against viral antigens in early HIV infection[4]; b) loss of antibodies in late HIV infection[5]; c) cross-reactivity to HIV2[6]; or (d) cross-reactivity due to autoantibodies or alloimmunization.[7] Similar indeterminate WB results have also been reported in vertically infected children[8] and correlated with impaired humoral response to HIV. It is unclear if lack of specific antibody bands depends on fast clearance, on poor production, or both. On the contrary, such reports are not available in children born to HIV-infected mothers who lose maternal antibodies. This report will focus on two children with indeterminate WB results persisting after 24 months of age despite no other evidence of HIV infection.

PATIENTS AND RESULTS

Forty-two children born to HIV-infected mothers were tested for the presence of anti-HIV serum antibodies by ELISA and WB every three months. The median age at clearance of maternal antibodies (i.e., ELISA and WB completely negative) was 14.9 months, ranging between 6.3 and 40 months. Five of the 42 children showed a late clearance (beyond 24 months), and two more children showed persistent WB reactivity for anti-p24 antibodies at 38 and 40 months of age, respectively, although all other tests for HIV infection (including PCR and virus culture) were persistently negative and the children were clinically and immunologically normal. In the follow-up, one of these two children lost his p24 WB reactivity at 40 months of age, while the other is persistently anti-p24 positive at 48 months of age, but asymptomatic.

COMMENTS

Persistence of an indeterminate WB seroreactivity in children who seroreverted after having been exposed to perinatal HIV infection may occur. This could be due to cross-reactivity or to the persistence of some HIV-associated antigen. Its meaning and prognostic value, if any, is still far from being clarified.

REFERENCES

1. GENESCA, J., B. W. JETT, J. S. EPSTEIN, J. W.-K. SHIH, I. K. HEWELETT & H. J. ALTER. 1989. What do Western blot–indeterminate patterns for human immunodeficiency virus mean in EIA-negative blood donors? Lancet ii: 1023–1025.
2. CENTERS FOR DISEASE CONTROL. 1989. Interpretation and use of the Western blot for serodiagnosis of human immunodeficiency virus type 1 infection. Morbid. Mortal. Wkly. Rpt. **38(S-7):** 1–7.
3. McDONALD, K. L., J. B. JACKSON & R. J. BROWMAN. 1989. Performance characteristics of serologic tests of human immunodeficiency virus type-1 antibody among Minnesota blood donors. Ann. Intern. Med. **110:** 617–621.
4. RANKI, A., M. KROHN, J. P. ALLAIN, G. FRANCHINI, S. L. VALLE & J. ANTONEN. 1987. Long latency precedes overt seroconversion in sexually transmitted human-immunodeficiency virus infection. Lancet **1:** 1249–1253.
5. FARZADEGAN, H., M. A. POLIS & S. M. WOLINSKY. 1988. Loss of human immunodeficiency virus antibodies with evidence of virus infection in asymptomatic homosexual men. Ann. Intern. Med. **108:** 785–790.
6. CENTERS FOR DISEASE CONTROL. 1989. Update: HIV-2 infection—United States. Morbid. Mortal. Wkly. Rpt. **33:** 572–580.
7. DOCK, N. L., S. H. KLEINMAN, M. A. RAIFIELD, et al. 1991. Human immunodeficiency virus infection and indeterminate Western blot patterns. Arch. Intern. Med. **151:** 525–530.
8. WALTER, E. B., R. E. MCKINNEY, B. A. LANE, K. J. WEINHOLD & C. M. WILFRED. 1990. Interpretation of Western blots specimens from children infected with human immunodeficiency virus type 1: Implications for prognosis and diagnosis. J. Pediatr. **117:** 255–258.

Analysis of the HIV-1 Envelope V3-Loop Sequences from Ten Mother–Child Pairs

GABRIELLA SCARLATTI,[a,b] THOMAS LEITNER,[c]
EVA HALAPI,[d] JOHAN WAHLBERG,[c]
MARIANNE JANSSON,[d] HANS WIGZELL,[d]
EVA MARIA FENYÖ,[b] JAN ALBERT,[e] MATHIAS UHLÉN,[c]
AND PAOLO ROSSI[d]

[b] *Department of Virology*
Karolinska Institute
105 21 Stockholm, Sweden

[c] *Department of Biochemistry and Biotechnology*
Royal Institute of Technology
100 44 Stockholm, Sweden

[d] *Department of Immunology*
Karolinska Institute
104 01 Stockholm, Sweden

[e] *Department of Virology*
National Bacteriological Laboratory
105 21 Stockholm, Sweden

It has been recently recognized that mother-to-child transmission of HIV-1 frequently occurs during delivery.[1] Little is known, however, about the pathway of the virus from the mother to the child. Mothers with low CD4+ lymphocyte counts and p24 antigenemia have been shown to have a higher risk of transmission.[2,3] The identification of specific molecular or antigenic features of the transmitted virus would be essential for a better understanding of the transmission process and thereby give some highlights for prevention trials. Because the V3 region of the viral envelope of HIV-1 has been described to harbor essential functions such as cellular tropism[4] and to be the principal target for neutralizing antibody re-

---

[a] Address for correspondence: Gabriella Scarlatti, Department of Virology, Karolinska Institute, c/o SBL, Lundagatan 2, 105 21 Stockholm, Sweden.

```
               281        291        301        311        321        331        341        351        361        371
               |          |          |          |          |          |          |          |          |          |
       age     EEEVVIRSENFTDNAKTIIVQLNESVEINCTRPNNNTRKSIHIGPGRAFYTTGEIIGDIRQAHCNISRAKWNNTLKQIVTKLREQF.?NKTIVFNQSSGG
      (months)

Child 1  (1)   -------------N-----------T---------------P-----------------------------------D------S------Q---------
                                                                                             V
Child 2  (2)   ----I---K----T-V---------------G-------------------A---------K---------D----------------Y.E----I-K----
Child 3  (3)   -------A-L------I--VH----IV-------S----QG--------F-----T----K-Y-V-T--DT-KK-AI-LG---.K----V---------
                                   x      v              r                            a    i  g     i           a
```

FIGURE 1. Amino acid V3 sequences of three HIV-1 infected children. The alignment sequence of the V3 loop is derived from the North American consensus, and the flanking sequence is taken from HIV-1 MN. Sequence heterogeneity is indicated by assigning two amino acids at the same position; large letters indicate amino acids in approximately equal amounts, while small letters indicate minor variants.

sponse,[5] selective changes in this region may weigh on mother-to-child transmission.

We have sequenced the V3 region from 10 seropositive mothers at delivery and compared those to the sequences obtained from the corresponding child (age: 0 to 4 months). Proviral DNA derived from peripheral blood mononuclear cells (PBMC) directly as well as from cultured PBMC and from viral RNA extracted from the serum was amplified by nested PCR with primers specific for the V3 region of gp120 *env* gene.[6] The PCR product was then used for direct solid-phase DNA sequencing.[7] Briefly, a further amplification step of the PCR product was performed with primers conjugated with biotin, and thereafter immobilized on streptavidin-coated magnetic beads (Dynal M280-Streptavidin, Dynal AS). Single-stranded DNA, obtained by denaturation, was subsequently sequenced from both directions with fluorescent primers. The product was loaded on a 6% polyacrylamide gel in an automated laser fluorescent (A.L.F.) sequencing apparatus (Pharmacia LKB Biotechnology AB, Uppsala, Sweden). Pairwise comparisons were performed to calculated inter- and intrapatient distances.

The amino acid sequence of the V3 region from each of the 10 children was homogeneous (examples in FIG. 1), as sequence variability within the V3 loop was observed only in one child (at 3 months of age). In contrast, the mothers showed varying degrees of heterogeneity. Nevertheless, sequence variability was present in the V3 region outside the cysteine loop in three additional children,

Pair		300 | EI<u>NCT</u>RPNNN	N-glycosylation site*
1-	mother	----I--N-- 　　　t　C	+/-
	child	----A--S--	-
2-	mother	A-N-T----- E h i v	+/-
	child	A--------	+
3-	mother	Q--------	+
	child	Q--------	+

FIGURE 2. Alignment of the amino acid sequences corresponding to the region with the N-linked glycosylation site (position 300) from mother–child pairs. Source of sequences: DNA from uncultured PBMC. Symbols as in figure 1, *N-linked glycosylation site: − absent, + present.

suggestive of a specific selective pressure on this region. Comparison of the children's sequences with those of the corresponding mothers showed that three mothers harbored mixed-virus populations with and without the N-glycosylation site in position 300 (according to HIV-1 MN[8]; FIG. 2). However, the virus variant with the mutation was only transmitted to one child.

In conclusion, infants harbor a homogeneous virus population. In contrast, their mothers have heterogeneous V3 sequences. The results thus indicate that selection of a certain HIV-1 variant occurs either at transmission or during initial replication in the child. No characteristic molecular features of the transmitted virus could be identified.

REFERENCES

1. GOEDERT, J. J., A. M. DULIÈGE, C. I. AMOS, S. FELTON & R. J. BIGGAR (for the International Registry of HIV-Infected Twins). 1991. Lancet **338:** 1471–1475.
2. SCARLATTI, G., V. LOMBARDI, A. PLEBANI, N. PRINCIPI, C. VEGNI, G. FERRARIS, A. BUCCERI, E. M. FENYÖ, H. WIGZELL, P. ROSSI & J. ALBERT. 1991. AIDS **5:** 1173–1178.
3. EUROPEAN COLLABORATIVE STUDY. 1992. Lancet **339:** 1007–1012.
4. SHIODA, T., J. A. LEVY & C. CHENG-MAYER. 1991. Nature **349:** 167–169.
5. PALKER, T. J., M. E. CLARK, A. LANGLOIS, T. J. MATTHEWS, K. J. WEINHOLD, R. R. RANDALL, D. P. BOLOGNESI & B. F. HAYNES. 1988. Proc. Natl. Acad. Sci. USA **85:** 1932–1936.
6. ALBERT, J. & E. M. FENYÖ. 1990. J. Clin. Microbiol. **28:** 1560–1564.
7. WAHLBERG, J., J. ALBERT, J. LUNDEBERG, A. VON GEGERFELT, K. BROLIDEN, G. UTTER, E. M. FENYÖ & M. UHLÉN. 1991. AIDS Res. Hum. Retrovir. **7:** 983–990.
8. MYERS, G., B. KORBER, J. A. BERZOFSKY, R. F. SMITH & G. N. PAVLAKIS. 1991. Human retroviruses and AIDS 1991. Los Alamos National Laboratory. Los Alamos, New Mexico.

The Presence of Cryptococcal Capsular Polysaccharide Increases the Sensitivity of HIV-1 Coculture in Children

MASSIMO PETTOELLO-MANTOVANI,[a] ARTURO CASADEVALL,[b,c] AND HARRIS GOLDSTEIN[a,b,d]

[a] Department of Pediatrics
[b] Department of Microbiology & Immunology
[c] Department of Medicine
Albert Einstein College of Medicine
Bronx, New York 10461

High concentrations of cryptococcal capsular polysaccharide (CCP) accumulate in the body fluids of AIDS patients infected with *Cryptococcus neoformans*.[1] Because HIV-1 infection can be modulated by the presence of polysaccharides such as dextran sulfate,[2] we investigated the effect of CCP on HIV-1 infection. We demonstrated that the presence of CCP significantly increased the production of p24 antigen after infection of H9 cells with HIV-infected H9 cells and after coculture of lymphocytes from an HIV-1-infected patient.[3] These results suggested that CCP has the capacity to enhance HIV-1 infection of cells and thereby accelerate the progression of AIDS in patients after cryptococcal infection. We postulated that the sensitivity of coculture for the isolation of HIV-1 from peripheral blood mononuclear cells (PBMC) could be increased by the addition of CCP.

MATERIALS AND METHODS

Cryptococcus neoformans serotype A (—ATCC 24064), the most common North American isolate, was grown in Sabouraud's broth; and the capsular polysaccharide was isolated, purified, and deproteinized from cultures as previously described.[4] Mononuclear cells were isolated from the blood of HIV-1-infected persons,[5] and the titer of HIV-1-infected peripheral PBMC, with or without added CCP (2 µg/ml), was determined as previously described.[6,7] After 14 days, an aliquot of the culture supernatant was assessed for the presence of p24 antigen using an antigen capture assay (Dupont-NEN, Wilmington, DE). The lowest number of

---

[d] Address for correspondence: Dr. Harris Goldstein, Albert Einstein College of Medicine, Forchheimer Building, Room 403, 1300 Morris Park Avenue, Bronx, NY 10461.

added PBMC that infected at least half of the quadruplicate cultures with HIV-1 was taken as the end point or tissue culture infective dose ($TCID_{50}$). Serum levels of p24 antigen were determined by an antigen capture assay as recommended by the manufacturer (Dupont-NEN).

RESULTS

To determine if the presence of CCP could enhance the sensitivity of coculture, fivefold dilutions of PBMC (1×10^6 to 1.6×10^2) from nine HIV-1-infected children ranging in age from 6 months to 10 years were cocultured with PHA-activated donor lymphocytes in the presence or absence of CCP. The presence of CCP significantly increased the sensitivity of coculture in all nine patients. In one child, HIV-1 was isolated from PBMC only when the coculture was performed in the presence of CCP, and in the other eight children HIV-1 was isolated from 5- to 10-fold fewer PBMC when the coculture was performed in the presence of CCP. Thus, the sensitivity of coculture for the detection of HIV-1 was increased when CCP was present during culture.

Because the measurement of serum levels of p24 antigen is frequently used as a marker of disease activity, we investigated whether the reciprocal titer of HIV-1-infected PBMC was related to the serum p24 antigen concentration. As shown in FIGURE 1, there was no correlation between the serum levels of p24 antigen and the number of HIV-1-infected PBMC. This may either be due to an artifact related to the inability of the assay used to measure p24 antigen complexed with antibody or may reflect the disparity between the levels of HIV-1 detected in peripheral blood and in lymphoid organs.[8]

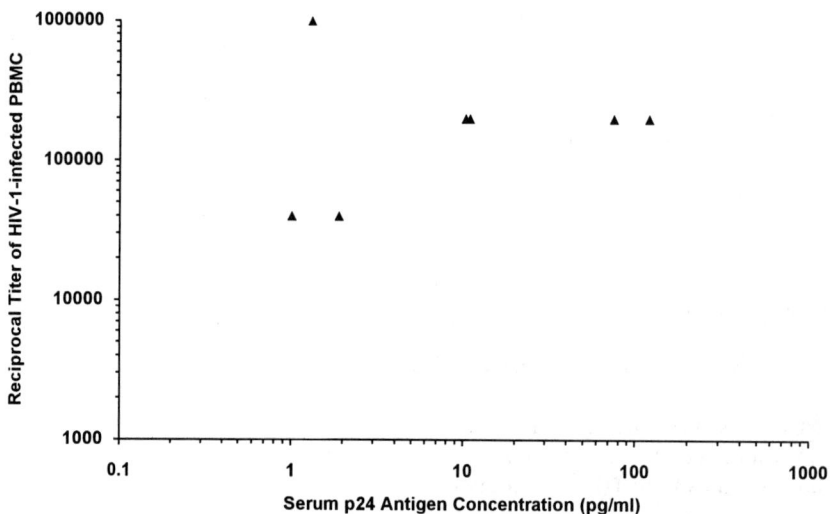

FIGURE 1. The serum concentration of p24 in HIV-1-infected children ($n = 7$) was determined and correlated with the reciprocal titer of HIV-1-infected PBMC.

DISCUSSION

The presence of CCP permitted the HIV-1 to be cocultured from significantly fewer PBMCs. Therefore, the addition of CCP to cocultures should increase their sensitivity for the detection of HIV-1. This may lead to earlier diagnosis of HIV-1 infection in children of HIV-1-infected mothers for whom residual maternal IgG makes serological tests nondiagnostic.

REFERENCES

1. MILLS, J. & H. MASUR. 1990. AIDS-related infections. Sci. Am. **263:** 50–57.
2. UENO, R. & S. KUNO. 1987. Dextran sulfate, a potent anti-HIV agent *in vitro* having synergism with zidovudine. Lancet **1:** 1379.
3. PETTOELLO-MANTOVANI, M., A. CASADEVALL, T. R. KOLLMANN, A. RUBINSTEIN & H. GOLDSTEIN. 1992. Enhancement of HIV-1 infection by the capsular polysaccharide of *Cryptococcus neoformans*. Lancet **339:** 21–23.
4. KOZEL, T. R. & R. CAZIN. 1971. Nonencapsulated variant of *Cryptococcus neoformans*. Infect. Immun. **3:** 287–295.
5. BOYUM, A. 1968. Isolation of mononuclear cells and granulocytes from human blood. Scand. J. Lab. Invest. **5:** 77–80.
6. HO, D. D., T. MOUDGIL & M. ALUM. 1989. Quantitation of human immunodeficiency virus type 1 in the blood of infected persons. N. Engl. J. Med. **321:** 1621–1625.
7. DIMITROV, D. H., J. L. MELNICK & F. B. HOLINGER. 1990. Microculture assay for isolation of human immunodeficiency virus type 1 and for titration of infected peripheral blood cells. J. Clin. Microbiol. **28:** 734–737.
8. PANTALEO, G., C. GRAZIOSI, J. F. DEMAREST, L. BUTINI, M. MONTRONI, C. H. FOX, J. M. ORENSTEIN, D.P. KOTLER & A. S. FAUCI. 1993. HIV infection is active and progressive in lymphoid tissue during the clinically latent stage of disease. Nature **362:** 355–358.

HCV Vertical Transmission in Infants Born to HIV-HCV Seropositive Mothers

A. MACCABRUNI,[a] D. CASELLI,[b] AND M. DEGIOANNI[a]

[a] *Institute of Infectious Diseases*
and
[b] *Pediatrics Department*
IRCCS Policlinico S. Matteo
University of Pavia
Pavia, Italy

We carried out an HCV serological study in HIV-seropositive mother–child pairs in order to evaluate the seroprevalence of HCV antibodies in HIV-seropositive mothers and the frequency of HCV vertical transmission from these women to their infants.

MATERIALS AND METHODS

We selected 42 HIV-infected mothers, who had been followed by us during pregnancy; afterwards, we detected in this group 28 HCV-seropositive women using the second-generation ELISA test.

RESULTS

Serological follow-up of the children born to these women showed two HCV-seropositive cases from birth until this report and two other cases who became HCV seronegative at 10 and 11 months and then became seropositive after another 4 and 6 months, respectively. All the other cases showed either HCV-seronegative results from birth or by an average age of 9.7 months.

The four HCV-seropositive children did not become HIV infected; their mothers were HIV-infected, but asymptomatic, with Ag p24 negative and $CD4^+$ lymphocytes counts $>400/mm^3$. They were or had been intravenous drug users.

CONCLUSION

Our preliminary data show agreement with the authors who assert that maternal coinfection with HIV-HCV does not appear to be an absolute requirement for vertical transmission of HCV.

This mode of transmission plays an important role in the spreading of HCV infection, particularly with reference to women at high risk for parenterally or sexually transmitted diseases such as mothers with a history of intravenous drug use. Vertical transmission of HCV from HIV-HCV coinfected mothers is possible even if maternal immunological parameters are satisfactory.

REFERENCES

1. GIOVANNINI, M., A. TAGGER, M. L. RIBERO, et al. 1990. Maternal–infant transmission of hepatitis C virus and HIV infections: A possible interaction. Lancet **335**: 1166.
2. THALER, M. M., C. K. PARK, D. V. LANDERS, et al. 1991. Vertical transmission of hepatitis C virus. Lancet **338**: 17–18.
3. PEREZ ALVAREZ, L., M. D. GURBINDO, T. HERNANDEZ-SAMPELAYO, et al. 1992. Mother-to-infant transmission of HIV and hepatitis C infections in children born to HIV-seropositive mothers. AIDS **6**: 427–428.

Preliminary Data on *Chlamydia pneumoniae* Seroprevalence in HIV-1 Infected Children

A. PLEBANI,[a] M. CLERICI SCHOELLER,[a] F. BLASI,[b] AND R. COSENTINI[b]

*[a] I Pediatric Clinic
and
[b] Institute of Respiratory Diseases
University of Milan
Milan, Italy*

HIV-1 infected patients are known to develop respiratory tract infections frequently. *Chlamydia pneumoniae* (CP) is a newly described species of the *Chlamydia* genus[1] and is drawing increasing attention toward the pathogenesis of respiratory tract infections in adult HIV-1 patients.[2,3] Nevertheless, to date, there are no data regarding the HIV-1 pediatric population.

In order to evaluate the CP seroprevalence in HIV-1 infected children, we studied three groups of patients:

1. 46 children with vertically transmitted HIV-1 infection (mean age 49.5 ± 29.4 months; median 51 months; range 5–111 months; 26 females and 20 males);
2. 37 seroreverted children born to HIV-1 positive mothers (mean age 28.5 ± 18.6 months; median 24 months; range 6–72 months; 18 females and 19 males); and
3. 42 healthy controls (mean age 54.8 ± 27 months; median 57 months; range 4–120 months; 23 females and 19 males).

The HIV-1 test (ELISA and WB) and the microimmunofluorescence test for IgG and IgM antibodies specific to CP antigen (Washington Research Foundation, Seattle) were performed on serum samples. For children under 15 months of age, HIV-1 infection was demonstrated by viral culture and polymerase chain reaction (at least two positive determinations). We used the CDC classification system for HIV-1 infection in the pediatric age group[4]; all 46 HIV-1 infected children were clinically symptomatic (P2).

CP-specific antibodies were found in 11 out of 46 (24%) children in group 1, 9 out of 37 (24%) children in group 2, and 3 out of 42 (7%) children in group 3 (see FIG. 1).

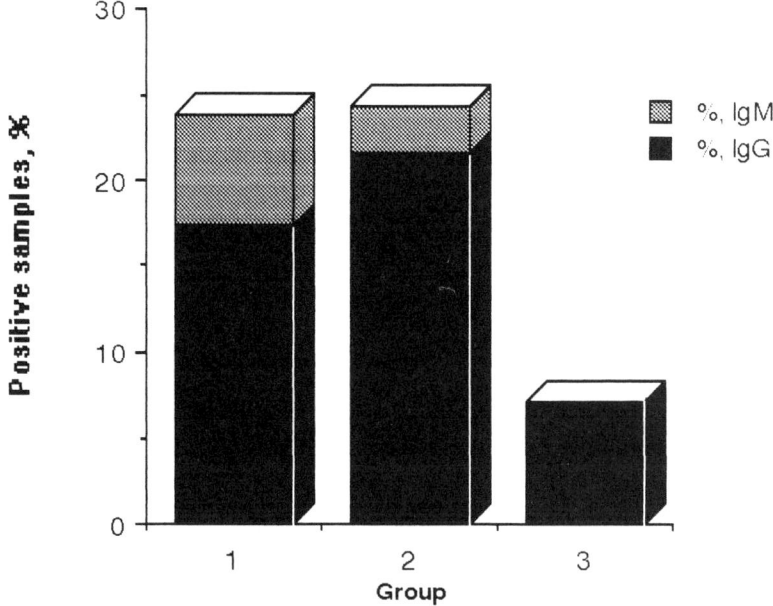

FIGURE 1. *Chlamydia pneumoniae* seroprevalence.

CP seroprevalence in children in groups 1 and 2 is higher, even though not significantly, compared to group 3. The similar results observed in the first two groups may be correlated to the shared family context (i.e., HIV-infected parents), thus increasing the risk of infections, including CP.[5] These data demonstrate that further studies on the pathogenetic role of CP in HIV-1 infected children are warranted.

REFERENCES

1. GRAYSTON, J. T., C. C. KUO, S.-P. WANG & J. ALTMAN. 1986. A new *Chlamydia psittaci* strain, TWAR, isolated in acute respiratory tract infections. N. Engl. J. Med. **315**: 161–168.
2. AUGENBRAUN, M. H., P. M. ROBLIN, K. CHIRGWIN, D. LANDMAN & M. R. HAMMERSCHLAG. 1991. Isolation of *Chlamydia pneumoniae* from the lungs of patients with HIV. J. Clin. Microbiol. **29**: 401–402.
3. CLARK, R., D. MUSHATT & B. FAZAL. 1991. Case report: *Chlamydia pneumoniae* in an HIV-infected man. Am. J. Med. Sci. **302**: 155–156.
4. CENTERS FOR DISEASE CONTROL. 1987. Classification system for human immunodeficiency virus (HIV) infection in children under 13 years of age. Morbid. Mortal. Wkly. Rpt. **36**: 225–36.
5. COSENTINI, R., F. BLASI, D. LEGNANI & A. LUPO. 1992. *Chlamydia pneumoniae* infection in HIV-1 positive intravenous drug abusers. VIII International Conference on AIDS; Amsterdam, the Netherlands, July 1992, Abstract Book, **38**: 19–24.

Mycobacterium avium Complex in HIV-Infected Children

DEBORAH GLEASON-MORGAN,[a,b] JOSEPH A. CHURCH,[a,b,d]
AND LAWRENCE A. ROSS[c,d]

[a] *Division of Allergy–Clinical Immunology*
[b] *Childrens AIDS Center*
[c] *Division of Infectious Diseases and Virology*
Childrens Hospital Los Angeles
Los Angeles, California 90027

[d] *Department of Pediatrics*
University of Southern California School of Medicine
Los Angeles, California 90033

As children with HIV infection survive longer, the risk of acquiring multiple opportunistic infections (OI) increases. *Mycobacterium avium* complex (MAC) is an OI that affects both adults and children with HIV infection and very low CD4$^+$ T-cell numbers.[1,2] Very little published data exists that describes MAC in children.[3] The purpose of this study was to describe the clinical and laboratory features of MAC in transfusion-acquired, HIV-infected children. The medical records of 34 children 5 years of age or greater with transfusion-acquired HIV infection were reviewed. In MAC-infected children ($n = 12$), the following were identified: age at MAC diagnosis, site of MAC, time from HIV-infecting transfusion to MAC diagnosis, and CD4$^+$ T-cell counts at the time of MAC diagnosis. The following features of MAC$^+$ and MAC$^-$ ($n = 22$) children were compared: age at last clinical evaluation, time from HIV-infecting transfusion to diagnosis of HIV infection, time from transfusion to last clinical evaluation, time from transfusion to death, CD4$^+$ T-cell counts at 5 years post HIV-infecting transfusion or at last clinical evaluation, bandemia, and hemoglobin and AST levels at last clinical evaluation. Presence of the following clinical symptoms were also examined: diarrhea (any mention in the 30 days before MAC diagnosis or at the last clinical evaluation), fever (any mention 38°C or greater in the 30 days before MAC diagnosis or at last clinical evaluation), abdominal pain or sweats (any mention in the 30 days before MAC diagnosis or last clinical evaluation).

Twelve children with MAC (7 males, mean age 8 years) and 22 children without MAC (12 males, mean age 9 years) were identified. Of the total, 15 children were Caucasian, 6 were African American, 12 were Latino, and 1 was Asian. MAC

TABLE 1. $CD4^+$ T Cells in MAC^+ versus MAC^- Children

	MAC^+ Mean ± SEM (Range)	MAC^- Mean ± SEM (Range)	p Value 2-Sample t-Test
$CD4^+$ T-cell percentage at 5 years post transfusion or last clinical evaluation	9 ± 2 (1–21)	20 ± 3 (1–45)	0.010
$CD4^+$ T-cell No. at 5 years post transfusion or last clinical evaluation	117 ± 39 (4–425)	451 ± 93 (5–1506)	0.015
$CD4^+$ T-cell percentage at MAC diagnosis or last clinical evaluation (MAC^-)	3 ± 1 (0–10)	14 ± 3 (1–64)	0.013
$CD4^+$ T-cell No. at MAC diagnosis or last clinical evaluation (MAC^-)	16 ± 6 (0–63)	214 ± 47 (4–674)	0.004

was cultured in the blood in nine cases and in the stool in three cases. The number of years from HIV-infecting transfusion to MAC diagnosis was 7 years. Mean $CD4^+$ T-cell count at the time of MAC diagnosis was $16/mm^3$. On comparison of the two groups, no statistical significance was found with regard to age at last evaluation, number of months from HIV-infecting transfusion to diagnosis of HIV infection, or months to last clinical evaluation or death. Significant differences were found in $CD4^+$ T-cell numbers (TABLE 1) as well as in three of four clinical features reviewed (TABLE 2). No significance was noted when comparing the laboratory values of bandemia, hemoglobin, or AST. In conclusion, MAC was found to be a frequent complication of long-term survival in HIV-infected children and occurred 3 to 11 years after HIV infection. It developed in children with profoundly decreased numbers of CD4 T cells. At comparable times from HIV infection, children who developed MAC had lower CD4 counts than children who remained MAC^-. Diarrhea, fever, and abdominal pain were more prevalent in children who developed MAC than in those who remained MAC^-. Sweats were uncommon in both groups. Circulating bandemia and elevated liver enzymes were more prevalent in children with MAC, and anemia was common in long-term survivors regardless of MAC status.

TABLE 2. Clinical Features of MAC^+ versus MAC^- Children

Clinical Feature	MAC^+ ($n = 12$)	MAC^- ($n = 22$)	Relative Risk (95% C.I.)[a]	p Value[b]
Diarrhea	11 (95%)	11 (50%)	1.8 (1.12, 3.01)	0.024
Fever	12 (100%)	7 (32%)	3.1 (1.73, 5.70)	<0.001
Abdominal pain	8 (67%)	5 (23%)	2.9 (1.25, 6.86)	0.025
Sweats	2 (17%)	0 (0%)	8.8 (0.46, 170.6)[c]	0.118

[a] Mantel Haenszel relative risk. C.I., confidence interval.
[b] Fisher's exact test.
[c] Logit estimate of relative risk.

REFERENCES

1. JACOBSON, M.A., P. C. HOPEWELL, D. M. YAJKO, *et al.* 1991. Natural history of disseminated *Mycobacterium avium* complex infection in AIDS. J. Infect. Dis. **164:** 994–998.
2. HAVLIK, J. A., C. R. HORSBURGH, B. METCHOCK, *et al.* 1992. Disseminated *Mycobacterium avium* complex infection: Clinical identification and epidemiologic trends. J. Infect. Dis. **165:** 577–580.
3. HOYT, L., J. OLESKE, B. HOLLAND, *et al.* 1992. Nontuberculous mycobacteria in children with acquired immunodeficiency syndrome. Pediatr. Infect. Dis. J. **11:** 354–360.

Peripheral B-Cell Activation and Immaturity in HIV-Infected Children[a]

C. RODRIGUEZ, E. RICHARD STIEHM, AND S. PLAEGER-MARSHALL

Department of Pediatrics
UCLA School of Medicine
Los Angeles, California 90024

HIV-infected children can manifest signs of B-cell activation such as polyclonal hypergammaglobulinemia from early in the course of disease. They may also develop autoimmune disease and unusual B-cell-related complications, for example, lymphocytic interstitial pneumonia and B-cell lymphomas. The purpose of our study is to compare the state of peripheral B lymphocyte activation of HIV$^+$ children in different stages of disease with that of healthy subjects and to characterize B-cell phenotypes that could serve as surrogate markers of infection (P0 infants), disease stage, progression, prognosis, or in the assessment of treatment response.

SUBJECTS AND METHOD

HIV-infected children included 10 P0 infants, median age 9 months (range: 2 days to 17 months), 6 P1 children, median age 3 years, 9 months (range: 3 months to 12 years), and 16 P2 children, median age 4 years, 4 months (range: 3 months–12 years). The controls were 13 healthy children, median age 3 years (range: 2 days–13 years). Also, age-adjusted reference ranges for serum immunoglobulin levels were used. Immunophenotyping of lymphocytes from whole blood was performed by two-color, laser-flow cytometry (FACScan, Becton-Dickinson) with the following panel of fluorescence-labeled (FITC or PE) monoclonal antibodies (Becton-Dickinson): (1) Lineage markers: CD19 and CD20 (pan B cell), CD5 (B-cell subset, producing auto-antibodies), L-selectin (resting B cells, lymph node homing receptor, Leu8), CD21 (EBV, CR2 receptor). (2) Activation markers: CD25 (IL-2 receptor), CD71 (transferrin receptor), CD23 (low-affinity IgE receptor). (3) Cell size was measured by forward-scatter mean channel number ratio (Fsc MCN subject/Fsc MCN day control). Quantification of immunoglobulins (IgG, IgA, IgM) was performed by nephelometry. Statistical analysis was by nonparametric Mann-Whitney U-rank sum test.

[a] This work was supported by a grant from the Fogarty International AIDS Training Program.

TABLE 1. Phenotype Changes in Peripheral B Lymphocytes of HIV-Infected Children versus Controls

Study Group	CD19 ABS.# (P90–P10)^a	Cell Size Fsc MCN RT	CD19/CD23 %(P90–P10)	CD19/L-Selectin %(P90–P10)
CT (13)	1158^b (2108–739)	0.925 (1–0.81)	81.5 (90–72)	91 (96–80)
P0 (7)	1419 (2788–437)	1.02 (1.19–0.97)*	77 (90–69)	92 (98–77)
P1 (6)	605 (1985–333)	0.95 (1.09–0.89)	73 (82–59)†	86 (92–67)
P2 (16)	487 (976–230)‡	1.11 (1.3–1.03)**	59 (80–40)§	71 (82–50)**

^{a} Percentile 90 and 10.
^{b} Median value.
STATISTICAL SIGNIFICANCE: * $p < 0.004$; † $p < 0.007$; ‡ $p < 0.0005$; § $p < 0.0004$; ** $p < 0.0001$.

SUMMARY OF RESULTS

Hypergammaglobulinemia, manifested by increased levels of IgG, IgA, and IgM, was evident in both P1 and P2 subjects, and to a lesser degree in P0 subjects. There was a decrease in the absolute B cell number in the patient groups, significant in P2, with respect to the control and P0 groups and a significant increase in cell size in the P2 and P0 group. Phenotypic differences observed between the HIV-infected subjects and the control group were a significant decrease of the median value of CD19/Leu8(+) in P2 subjects, and CD19/CD23(+) in P2 and P1, but no differences in the other phenotypes, including the "classical" activation markers CD71 and CD25 (TABLE 1, FIG. 1). The differences in B-cell number, size, and proportion of CD23 and L-Selectin persist between a group of 8 P2 patients and 8 age-matched controls.

CONCLUSIONS

These preliminary observations suggest that B-cell activation manifested as hypergammaglobulinemia in HIV-infected children may not be directly expressed by an increase in peripheral B-cell activation markers, at least in early stages of disease, but only indirectly by a decrease of L-Selectin (+) resting B cells as seen in the symptomatic stage (P2). Additionally, peripheral B cells manifest a significant decrease in the expression of CD23 even during the asymptomatic stage (P1). Although the mechanism of this change is not yet clear, we believe that the proportion of CD19/CD23(+) cells could serve as a marker of disease progression. The significant increase in B-cell size along with the decrease in CD23 and L-Selectin could be due to an increase in the proportion of immature circulating B cells; further characterization of these cells is required. The cause of the significant decrease in cell number in the sicker patients is unknown, but it may be due to stem cell "fatigue" or to an elimination of mature B cells. Finally, the above changes persist if P2 patients are compared to age-matched controls. In the P0 group, though, further follow-up is required to determine if the differences in phenotype are age or disease related.

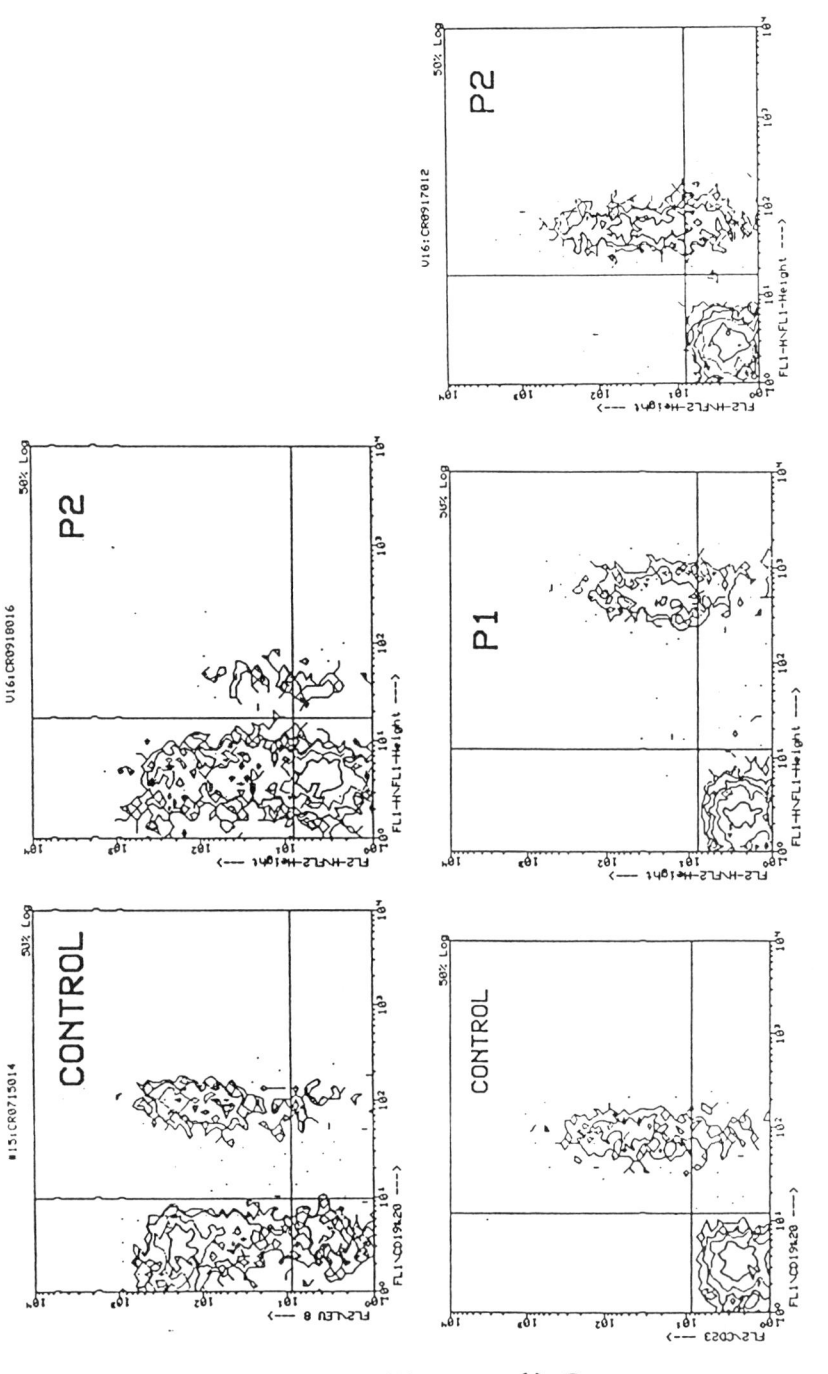

FIGURE 1. CD19/CD23(+) and CD19/L-Selectin(+) cells in HIV-infected children versus controls. The two-color flow cytometry contour graphs show a decrease in the double-positive CD19/L-Selectin cells (*upper row*) and CD19/CD23 cells (*lower row*) as well as total CD19 with disease progression.

REFERENCES

1. MARTINEZ-MAZA, O., et al. 1987. J. Immunol. **138(11):** 3720–3724.
2. YARCHOAN, R., et al. 1986. Clin. Invest. **78(2):** 439–447.
3. PAHWA, S., et al. 1985. Proc. Natl. Acad. Sci. USA **82:** 8198–8202.
4. PAHWA, S. 1990. Crit. Care Med. **18(2):** S138–S143.
5. STIEHM, E. R. 1990. Immunology of HIV. *In* Pediatric AIDS: The Challenge of HIV Infection in Infants, Children and Adolescents. P. A. Pizzo & C. M. Wilfert, Eds.: 95–112. William and Wilkins. Philadelphia.
6. HAMET, I. 1992. Immunol. Today **13:** 215–218.

Central Nervous System in Pediatric AIDS

Results from Neuropathologic Pediatric AIDS Registry[a]

P. B. KOZLOWSKI,[b] J. H. SHER,[c] C. RAO,[c] P. A. ANZIL,[c]
M. A. WRZOLEK,[c] L. SHARER,[d] E-S. CHO,[d] D. W.
DICKSON,[e] K. M. WEIDENHEIM,[e] J. F. LLENA,[e]
S. J. NELSON,[f] AND M. D. KANZER[g]

The Neuropathologic Registry of Pediatric AIDS (Registry) was established in 1990 to collect and analyze data from cases from several medical centers, each with only a limited number of pediatric AIDS cases. The Registry's database includes detailed neuropathological data, general clinical data (risk factors, gestation, symptoms), and autopsy data (general findings, specific organ abnormalities, infections) of children up to age 13 that died of AIDS. All data are confidential. The database does not contain names, addresses, or identifying numbers. The only number is a linking laboratory number assigned by the referring physician.

The Registry currently contains data from 156 pediatric AIDS cases. The most common mode of transmission of HIV was maternal–fetal, with only 13 transfusion-related cases, including two hemophiliacs. In only six of 156 cases was the central nervous system normal grossly and histologically. In the remaining 150 cases (96.1%), the central nervous system showed abnormalities, with several lesions occurring in combination in many of these cases.

Microencephaly/brain atrophy was seen in 99 cases (63.5%), and a brain-weight deficit of 5% or more was seen in 83 out of 113 cases for which the brain weight was reported. HIV encephalitis was seen in 60 (38.5%) cases.

CNS infection with secondary pathogens was seen in 16 cases (10.2%) including 11 cases of CMV, 3 cases of *Candida,* and one each of *Aspergillus, M. tuberculo-*

[a] This work was supported in part by National Institutes of Health Grant HD 24884 and by the New York State Office of Mental Retardation and Developmental Disabilities.
[b] New York State Institute for Basic Research, Staten Island, NY 10314.
[c] State University of New York Health Science Center at Brooklyn, Brooklyn, NY 11203.
[d] New Jersey Medical School, Newark, NJ 07103.
[e] Albert Einstein College of Medicine, Bronx, NY 10461.
[f] University of Miami, Fort Lauderdale, FL 33312.
[g] Medical Center of Delaware, Newark, DE 19718.

sis, M. avium intracellulare, Pseudomonas, Streptococcus, and measles virus inclusion body infection.

Vascular pathology (total 30 cases) included 14 cases of infarcts, 4 of hemorrhages, 7 of arteritis/vasculitis, and 13 of microscopic infarcts. There were eight cases of the CNS lymphoma (five primary and three secondary), and one case of metastatic Leiomyosarcoma. Spinal cord abnormalities included 16 cases of corticospinal tract degeneration, and six cases of vacuolar myelopathy. Basal ganglia mineralizations were seen in 101 (64.7%) cases. Miscellaneous pathology included one case of acute Wernicke's encephalopathy, one case of major CNS malformation, and two cases of subacute necrotizing encephalopathy.

Despite the rapid increase of pediatric AIDS cases, the number of autopsies remains constant or has fallen in some centers. This trend is quite disturbing because it limits our knowledge of the disease, and it will compromise verification of efficacy of new treatments. The neuropathology of AIDS in children presents with phenomena different from those seen in adults, including more common CNS involvement by HIV-related pathology, severe microencephaly, and relative rarity of opportunistic infections in the CNS. Collection of large numbers of pediatric AIDS cases allows for more meaningful statistical analysis of the observations made by individual contributors.

For information concerning the Registry, please contact Dr. Piotr B. Kozlowski, New York State Institute for Basic Research in Developmental Disabilities, 1050 Forest Hill Road, Staten Island, NY 10314; Telephone: (718) 494-5161 or 5354; FAX: (718) 494-5347 or (718) 494-5347.

Image Analysis of Myelination in Second-Trimester Human Fetal Spinal Cords at Risk for HIV-1 Infection[a]

K. M. WEIDENHEIM,[b,c] I. EPSHTEYN,[b]
W. K. RASHBAUM,[c] J. F. McGURK,[d] AND W. D. LYMAN[b]

[b] *Department of Pathology (Neuropathology)*
[c] *Department of Obstetrics and Gynecology, and*
[d] *Department of Neuroscience*
Albert Einstein College of Medicine
Bronx, New York 10461

White matter changes, including diffuse pallor and corticospinal tract degeneration, are a major part of the neuropathology of pediatric AIDS.[1] Interference with normal myelination may occur in infected children.[2] Because significant numbers of HIV-1-positive children are believed to have been infected during gestation[3] and this is a time of significant nervous system development, this project examined the theory that vertical transmission of HIV-1 can affect myelination. To elucidate this problem, expression of the myelin-associated protein myelin basic protein (MBP) in the dorsal columns of 42 normal second-trimester human fetal spinal cords (HFSC) and 13 at-risk HFSC was compared using a computerized image-analysis system. Vibratome sections of lumbosacral spinal cord sections were stained using an immunocytochemical method for MBP.[4] The percentage of area of the dorsal funiculi occupied by reaction product was calculated for each specimen using the Quantimet image-analysis system. Control specimens were used to construct a normal curve of MBP expression versus gestational age, to which at-risk specimens could be compared.

---

[a] This work was supported by United States Public Health Service Grants MH 47667, MH 46815, and DA 05583.

[c] Address for correspondence: Karen M. Weidenheim, M.D., Department of Pathology (Neuropathology), Building K, Room 439, Albert Einstein College of Medicine, 1300 Morris Park Avenue, Bronx, New York 10461.

RESULTS

MBP expression increased between 10 to 24 gestational weeks (GW) (FIG. 1). Marked variability could be found among control specimens of the same gestational age (FIG. 1). No significant differences were found between control and at-risk specimens (FIG. 2).

DISCUSSION

In the HFSC, MBP expression in the dorsal columns increases rapidly between 10 and 24 GW. Variability is marked among specimens of similar gestational age. Some of this variability may be due to variation in fetal size, which produced inaccuracy in determining precise fetal age. We believe that foot length can be used to estimate gestational age correctly within approximately 1 to 2 weeks. The dilatation and extraction procedure used for pregnancy termination begins to disrupt the maternal–fetal unit at least 24 hours before specimen collection and could affect MBP integrity. In addition, technical variations in the immunocytochemical staining procedure may have produced some variability. Similar variability was observed in the at-risk population.

The at-risk population studied here includes fetuses of mothers who are HIV-1 positive (7/13), five of whom admitted previous drug abuse, as well as those at risk because of heterosexual activity (multiple partners or a partner who abused intravenous drugs). Four of four fetal specimens tested for HIV-1 by PCR were

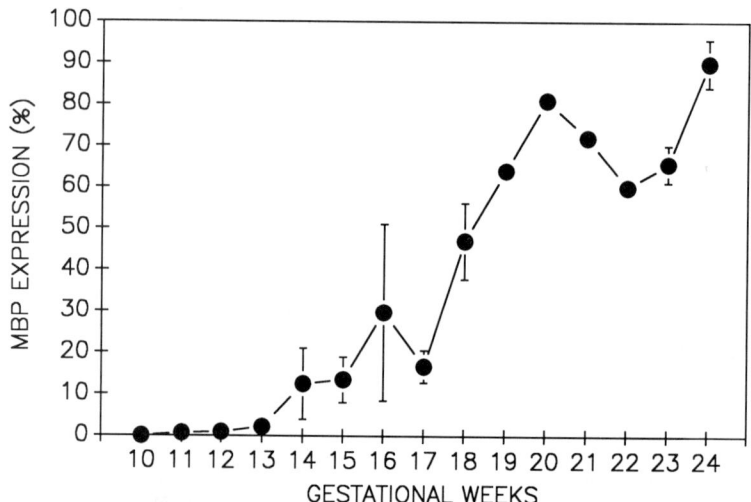

FIGURE 1. Measure of myelination: This standard curve depicts the increase in MBP expression in the dorsal columns of the lumbosacral spinal cord between 10 and 24 GW. Error bars represent standard deviation.

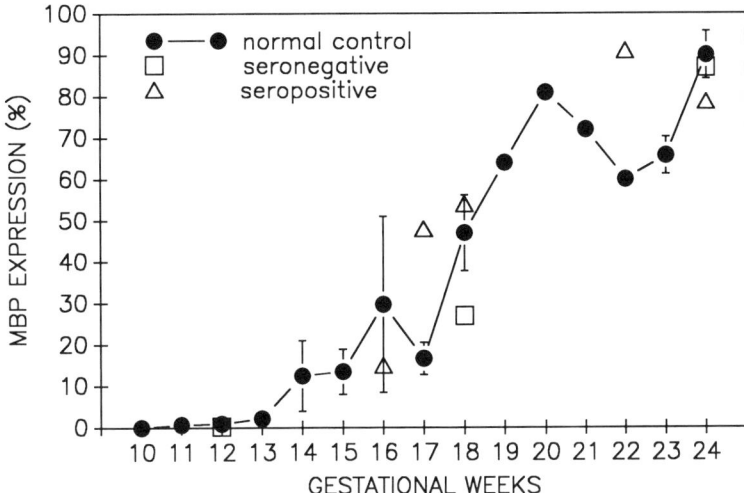

FIGURE 2. **Measure of myelination:** Comparison of MBP expression in control specimens with MBP expression in specimens from seronegative and seropositive women. No significant differences are observed at 12, 16, or 24 GW. At 17 and 22 GW, MBP expression appears increased in a single specimen from a seropositive woman. At 18 GW, MBP expression appears decreased in a specimen from a seronegative woman and within the control range for a specimen from a seropositive woman. Control values are calculated from six specimens at 12 GW, four at 16 GW, three at 17 GW, three at 18 GW, one at 22 GW, and three at 24 GW. Three specimens from seropositive females were available at 24 GW. Error bars represent standard deviation.

negative; results for the remaining specimens were not available. It is therefore unsurprising that no significant differences between control and at-risk specimens were found. Results from specimens of 17, 18, and 22 GW suggest that an apparent increase in MBP expression may occur in fetuses of seropositive mothers. Increased expression might reflect activation of oligodendrocytes by a cytokine present in infected women or may indicate alterations in the neuropil itself, perhaps induced by loss of water or cord parenchyma as a consequence of maternal HIV-1 infection. Study of additional infected and uninfected specimens is necessary to confirm this trend.

REFERENCES

1. DICKSON, D.W., et al. 1989. APMIS Suppl. **8:** 40–57.
2. WEIDENHEIM, K. M., et al. 1990. In Brain in Pediatric AIDS. P. B. Kozlowski, D. A. Snider, P. M. Vietze & H. M. Wisniewski, Eds.: 170–182. Karger. Basel.
3. SOEIRO, R., et al. 1992. J. Infect. Dis. **166:** 699–703.
4. WEIDENHEIM, K. M., et al. 1992. J. Neuropathol. Exp. Neurol. **51:** 142–149.

Administration of Aerosolized Pentamidine to HIV-Infected Infants

IVAN L. HAND,[a] ANDREW WIZNIA, AND MAURA PORRICOLA

Bronx Lebanon Hospital Center
Albert Einstein College of Medicine
Bronx, New York 10457

The aim of this study is to evaluate the safety of administering aerosolized pentamidine (AP) to HIV-infected infants. Aerosolized pentamidine has been effectively used as a prophylaxis for *Pneumocystis carinii* pneumonia (PCP) in HIV-infected patients.[1] Currently, HIV-infected infants are being treated primarily with trimethaprim-sulfamethoxazole (Bactrim) as a PCP prophylaxis[2] despite the presence of serious side effects such as allergic reactions and bone marrow suppression. AP offers the advantages of avoidance of systemic toxicity by direct deposition at the alveolar level as well as relatively long tissue half-life levels.[3]

Seven infants, aged 3.5 to 11 months at entry, were treated with AP, using a Respigard II nebulizer (Marquest Medical Products, Englewood, CO) and an appropriately sized infant face mask, after the infants were sedated with chloral hydrate (50 to 100 mg/kg). The dosage of AP was calculated by the subject's weight and per minute ventilation and was based on an adult-equivalent dose of 300 mg of pentamidine. Pulmonary function measurements were obtained using the passive expiratory flow technique (Sensormedics 2600, Yorba Linda, CA). Through the use of a dual-piston occlusion valve, we were able to alternate between aerosol administration and the measurement of pulmonary function.

Preliminary data demonstrates no clinical side effects in 77% (28/36) of the treatments given. Observed side effects included coughing (6), mild wheeze (1), and transient O_2 desaturation (1); none required cessation of treatment. There was a significant increase in tidal volume ($p < 0.01$) and pulmonary resistance ($p < 0.05$) after administration of aerosolized pentamidine (TABLE 1). There was no significant change in compliance or the percent of expired volume at the time of peak tidal flow, a measure of airflow obstruction.[4]

This study demonstrates that it is possible to administer AP to infants and that it is generally well tolerated with side effects similar to those seen in the adult

---

[a] Address for correspondence: Ivan L. Hand, M.D., Department of Pediatrics, Bronx Lebanon Hospital Center, 1650 Grand Concourse, Bronx, New York 10457.

TABLE 1. Pulmonary Function Measurements before and after Administration of Aerosolized Pentamidine

	Before Pentamidine	After Pentamidine	p Value[a]
Tidal volume (ml/kg)	8.53 ± 1.8	9.00 ± 1.8	$p < 0.01$
% volume/PTEF[b]	0.26 ± 0.09	0.28 ± 0.12	NS
Compliance (ml·cmH$_2$O·kg)	1.54 ± 0.53	1.49 ± 0.48	NS
Resistance (cmH$_2$O·ml·sec)	0.041 ± 0.02	0.046 ± 0.02	$p < 0.05$

[a] Two-tailed Wilcoxon paired sample test.
[b] Percent volume at peak tidal flow.

population. Further study is needed to determine the safety and efficacy of this regimen in infants.

REFERENCES

1. LEOUNG, G. S., D. W. FEIGAL, A. B. MONTGOMERY, et al. 1990. Aerosolized pentamidine for prophylaxis against *Pneumocystis carinii* pneumonia. N. Engl. J. Med. **323:** 769–775.
2. Guidelines for Prophylaxis against *Pneumocystis carinii* Pneumonia for Children Infected with the human Immunodeficiency Virus. 1991. Morbid. Mortal. Wkly. Rpt. **40:** 1–13.
3. MONTGOMERY, A. B., R. J. DEBS, J. M. LUCE, et al. 1988. Selective delivery of pentamidine to the lung by aerosol. Am. Rev. Respir. Dis. **137:** 477–478.
4. MORRIS, M. J. & D. J. LANE. 1981. Tidal expiratory flow patterns in airflow obstruction. Thorax **36:** 135–142.

Pharmacokinetics of Trimetrexate Glucuronate in Infants with AIDS and *Pneumocystis carinii* Pneumonia

BISHARA J. FREIJ,[a,b] RAOUL L. WIENTZEN, JR.,[c]
GAYLE HAYEK,[c] AND LLOYD R. WHITFIELD[d]

[a] Department of Pediatrics
William Beaumont Hospital
Royal Oak, Michigan 48073

[c] Department of Pediatrics
Georgetown University Hospital
Washington, D.C. 20007

[d] Parke-Davis Pharmaceutical Research
A Division of Warner-Lambert Company
Ann Arbor, Michigan 48105

Pneumocystis carinii pneumonia (PCP) is the most commonly encountered opportunistic infection in HIV-infected children. At present, only trimethoprim-sulfamethoxazole (TMP/SMX) and pentamidine isethionate are approved for its treatment; both have moderate efficacies but significant toxicities.

Trimetrexate is an anti-cancer drug that is 1,500-fold more potent than TMP against *P. carinii*. Its major mechanism of action is inhibition of the enzyme dihydrofolate reductase (DHFR). The dose-limiting adverse effect of trimetrexate is myelosuppression. Trimetrexate, with leucovorin rescue, has been shown to be safe and effective for initial therapy of adult AIDS patients with PCP, and in those intolerant of or unresponsive to standard drugs.[1]

MATERIALS AND METHODS

We studied the pharmacokinetics of trimetrexate in two infants with AIDS and PCP (confirmed by lung biopsies) who had failed conventional therapy. Patient

---

[b] Address for correspondence: Bishara J. Freij, M.D., Department of Pediatrics, William Beaumont Hospital, 3535 West Thirteen Mile Road, Royal Oak, Michigan 48073-6706.

A was a 4-month-old white boy who failed to respond to 7 days of intravenous (i.v.) TMP/SMX, followed by 16 days of pentamidine. Patient B was a 6-month-old African-American girl who was refractory to 10 days of i.v. TMP/SMX, followed by 7 days of pentamidine. Neither infant had other opportunistic pathogens.

Trimetrexate glucuronate was infused once daily as an i.v. infusion over 60 min at a dose of 30 mg/m^2 for 21 days. Leucovorin, a reduced folate that bypasses trimetrexate-induced DHFR blockade in mammalian (but not protozoan) cells, was given i.v. every 6 hours at a dose of 20 mg/m^2 for 24 days. Blood was collected before the first dose, and again at 15 min, 30 min, 1 hr, 1.5 hr, 2 hr, 4 hr, 8 hr, 12 hr, and 18 hr. Peak and trough trimetrexate plasma concentrations were measured on days 2, 3, 5, and 14. Multiple blood samples were obtained on day 21 at times 0, 15 min, 30 min, 1 hr, 1.5 hr, 2 hr, 4 hr, 8 hr, 12 hr, 18 hr, 24 hr, 36 hr, 48 hr, and 72 hr. Safety monitoring included serial complete blood counts, platelet counts, renal panels, and liver enzyme measurements. Trimetrexate plasma levels were measured by high-pressure liquid chromatography with UV detection. Pharmacokinetic data were obtained by noncompartmental pharmacokinetic methods with the aid of the LAGRAN computer program.

RESULTS

The plasma trimetrexate concentration–time plots for patients A and B are depicted in FIGURE 1, and the pharmacokinetic data are summarized in TABLE 1. Total plasma clearance (CL_p) values for both infants on day 1 of therapy were low compared with the previously reported mean CL_p value of 40.1 ml/(min·m^2) in children with cancer.[2] CL_p increased by 144% and 63% for infants A and B, respectively, over the 21-day study period but still remained lower than the mean observed for children with malignancies. Volume of distribution at steady state (VDss) values were half the mean VDss values for pediatric cancer patients. VDss increased during the course of the study to reach values similar to the reported mean by day 21. Elimination half-lives on days 1 and 21 were comparable to those for children with cancer. No hepatic, renal, or hematologic adverse effects were noted during trimetrexate therapy.

TABLE 1. Trimetrexate Pharmacokinetic Parameters for Infants with AIDS and PCP[a]

	AUC	CL_p	VDss	$T_{1/2}$
A/Dose 1	47.7	10.5	6.0	7.2
A/Dose 21	19.5	25.6	14.6	12.1
B/Dose 1	21.8	23.0	6.5	4.4
B/Dose 21	13.3	37.6	11.1	4.1

[a] Abbreviations: AUC = area under the plasma concentration–time curve [μg/(hr·ml)]; CL_p = plasma clearance [ml/(min·m^2)]; VDss = steady-state volume of distribution (l/m^2); and $T_{1/2}$ = apparent elimination half-life (hr).

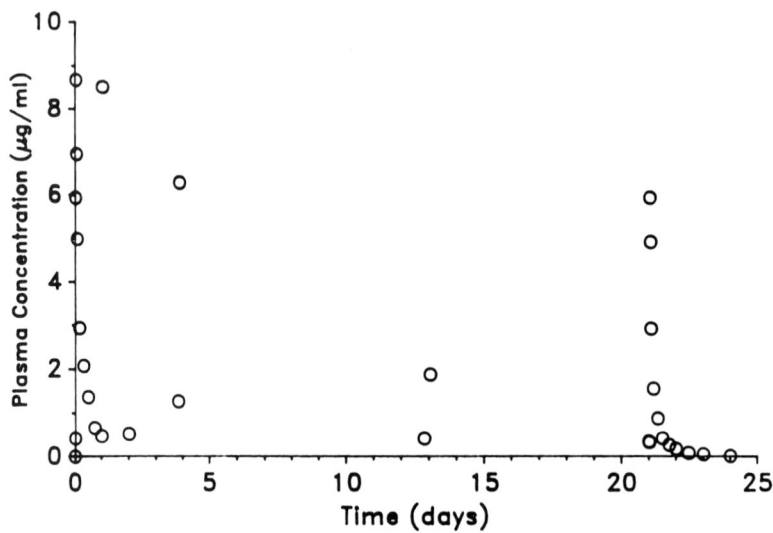

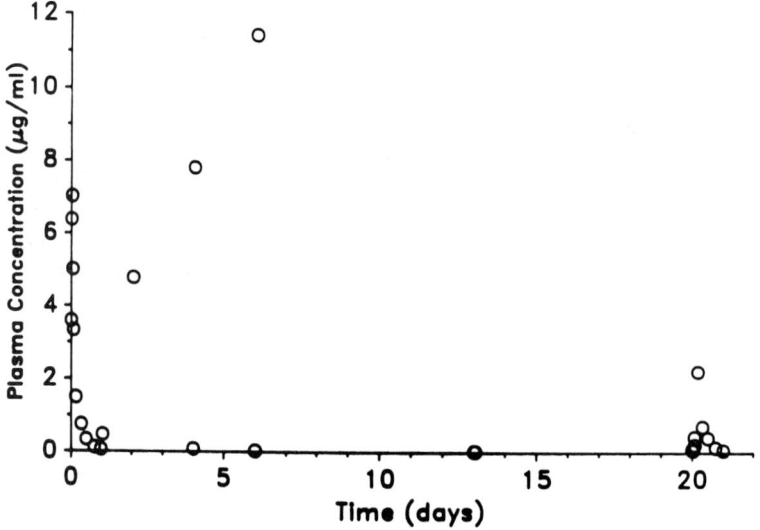

FIGURE 1. Plasma trimetrexate concentration–time plots for patient A *(upper panel)* and patient B *(lower panel)*.

CONCLUSIONS

Trimetrexate pharmacokinetics were nonlinear and changed over the 21 days of therapy. The drug's pharmacokinetic behavior differed in seriously ill infants with AIDS and PCP from that which has been observed in pediatric and adult patients with cancer, but is similar to that of the 7-month-old boy with severe combined immunodeficiency and refractory PCP reported by Smit et al.[3] The drug was well tolerated and caused no adverse effects at the dosage level used in this study.

REFERENCES

1. ALLEGRA, C. J., B. A. CHABNER, C. U. TUAZON, D. OGATA-ARAKAKI, B. BAIRD, J. C. DRAKE & H. MASUR. 1988. Semin. Oncol. **15(Suppl. 2):** 46–49.
2. BALIS, F. M., R. PATEL, E. LUKS, K. M. DOHERTY, J. S. HOLCENBERG, C. TAN, G. H. REAMAN, J. BELASCO, L. J. ETTINGER, S. ZIMM & D. G. POPLACK. 1987. Cancer Res. **47(18):** 4973–4976.
3. SMIT, M. J. M., R. DE GROOT, J. J. M. VAN DONGEN, E. VAN DER VOORT, H. J. NEIJENS & L. R. WHITFIELD. 1990. Pediatr. Infect. Dis. J. **9(3):** 212–214.

Evaluation of Anti-HIV Agents *in Vitro* by Quantitative PCR

BHARAT JOSHI, JAY EPSTEIN, SHERWIN F. LEE,
RON MAYNER, AND INDIRA K. HEWLETT[a]

Laboratory of Retrovirology
Division of Transfusion Science
Center for Biologics Evaluation and Research
Food and Drug Administration
Bethesda, Maryland 20892

We have investigated the anti-HIV activity of the combination of AZT and rIFN-a2B *in vitro* by quantitative PCR analysis of viral DNA and RNA in infected H9 and U937 cells in order to obtain a more accurate and quantitative estimate of the extent of viral inhibition and the stages at which this inhibition occurs. H9 and U937 cells in the logarithmic phase of growth were infected with HIV-1 (100 ng of p24 per 100 × 10^6 cells, IIIB strain), washed with PBS, and subsequently transferred to fresh medium or medium containing AZT (10 µg/ml) or rIFNa (50 U/ml) alone or a combination of AZT and rIFNa at the same concentration. Cells were sampled at various time points for viral DNA and RNA analysis by PCR and culture supernatant for viral antigen. Fresh medium containing the various drugs was added to ensure their constant presence and uniform concentration during the course of the experiment. PCR products were quantitated by densitometry.

In both H9 and U937 cells, greater than 95% inhibition of RT activity in the supernatant was observed with AZT and the combination of AZT and rIFNa (FIG. 1). rIFNa exerted less of an inhibitory effect on U937 cells, that is, 65% and 30% at days 9 and 12, respectively. Viral antigen (p24) was inhibited by greater than 95% by both AZT and the combination of AZT and rIFNa (data not shown). By PCR, however, a different pattern was observed. Levels of viral DNA detected by PCR were decreased by 90% in H9 cells treated with the combination of AZT and rIFNa in the early phase of the infection, whereas only 35 to 40% inhibition was observed in cells treated with either AZT and rIFNa alone. A greater degree of sustained inhibition (70%) was also seen with the combination of AZT and rIFNa (FIG. 2A, B). HIV RNA synthesis did not appear to be significantly inhibited by either AZT or rIFNa alone. Combination treatment with AZT and rIFNa re-

---

[a] To whom correspondence should be addressed.

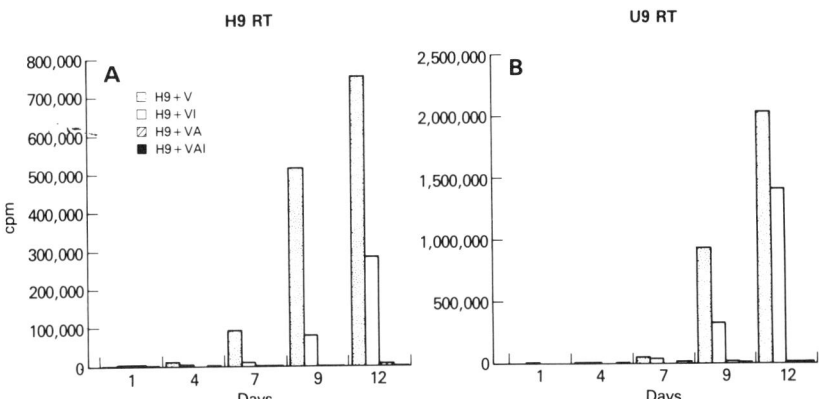

FIGURE 1. Reverse transcriptase activity in the supernatant of H9 and U937 cells infected with HIV-1 (v) and treated with rIFNa2B (VI) or AZT (VA) or AZT + rIFNa (VAI).

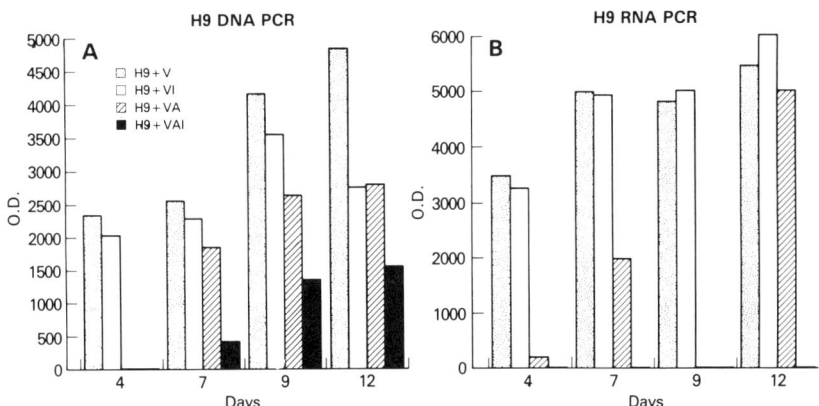

FIGURE 2. Bar graph representation of DNA (**A**) and RNA (**B**) levels detected by PCR in infected and drug-treated cultures of H9 cells. Note: RNA for the 9-day sample was not done.

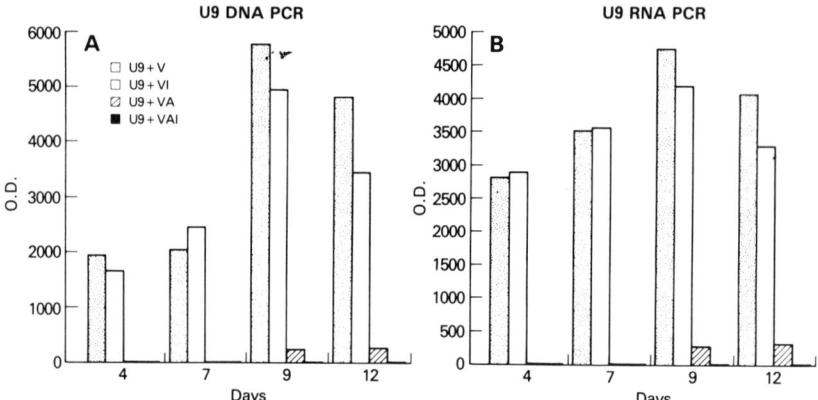

FIGURE 3. Bar graph representation of DNA (**A**) and RNA (**B**) levels detected by PCR in infected and drug-treated cultures of U937 cells.

sulted in undetectable levels of viral RNA in infected cells (FIG. 1B). In U937 cells, both AZT and the combination of AZT and rIFNa effectively inhibited both DNA and RNA (90%) synthesis (FIG. 3A,B). Treatment with rIFNa alone did not result in inhibition early in infection, although some effect on viral DNA (40%) synthesis was observed around 12 days post infection and treatment. Cell viability of both cultures ranged from 70 to 90%.

Similarly, combination treatment with ddC and rIFNa also resulted in significant inhibition (95%) of HIV DNA and RNA synthesis in H9 cells with minimal cellular toxicity (data not shown). In conclusion, both AZT and DDC singly and the combination of AZT or DDC with rIFNa effectively inhibited virus production from infected H9 and U937 cells as indicated by p24 antigen and RT assays, especially in the early phase of treatment and infection. Combination treatment, however, was more effective in inhibiting virus expression at the nucleic acid level in a sustained manner. These results suggest that quantitative PCR may be of use in measuring virus burden and expression in infected cells.

REFERENCES

1. HARTSHORN, K. L., M. W. VOGT, T. C. CHOU, R. S. BLUMBERG, R. BYINGTON, R. T. SCHOOLEY & M. S. HIRSCH. 1987. Synergistic inhibition of human immunodeficiency virus *in vitro* by azidothymidine and recombinant interferon alpha A. Antimicrob. Agents Chemother. **31:** 168–172.
2. SCHOCHETMAN, G., C-Y. OU & W. K. JONES. 1988. Polyerase chain reaction. J. Infect. Dis. **158:** 1154–1157.

Immunoregulation of Tumor Necrosis Factor Production by HIV-1 gp-120 in Neonates and Adults[a]

MADHAVAN P. N. NAIR, ANN M. SWEET, AND
STANLEY A. SCHWARTZ

*Department of Medicine
Division of Allergy and Immunology
State University of New York at Buffalo
Buffalo, New York 14203*

The mechanisms that contribute to the activation of latent HIV infection to progression of disease and to the development of clinical AIDS are not clearly understood. Recent studies have shown that the pathogenesis of HIV-1 infection was mediated through secretion of viral proteins or viral induction of cytokines. Earlier studies showed that tumor necrosis factor (TNF) acts as a potent activator of HIV production.[1] Although significant progress has been made in studying the natural history of HIV infection in adults, understanding the natural history of infection in neonates still remains unclear. The present study examines the effects of gp-120 on the production of TNF by normal cord blood compared to adult blood *in vitro*.

EXPERIMENTAL DESIGN

Neonatal umbilical cord blood samples were collected in heparinized tubes (20 U/ml) under sterile conditions from healthy term infants at vaginal delivery before the expulsion of the placenta. Peripheral blood was obtained simultaneously from healthy, unrelated adult volunteers of either sex (20–40 yr). Donors or their parents were apprised of the study, and consents were obtained consistent with the policies of the University at Buffalo and the NIH. One-milliliter blood samples were aliquoted rapidly into sterile Eppendorf tubes. Triplicates of blood samples received HIV-1 gp-120 at 0, 1, 10, 50, and 100 ng/ml concentrations. Triplicates of cultures also received these concentrations of gp-120 plus lipopolysaccharide (LPS, 10 μg/ml). Control and treated blood samples were incubated at 37 °C for 4 to 6 hr in a

---

[a] This work was supported in part by National Institutes of Health Grant 1 R01 MH 47225.

5% CO_2 and 95% air incubator. The TNF activities of the treated and control blood plasma samples were determined by a cytotoxicity assay using the TNF-sensitive WEHI 164 subclone 13 cell line as described.[2]

RESULTS AND DISCUSSION

The data presented in TABLE 1 show that gp-120 produced a dose-dependent induction of TNF by cord blood as well as adult peripheral blood compared to untreated blood samples. Aliquots of cord blood samples incubated with 1, 10, 50, and 100 ng/ml of gp-120 produced 57, 100, 175, and 207 ng/ml of TNF control. Adult peripheral blood incubated with gp-120 produced increased levels of TNF compared to that of cord blood, the values being 96, 186, 210, and 360 ng/ml, respectively, for 1, 10, 50, and 100 ng concentrations of gp-120 compared to 48 ng of TNF produced by control blood culture. Cord blood cultured with 10 μg/ml of LPS demonstrated 400 ng of TNF (TABLE 2). Gp-120 produced a dose-dependent suppression of LPS-induced TNF production, the values being 408, 325, 285, and 254, respectively, for 1, 10, 50, and 100 ng/ml of gp-120, compared to 400 ng of TNF produced by LPS alone. Adult blood cultured with 10 μg/ml of LPS produced a significantly higher level of TNF (525 ng/ml). Gp-120 also produced a dose-dependent inhibition of LPS-induced TNF production by adult blood, the values being 506, 403, 385, and 329 compared to 525 ng/ml of TNF produced by LPS alone. Although cord blood produced a lower level of TNF compared to adult blood, gp-120-induced suppression of TNF was similar to that of adult blood. Because TNF is known to be involved in host defense mechanisms against tumors and infectious and inflammatory diseases, gp-120-induced inhibition of TNF production may increase the susceptibility of the host to various infections and tumors. On the other hand, since TNF is known to play a significant role in the activation of latent HIV infection to active disease, gp-120-induced TNF may facilitate the progression of the HIV disease. This seemingly contrary

TABLE 1. Gp-120 Induces the Production of TNF by Normal Cord Blood and Adult Peripheral Blood[a]

Concentration of gp-120	TNF (ng/ml)	
	Cord Blood	Adult Blood
0	26.3 ± 11.29[b]	48.3 ± 7.9
1 ng/ml	57.4 ± 12.8 ($p < 0.1$)[c]	96.7 ± 19.6 ($p < 0.5$)
10 ng/ml	100.8 ± 21.7 ($p < 0.02$)	186.3 ± 28.6 ($p < 0.001$)
50 ng/ml	175.6 ± 19.8 ($p < 0.001$)	210.4 ± 39.7 ($p < 0.001$)
100 ng/ml	207.3 ± 35.9 ($p < 0.001$)	360.5 ± 47.8 ($p < 0.001$)

[a] Normal cord blood and adult peripheral blood samples were cultured with different concentrations of HIV-I gp-120 proteins for 4 to 6 hr, and the plasma TNF was determined by cytotoxic assay using WEHI 164 subclone #13 cell line.

[b] TNF values are expressed as mean ± SD of five separate experiments using five different blood samples run in triplicate.

[c] Statistical evaluations between control and treated blood groups were determined by Student's t test.

TABLE 2. Gp-120 Suppresses LPS-Induced Production of TNF by Whole Blood[a]

	TNF (ng/ml)	
Concentration of LPS and gp-120	Cord Blood	Adult Blood
LPS (10 μg/ml)	400.8 ± 51.8[b]	525.0 ± 58.6
LPS (10 μg/ml) + gp-120 (1 ng/ml)	408.3 ± 47.6 ($p < 0.2$)[c]	506.8 ± 46.0 ($p < 0.8$)
LPS (10 μg/ml) + gp-120 (10 ng/ml)	325.8 ± 30.3 ($p < 0.2$)	403.9 ± 39.2 ($p < 0.1$)
LPS (10 μg/ml) + gp-120 (50 ng/ml)	285.0 ± 29.9 ($p < 0.05$)	385.6 ± 29.8 ($p < 0.05$)
LPS (10 μg/ml) + gp-120 (100 ng/ml)	254.8 ± 21.7 ($p < 0.02$)	329.5 ± 28.9 ($p < 0.01$)

[a] Normal cord blood and adult peripheral blood samples were cultured with either LPS alone or LPS plus different concentrations of gp-120, and the plasma TNF values were determined as stated in the footnote for TABLE 1.
[b] Values are expressed as mean ± SD of five experiments using the same blood samples employed for the experiments in TABLE 1.
[c] Statistical evaluations between LPS TNF values and LPS plus gp-120 TNF values were determined by Student's t test.

effect of gp-120 on TNF production may support a model of immunopathogenesis mediated by specific HIV peptides. Further studies on the mechanisms of gp-120-induced TNF in neonates of HIV-infected mothers may provide a basis for a better understanding of the differential natural course of disease, the early and late development of disease in neonates, and for devising therapeutic strategies aimed at counteracting the specific production or overproduction of TNF.

ACKNOWLEDGMENTS

We wish to express our appreciation to Carol Sperry and Gerry Sobkowiak for their expert secretarial assistance.

REFERENCES

1. MERRILL, J. E. & I. S. CHEN. 1991. FASEB J. 5: 2391–2397.
2. NAIR, M. P. N., S. A. SCHWARTZ, Z. A. KRONFOL & J. F. GREDEN. 1993. Alcoholism. Clin Exp. Res. In press.

Different Strains of HIV-1 Infect Distinct Human Fetal Neural Cells

WILLIAM C. HATCH, E. POUSADA, L. LOSEV,
AND W. D. LYMAN

*Department of Pathology
Albert Einstein College of Medicine
Bronx, New York 10461*

The number of children infected with HIV-1 continues to increase.[1] In addition to severe immunodeficiencies, children infected by HIV-1 demonstrate nervous system disease.[2,3] This neurological dysfunction is manifested as disruptions in the attainment of developmental milestones, intellectual deterioration, motor weakness, and impaired brain growth.[2,3] Because some children are believed to be infected during gestation and it is thought that HIV-1 may infect neural cells, this work tested the hypothesis that different tropic strains of HIV-1 infect cells of the developing human fetal central nervous system (CNS) and, as a result, this infection contributes to AIDS neuropathology.

It is thought that isolates of HIV-1 from the brain may represent a distinct population of AIDS virus.[4] Variations in HIV isolates from the CNS may also be responsible for determining neurological disease manifestations during AIDS.[5] HIV-1 isolates from the CNS of AIDS dementia patients preferentially replicate in cells of the monocyte/macrophage lineage (M-tropic) compared with isolates obtained from the blood (L-tropic).[4] One mechanism of HIV entry into the CNS is via infected T cells and/or monocytes, resulting in resident CNS cells including tissue macrophages being infected (Trojan horse theory).[6]

To examine the ability of different of HIV-1 isolates to infect the human fetal CNS cells, we have established organotypic cultures (OTC) of human fetal CNS tissue as a model of the developing brain. Tissue from either cortical germinal matrix or dorsal spinal cord was dissected into 1-mm^3 sections and cultured in 24-well Falcon Primaria tissue culture plates. These cultures, which have been maintained for up to 12 weeks, are characterized by a central tissue core surrounded by an outgrowth area of rapidly growing neural cells. Immunocytochemical, ultrastructural, and Western blot analyses of these cultures have identified neurons, astrocytes, microglia, oligodendrocytes, and endothelial cells that represent all the major cell types found in the CNS.

CNS OTC were exposed to either lymphocytotropic (L-tropic [RF and MN])[7] or monocytotropic (M-tropic [JRFL and JRCSF]) HIV-1 isolates.[5] The HIV-1 inoculum was removed after two days, and the cultures were washed and monitored for viral infection. Viral titration experiments have determined that the minimal infectious dose of HIV-1 capable of infecting these cultures is below the viral titers detected in the plasma of AIDS patients. HIV-1 RNA has been localized by *in situ* hybridization in the cytoplasm of CNS cells. Analysis of CNS OTC has identified viral DNA in HIV-1 exposed cultures after the application of the polymerase chain reaction (PCR). Immunocytochemical analysis with anti-HIV-1 gp41, gp120, *nef,* and p24 antibodies have identified viral proteins in cells in both the tissue body and outgrowth area. Both media-exposed and heat-inactivated HIV-1 exposed control cultures were negative by all these criteria. Double-label immunocytochemistry has identified that both L- and M-tropic HIV-1 isolates infect microglia. In contrast, only L-tropic HIV-1 isolates (MN and RF) appear to infect astrocytes within CNS OTC.

These results demonstrate that both monocytropic and lymphocytropic HIV-1 isolates appear to infect microglia in CNS OTC. HIV-1 appeared to infect astrocytes in CNS OTC only after exposure to lymphocytotropic isolates. In summary, this CNS OTC model system permits further examination of the interaction of HIV-1 with the developing human CNS and possibly identification of the mechanisms of AIDS neuropathology.

REFERENCES

1. Consensus Workshop S., Italy, January 17–18. 1992. Maternal factors involved in mother-to-child transmission of HIV-1. J. AIDS **5:** 1019–1029.
2. Epstein, L. 1992. AIDS and the central nervous system in children. *In* Fetal and Perinatal Neurology. John R. Smythies & Ronald J. Bradley, Eds.: 320–328. S. Karger. Basel, Switzerland.
3. Brenneman, D. E. & S. K. McCune. 1990. Acquired immune deficiency syndrome and the developing nervous system. *In* International Review on Neurobiology. Y. Fukuyama, Y., Suzuki, S. Kamoshita & P. Casaer, Eds.: Vol. 32: 305–353. Academic Press, Inc., San Diego.
4. Cheng-Mayer, C., C. Weiss, D. Seto & J. A. Levy. 1989. Isolates of human immunodeficiency virus type 1 from the brain may constitute a special group of the AIDS virus. Proc. Natl. Acad. Sci. USA **86:** 8575–8579.
5. Koyanagi, Y., S. Miles, R. T. Mitsuyasu, J. E. Merrill, H. V. Vinters & I. S. Y. Chen. 1987. Dual infection of the central nervous system by AIDS viruses with distinct cellular tropisms. Science **236:** 819–822.
6. Sharpless, N. E., W. A. O'Brien, E. Verdin, C. V. Kufta, I. S. Y. Chen & M. Dubois-Dalcq. 1992. Human immunodeficiency virus type 1 tropism for brain microglial cells is determined by a region of the *env* glycoprotein that also controls macrophage tropism. J. Virol. **66:** 2588–2593.
7. Reitz, Jr., M. S., G.-G. Guo, J. Oleske, J. Hoxie, M. Popovic, E. Read-Cannole, P. Markham, H. Streicher & R. C. Gallo. 1992. On the historical origins of HIV-1 (MN) and (RF). AIDS Res. Hum. Retrovir. **8:** 1539–1541.

Productive Infection of Human Fetal Microglia *in Vitro* by HIV-1[a]

SUNHEE C. LEE, WILLIAM C. HATCH, WEI LIU,
CELIA F. BROSNAN, AND DENNIS W. DICKSON

*Department of Pathology (Neuropathology)
Albert Einstein College of Medicine
Bronx, New York 10461*

Central nervous system (CNS) involvement is frequent in both pediatric and adult AIDS.[1] Microglia have been shown to be the primary target for HIV-1 infection in the CNS *in vivo*.[2,3] *In vitro* studies concerning susceptibility of human microglia to HIV-1 infection reported conflicting results: Microglia from adult brain showed productive infection by HIV-1,[4] whereas microglia from fetal brain did not.[5] We have prepared highly purified human microglial cell cultures from abortuses of 16 to 24 weeks' gestation[6] and exposed them to both moncytotropic (HIV-1_{JR-FL} and HIV-1_{JR-CSF}) and lymphocytotropic (HIV-1_{MN}) isolates of HIV. Culture supernatants were examined for p24 antigen expression for a four-week period following viral exposure. Concurrently, cytopathic effects and cellular viral antigen expression (gp41 and p24) were examined by immunocytochemistry. The results showed that human fetal microglia are productively infected by HIV, as reflected by p24 levels (FIG. 1) and syncytia formation and expression of gp41 and p24 immunoreactivity. Electron microscopy of the HIV-1_{JR-FL} exposed microglia showed numerous viral particles in association with internal membranes as well as cell surfaces (FIG. 2). Control cultures or astrocytes overgrown in the microglia cultures did not show evidence of infection under identical experimental conditions. These data demonstrate that the human fetal microglia, like their adult counterparts, are susceptible to HIV-1 infection *in vitro* and can support the production of virus. This further proves that microglial cells in the CNS have specific susceptibility for HIV-1 and may be the key cell type in the pathogenesis of the CNS dysfunction in AIDS.

---

[a] This work was supported by National Institute of Mental Health Grant MH 47667.

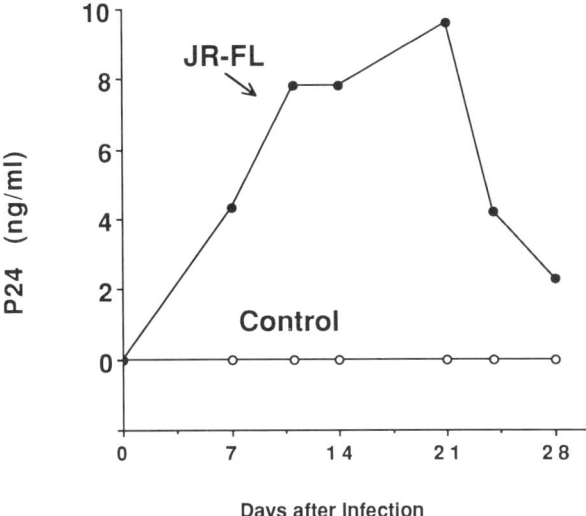

FIGURE 1. p24 *gag* antigen capture assay in human fetal microglial culture. Highly enriched microglia cultures were prepared as described.[6] Microglia seeded at 0.1 million cells/mm^2 in 24-well plates were exposed to HIV-1$_{JR-FL}$ or medium only (control) for 16 hr. Culture supernatants were collected at indicated time points, and p24 levels were measured using a commercial ELISA kit (DuPont, Wilmington, DE).

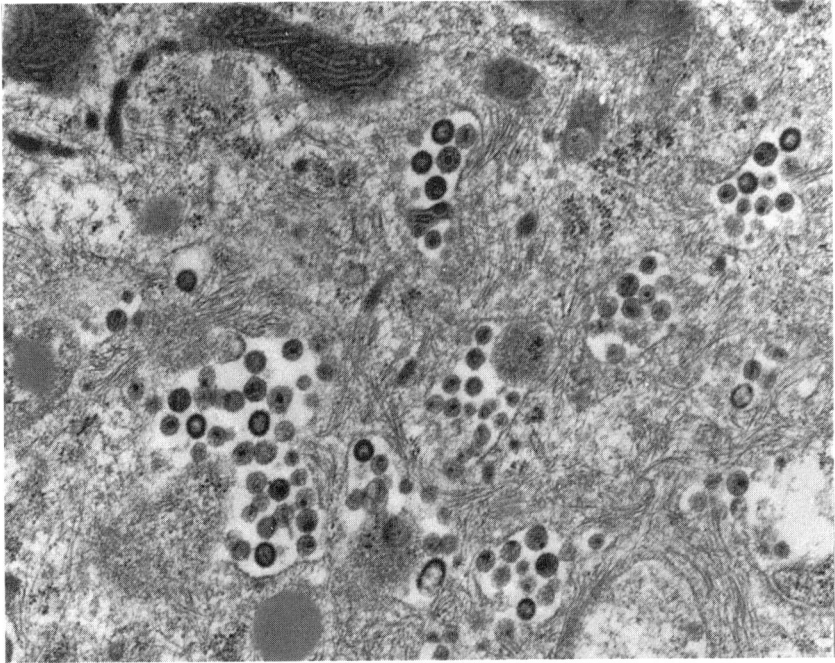

FIGURE 2. Electron microscopy of human fetal microglial culture infected with HIV-1$_{JR-FL}$. Mature and immature viral particles with structure characteristic of HIV are present within membrane-bound spaces of a microglial cell ($\times$30,000, reduced by 30%).

REFERENCES

1. NAVIA, B. A., *et al.* 1986. Ann. Neurol. **19:** 517.
2. NAVIA, B. A., *et al.* 1986. Ann. Neurol. **19:** 525.
3. KURE, K., *et al.* 1991. Hum. Pathol. **22:** 700.
4. WATKINS, B. A., *et al.* 1990. Science **249:** 549.
5. PEUDENIER, S., *et al.* 1991. Ann. Neurol. **29:** 152.
6. LEE, S. C., *et al.* 1992. Lab. Invest. **67:** 465.

HIV Infection of Human Cortical Neuronal Cells

Enhancement by Differentiating Growth Factor[a]

R. RODRIGUEZ,[b] S. RENNE,[b] D. J. VOLSKY,[b]
AND Y. MIZRACHI[c]

[b] Columbia University
St. Luke's–Roosevelt Hospital
New York, New York 10019

[c] Division of Allergy and Immunology
Albert Einstein College of Medicine
of Yeshiva University
Bronx, New York 10461-1602

The mechanism whereby HIV-1 contributes to the damage of neuronal cells is unknown.[1,2] HIV-1 displays a different pattern of infection in CD4-negative neural cells *in vitro* than that in T lymphocytes: In neural cells, the levels of viral DNA and RNA are low, the virus replicates poorly and transiently, and no cytopathic effects are apparent.[3-6] Recent reports indicate that HIV-1 may cause structural and functional damage to target cells in the absence of cytocidal infection.[7-10] Many of these impairments may be attributed to the interaction between HIV-1 and target cell membranes during virus binding and entry. This stage has a destabilizing effect on target cell membrane and cellular integrity.[11] Incubation of neural cells with HIV-1 or with purified HIV-1 envelope glycoprotein (gp120) *in vitro* reduces the response of neural cells to growth factors,[12] induces Ca^{2+} influx,[13] and may cause cell death.[14] These data suggest that gp120 recognizes specific receptors on CD4-negative neural cells.

A proliferating immature neuronal cell line[15] established from a unilateral megalocephaly, a disorder associated with continued proliferation of cortical neurons, provided us with a model system to study functional interactions between HIV-1 and neuronal cells. These cells demonstrate more differentiated characteristics than those of the neuroblastoma cells and are more susceptible to neuronal growth

---

[a] Portions of this work were supported by PAF/AmFAR Grants 50094-9-PG and 500168-11-PG to Y. Mizrachi.

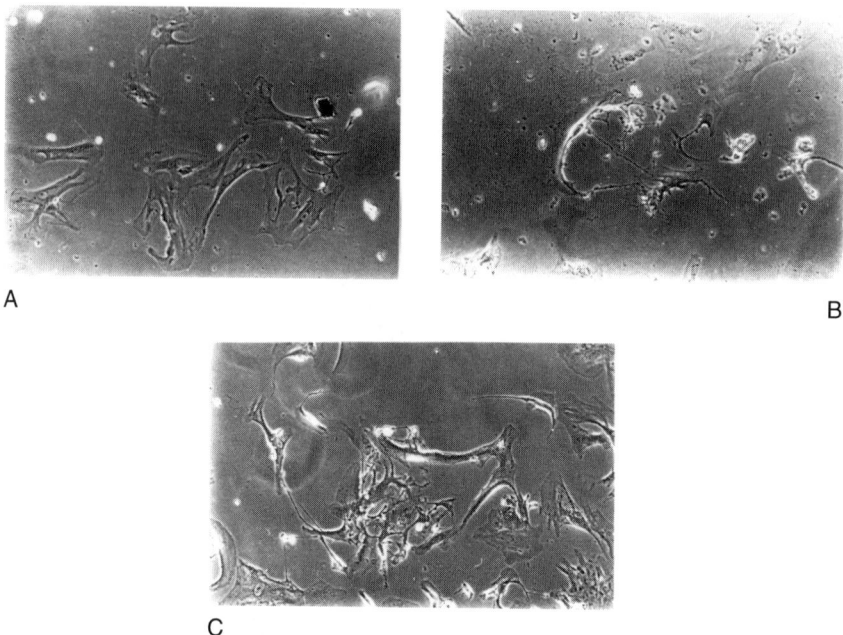

FIGURE 1. Infection of human cortical neurons with HIV-1. (**A**) Noninfected cells. (**B**) HIV-1 infection of human cortical neurons. (**C**) HCN-1A cells were treated with FGF three days before and during infection. Micrograph taken 24 hours after infection.

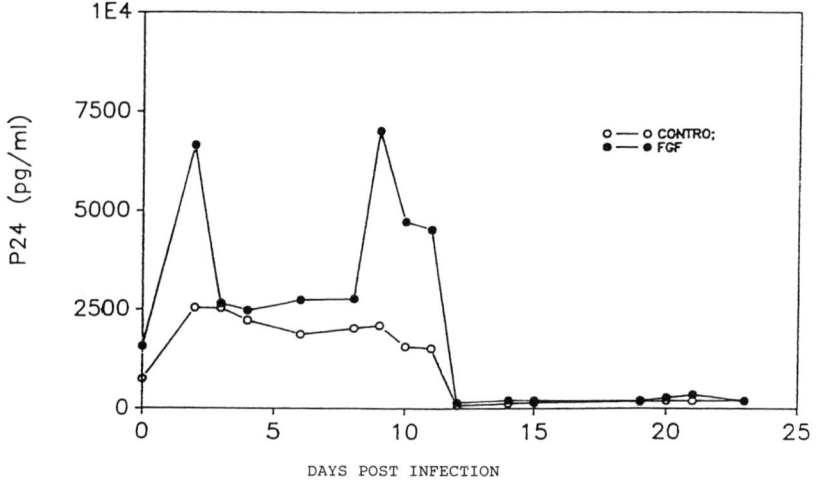

FIGURE 2. Enhancement of HIV-1 expression in human neuronal cells by neuronal growth factors. Human cortical neurons were treated with 100 ng/ml FGF for three days before infection. The cultures were supplemented every three days with the growth factors.

factor activation than the neuroblastoma cells. Twenty-four hours after virus addition to the human cortical neurons, pronounced morphological changes were observed. The cells diminished in size and small neurites could be observed. These neurites became more pronounced during the following several days. A representative micrograph nine days following HIV-1 infection of HCN-1A cells in comparison to uninfected HCN-1A cells is shown in FIGURE 1. These morphological changes observed are indicative of neuronal differentation. The extent of viral production in the proliferating immature human cortical neurons was low and similar to that observed in cultured neuroblastoma and glioma cells unlike the high level of virus production in CD4-transfected H4[16] and HELA[17,18] cells.

The extent of HIV-1 expression following infection in the human cortical neurons was found to depend on the differentiation state of these cells. Pretreatment of these cells with fibroblast growth factor (FGF; FIG. 2) enhanced virus production about three times while a proliferative growth factor, the epidermal growth factor, had no effect on the extent of viral production in these human cortical neurons.

These results indicate that HIV-1 infection of neural cells may alter the physiological state of the cells. Moreover, the physiological state of the cells may affect the extent of HIV-1 infection and its expression in neural cells.

REFERENCES

1. KETZLER, S., S. WEIS, H. HANG & H. BUDKA. 1990. Acta Neuropathol. (Berlin) **80:** 92–94.
2. MIZRACHI, Y., M. ZEIRA, M. SHAHABUDDIN, G. LI, F. SINANGIL & D. J. VOLSKY. 1991. Bull. Inst. Pasteur **89:** 81–96.
3. DEWHURST, S., K. SAKAI, J. M. STEVENSON, M. J. EVINGER-HODGER & D. J. VOLSKY. 1987. J. Virol. **61:** 3774–3782.
4. WIGDAHL, B. & C. KUNSCH. 1990. Prog. Med. Virol. **37:** 1–46.
5. LI, X. L., T. MOUDGIL, H. V. WINTERS & D. D. HO. 1990. J. Virol. **64:** 1383–1387.
6. CHENG-MAYER, C., J. RUTKA, M. L. ROSENBLUM, T. MCHUGH, D. P. STITES & J. A. LEVY. 1987. Proc. Natl. Acad. Sci. USA **84:** 3526–3530.
7. GUPTA, S. & B. VAYUVEGULA. 1987. J. Clin. Immunol. **7:** 486–489.
8. LYNN, W. S., A. TWEEDALE & M. CLOYD. 1988. Virology **163:** 43–51.
9. LIFSON, J. D., G. R. REYES, M. S. MCGRATH, B. S. STEIN & E. G. ENGLEMAN. 1986. Science **232:** 1123–1127.
10. GARRY, R. F., A. A. GOTTLIEB, K. P. ZUCKERMAN, J. R. PACE, T. W. FRANK & D. A. BOSTICK. 1988. Bioscience **8:** 35–47.
11. SINANGIL, F., A. LOYTER & D. J. VOLSKY. 1988. FEBS Lett. **239:** 88–92.
12. MIZRACHI, Y. 1989. J. Neurosci. Res. **23:** 217–224.
13. DREYER, E. B., P. K. KAISER, J. T. OFFERMANN & S. A. LIPTON. 1990. Science **248:** 364–367.
14. BRENNEMAN, D. E., G. L. WESTBROOK, S. P. FITZGERALD, D. L. ENNIST, K. L. ELKINS, M. R. RUFF & C. B. PERT. 1988. Nature **335:** 639–642.
15. RONNETT, G. V., L. D. HESTER, J. S. NYE, K. CONNORS & S. H. SNYDER. 1990. Science **248:** 603–605.
16. VOLSKY, B., K. SAKAI, M. M. REDDY & D. J. VOLSKY. 1992. Virology **186:** 303–308.
17. KLATZMANN, D., E. CHAMPAGNE & S. CHAMARET. 1984. Nature **312:** 767.
18. MADDON, P. J., A. G. DALGLEISH, J. S. MCDOUGAL, P. R. CLAPHAM, R. A. WEISS & R. AXEL. 1986. Cell **47:** 333–348.

Neural Cell Receptor for HIV-1

Initial Biochemical Characterization[a]

Y. MIZRACHI

Division of Allergy and Immunnology
Albert Einstein College of Medicine
of Yeshiva University
Bronx, New York 10461-1602

Acquired immune deficiency syndrome (AIDS) is associated with a wide spectrum of nervous system disorders. The mechanism whereby HIV-1 contributes to the damage of neuronal cells is unknown. We hypothesize that the binding and fusion of HIV-1 with neural cells alters or impairs neural cell function. We have found that gp120 interacts specifically and with high affinity with neural cells. This binding was found to be independent of CD4.

CD4 is the well-characterized receptor for HIV-1 on T lymphocytes and macrophages[1,2]; however, soluble CD4 does not block HIV-1 infection in neural cells,[3-5] suggesting that the HIV-1 receptor on neural cells is different from CD4. Our studies[6] support this suggestion by demonstrating that gp120 binds to CD4-negative neural cells and that HIV-1 fusion with neural cells is independent of CD4 but requires gp120. The ability of HIV-1 to use more than one cell surface receptor may explain the large number of host cells that this virus infects.[7,8]

We have previously demonstrated that HIV-1 fusion with neural cells was independent of CD4[6] in contrast to HIV-1 fusion with T lymphocytes. We also have found that ^{125}I-labeled gp120 binding to neural cells such as the SKNMC neuroblastoma and H4 astroglioma cells was not inhibited by sCD4 and thus is independent of CD4, while gp120 binding to T lymphoctyes could be efficiently inhibited by sCD4 (data not shown).

SENSITIVITY TO TRYPSINIZATION OF gp120-BINDING MOLECULE ON NEURAL CELLS

^{125}I-labeled gp120 binding to galactocerebrosides (GC) and the inhibition of this binding with antibodies to GC were recently described.[9,10] GC may not be the

---

[a] Portions of this work were supported by PAF/AmFAR Grants 50094-9-PG and 500168-11-PG.

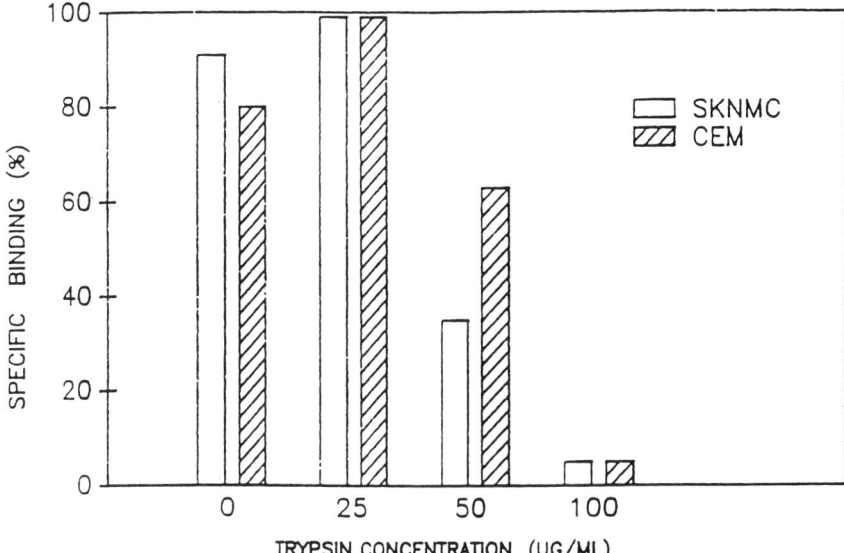

FIGURE 1. Sensitivity to trypsinization of gp120-binding molecule on neural cells. SKNMC neuroblastoma cell membranes were trypsinized with 50, 100, and 200 µg/ml of trypsin for 10 min. Specific binding of ^{125}I-labeled gp120 diminished in both CD4-bearing T cells and neural cells in a dose-dependent manner.

sole alternative to CD4. SKNMC neuroblastoma cell membranes were trypsinized with 50, 100, and 200 µg/ml of trypsin for 10 min. Specific binding of ^{125}I-labeled gp120 diminished in both CD4-bearing T cells and neural cells (FIG. 1) in a dose-dependent manner. Thus, it may be that both GC and a protein molecule are involved in gp120 binding. Such cooperation between glycolipid and protein molecules in ligand binding have been described previously.[11]

IDENTIFICATION OF THE gp120 BINDING PROTEIN ON NEURAL CELLS

Initial immunoprecipitation was performed from extracts prepared from 5×10^8 cells incubated with gp120, sheep anti-gp120, and PGS sequentially. The receptor bound to protein G Sepharose (PGS) was eluted with high-salt (750 mM) NaCl, desalted, and then concentrated using centricon membranes. This preparation was subjected to immunoblotting. After blocking of the membranes with 2.5% bovine serum albumin, identification of the gp120-binding protein was performed by incubating the membrane with gp120, followed by sheep anti-gp120 antibodies, and then by anti-sheep IgG labeled with alkaline phosphatase. The detection of the alkaline phosphatase tag was performed according to the manufacturer's instruc-

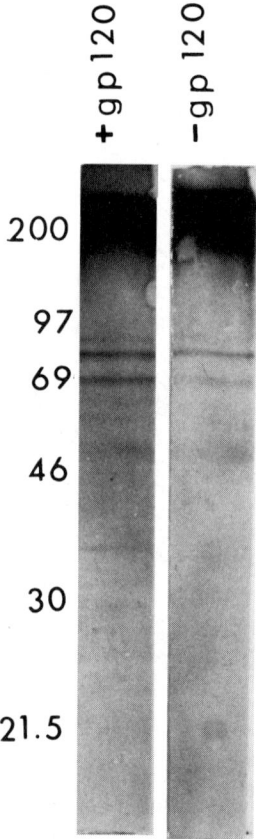

FIGURE 2. Detection of the 69-kDa gp120-binding protein on neural cells. See text for details.

tions. As shown in FIGURE 2, enrichment of the band at 69 kDa could be seen. No such enrichment could be seen for the nonspecific band detected at 72 kDa. The control included all the other components used in the process of identification except for gp120. Further experiments are being conducted to verify the identity of the gp120-binding protein.

Characterization of the HIV-1 receptor expressed on CD4-negative cells will be crucial in attempts to control HIV-1 infection in these cells. Lately, it has been described[9,10] that antibodies to GC inhibit HIV-1 infection of neural cells; however, our data suggest the existence of a gp120-binding protein. It is possible that both are components of the same complex controlling HIV-1 entry into CD4-negative cells. Such cooperation between proteins and glycolipids for ligand binding have been previously described for tetanus toxin.[11]

REFERENCES

1. CLAPHAM, P. R., J. M. WEBER, J. WHITBY, K. MCINTOSH, G. DALGLEISCH, P. J. MADDON, K. C. DEEN, R. W. SWEET & R. A. WEISS. 1989. Nature 337: 368–370.
2. HAROUSE, J. M., C. KUNSCH, V. T. HARTLE, V. A. LAUGHLIN, J. A. HOXEI, B. WIGDAHL & F. GONZALEZ-SCARANO. 1989. J. Virol. 63: 2527–2533.
3. WIGDAHL, B. & C. KUNSCH. 1990. Human immunodeficiency virus infection and neurologic dysfunction. Prog. Med. Virol. 37: 1–46.
4. LI, X. L., T. MOUDGIL, H. V. WINTERS & D. D. HO. 1990. J. Virol. 64: 1383–1387.
5. TATENO, M., F. GONZALEZ-SCARANO & J. A. LEVY. 1989. Proc. Natl. Acad. Sci. USA 86: 4287–4290.
6. MIZRACHI, Y., M. ZEIRA, M. SHAHABUDDIN, G. LI, F. SINANGIL & D. J. VOLSKY. 1991. Bull. Inst. Pasteur 89: 81–96.
7. ADACHI, A., H. E. GENDELMAN, S. KOENIG, T. FOLKS, R. WILLEY, A. RABSON & M. A. MARTIN. 1986. J. Virol. 59: 284–291.
8. ZUCKER-FRANKLIN, D., S. SEREMETIS & Z. Y. Zheng. 1990. Blood 75: 1920–1923.
9. HAROUSE, J. M., S. BHAT, S. L. SPITALINIK, M. LAUGHLIN, K. STEFANO, D. H. SILBERBERT & F. GONZALEZ-SCARANO. 1991. Science 253: 320–322.
10. BHAT, S., S. L. SPITALNIK, F. GONZALEZ-SCARONO & D. H. SILBERBERG. 1991. Proc. Natl. Acad. Sci. USA 88: 7131–7134.
11. YAVIN, E. & A. NATHAN 1986. Eur. J. Biochem. 154: 403–407.

HIV-1 mRNA Transcripts from Persistently Infected Human Fetal Astrocytes

WALTER J. ATWOOD, CARLO S. TORNATORE,
KAREN MEYERS, AND EUGENE O. MAJOR[a]

Laboratory of Viral and Molecular Pathogenesis
Section on Molecular Virology and Genetics
National Institute of Neurological Disorders and Stroke
National Institutes of Health
Bethesda, Maryland 20892

In vitro HIV-1 infection of human fetal astrocytes initiates a noncytopathic, productive infection that results in a long-term persistence during which the viral genome remains latent.[1] The cytokines TNF-α and IL-1β can activate HIV-1 gene expression from these cells, which results in the production of infectious virus.[1]

In this report we have investigated the temporal regulation of HIV-1 gene expression in human fetal astrocytes at the transcriptional level. At two days posttransfection (PT), three species of HIV-1 mRNA transcripts can be detected by Northern blot. The transcripts are 9, 4, and 2 kb in size and represent multiply spliced HIV-1 mRNA that are known to code for the HIV-1 regulatory proteins *tat, rev,* and *nef*. By 15 days PT only the 2-kb transcript remains. Treatment of the cells with TNF-a or IL-1b at 15 or 27 days PT causes an increase in the 2-kb transcript. The 9- and 4-kb transcripts are no longer detectable by Northern blot. To more precisely define the HIV-1 specific transcripts that are produced in these cells, we amplified cDNA that was reverse transcribed from HIV-1 RNA isolated at two days post transfection. The primers that were chosen were in the first and seventh exon of the HIV-1 genome and amplify multiply spliced HIV-1 mRNA. The PCR products were resolved on 1.4% agarose gels, blotted to nylon filters, and hybridized to an HIV-1 specific probe. At least six multiply spliced transcripts hybridized to our probe. To determine which exons each of the six bands represented, we stripped the filters and reprobed them with oligonucleotides representing each of the five exons in the HIV-1 genome. Transcripts representing *tat, rev,* and *nef* hybridized to these probes. Using this method, we were able to determine that treatment of the cells with TNF-α or IL-1β resulted in an induction of *tat, rev,* and *nef* specific transcripts. We further demonstrate that this induction can

---

[a] To whom correspondence should be addressed.

occur in the absence of the viral transactivator *tat*, inasmuch as the same cytokines increase expression of the reporter gene chloramphenicol acetyl-transferase (CAT), which is under the control of the HIV-1 5' long terminal repeat (LTR).

These results demonstrate that HIV-1 mRNA transcripts can be detected in persistently infected cultures of human fetal glial cells following induction with cytokines as late as 28 days posttransfection. The mRNA transcripts are multiply spliced and code for *tat, rev,* and *nef*. The fact that the *nef* transcript is most readily detectable at later time points may reflect its putative role as a negative regulator of HIV-1 gene expression. The difficulty in detecting HIV-1 in astrocytes *in vivo* may in part be due to the virus's demonstrated ability to establish long-term persistent infections in culture during which the virus remains latent. The latent infection in astrocytes is not a dead end for the virus, as several cytokines known to be produced by cells of the CNS can reactivate virus production from these cells.

REFERENCES

1. TORNATORE, C., A. NATH, K. AMEMIYA & E. O. MAJOR. 1991. Persistent HIV-1 infection in human fetal glial cells reactivated by T-cell factors or by the cytokines TNF-α and IL-1β. J. Virol. **65:** 6094–6100.

Index of Contributors

Achilli, G., 275–276
Albert, J., 277–280
Althaus, B., 194–201
Alvarado, L., 249–251
Ammann, A. J., 178–185
Anzil, P. A., 295–296
Aricò, M., 262–263, 275–276
Ascher, D. P., 258–261
Atwood, W. J., 324–325

Barnes, S., 255–257
Belman, A. L., 107–122
Blankenship, C., 20–34
Blasi, F., 286–287
Bossi, G., 262–263, 275–276
Brambilla, D., 123–140, 245–248
Brosnan, C. F., 314–316
Brunell, P. A., 9–13
Bryson, Y. J., 14–19
Bussel, J. B., 20–34

Caldwell, M. B., 4–8
Calvelli, T., 151–157
Casadevall, A., 281–283
Caselli, D., 262–263, 275–276, 284–285
Cervia, J. S., 20–34
Chen, C. (X), 20–34
Cho, E-S., 295–296
Church, J. A., 288–290
Cosentini, R., 286–287
Coughlin, R. T., 268–271, 272–274
Coulter, D., 123–140
Cryz, S. J., Jr., 194–201
Cunningham-Rundles, S., 20–34

da Cunha, A., 229–244
Degioanni, M., 275–276, 284–285
Deicas, A., 275–276
Denny, T. N., 35–51
Diaz, C., 245–248
Dickson, D. W., 93–106, 295–296, 314–316

Edelson, P., 20–34
Ehrhardt, A., 249–251
Eiden, L. E., 229–244
Epshteyn, I., 297–299
Epstein, J. S., 264–267, 306–308

Feldman, J., 249–251
Fennell, E. B., 141–150
Fenyö, E. M., 277–280

Fischer, G. W., 258–261
Fowler, A. K., 258–261
Fox, H., 245–248
Fratazzi, C., 213–228
Frederick, W., 255–257
Freij, B. J., 302–305
Fürer, E., 194–201

George, J. R., 268–271, 272–274
Gershon, A. A., 166–177
Gleason-Morgan, D., 288–290
Goldberg, D., 258–261
Goldstein, H., 194–201, 281–283
Green, K., 245–248
Greene, M. F., 213–228
Gwinn, M. L., 4–8

Halapi, E., 277–280
Hand, I. L., 300–301
Hasler, T., 194–201
Hatch, W. C., 202–212, 312–313, 314–316
Havens, J., 249–251
Hayek, G., 302–305
Hewlett, I. K., 264–267, 306–308
Heyes, M., 229–244
Hinds, T., 20–34
Huang, D.-P., 255–257
Hung, C.-H., 268–271, 272–274
Hutto, C., 65–70

Jansson, M., 277–280
Joshi, B., 264–267, 306–308
Joshi, V. V., 71–92

Kairam, R., 123–140
Kanzer, M. D., 295–296
Kline, J., 123–140
Korber, B. T. M., 65–70
Kozlowski, P. B., 295–296
Kuban, K., 123–140

Lambert, J. S., 186–193
Lansky, L., 123–140
Larocca, J. N., 202–212
Laurence, J., 52–64
Lee, S. C., 314–316
Lee, S. F., 306–308
Leitner, T., 277–280
Levin, B., 123–140
Liu, W., 314–316
Llena, J. F., 93–106, 295–296

Losev, L., 312–313
Luzuriaga, K., 14–19
Lyman, W. D., xi–xii, 202–212, 297–299, 252–254, 312–313

Maccabruni, A., 262–263, 275–276, 284–285
Major, E. O., 324–325
Manak, M. M., 255–257
Marconi, M., 262–263
Marshall, P., 123–140
Martin, N. L., 14–19
Mayner, R., 306–308
McGurk, J. F., 297–299
Mendez, H., 245–248
Meyers, K., 324–325
Mizrachi, Y., 317–319, 320–323
Mofenson, L. M., 35–51, 245–248
Moriarty, R. A., 258–261
Muñoz, J. L., 65–70
Murray, E. A., 229–244

Nair, M. P. N., 309–311
Nelson, S. J., 93–106, 295–296
NHLBI P^{2}C^2 Pediatric Pulmonary and Cardiac Complications of HIV Infection Study Group, 35–51
NICHD IVIG Clinical Trial Group, 35–51
Nohr, D., 229–244
NYC Perinatal HIV Transmission Collaborative Study Group, 268–271, 272–274

Parekh, B. S., 268–271, 272–274
Parks, W. P., 65–70
Pasinetti, G., 262–263
Penninck, D., 213–228
Petersen, D., 255–257
Pettoello-Mantovani, M., 281–283
Plaeger-Marshall, S., 291–294
Plebani, A., 286–287
Pollock, L., 264–267
Porricola, M., 300–301
Pousada, E., 312–313

Que, J. U., 194–201

Rao, C., 295–296
Rashbaum, W. K., 202–212, 252–254, 297–299
Raszka, W. V., Jr., 258–261
Rausch, D. M., 229–244
Renne, S., 317–319
Rich, K., 245–248
Riordan, G., 264–267

Robb, M. L., 258–261
Roberts, C. R., 258–261
Rodriguez, C., 291–294
Rodriguez, E. M., 123–140, 245–248
Rodriguez, R., 317–319
Rogers, M., 272–274
Rogers, M. F., 4–8
Rosenblatt, H. M., 35–51
Ross, L. A., 288–290
Rossi, P., 277–280
Rubinstein, A., 1–3, 151–157, 194–201
Rubinstein, R., 151–157
Ruprecht, R. M., 213–228

Sanders-Laufer, D., 20–34
Scarlatti, G., 277–280
Schluchter, M. D., 35–51
Schochetman, G., 268–271, 272–274
Schoeller, M. C., 286–287
Schwartz, S. A., 309–311
Shaffer, N., 268–271, 272–274
Sharer, L., 229–244, 295–296
Sharma, P. L., 213–228
Shearer, W. T., 35–51
Sheon, A., 245–248
Sher, J. H., 295–296
Simonds, R. J., 4–8
Snider, J. V., 255–257
Stiehm, E. R., 186–193, 291–294
Stronati, M., 262–263
Sullivan, J. L., 14–19
Sweet, A. M., 309–311

Tornatore, C. S., 324–325

Uhlén, M., 277–280

Van Dyke, R. B., 158–165
Veber, M. B., 20–34
Velez-Borras, J., 123–140
Volsky, D. J., 317–319

Waecker, N. J., 258–261
Wahlberg, J., 277–280
Wara, D. W., 14–19
Weidenheim, K. M., 93–106, 295–296, 297–299
Weihe, E., 229–244
Whitaker, A., 249–251
Whitfield, L. R., 302–305
Wientzen, R. L., Jr., 302–305
Wigzell, H., 277–280
Wiznia, A., 300–301
Wolinsky, S. M., 65–70
Wrzolek, M. A., 295–296
Wyand, M., 213–228